Essentials of Oral Pathology

Essentials of Oral Pathology

Editor: Philip Chiders

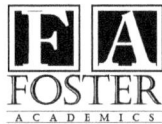

FA
FOSTER
ACADEMICS

www.fosteracademics.com

www.fosteracademics.com

FA FOSTER
ACADEMICS

Cataloging-in-Publication Data

Essentials of oral pathology / edited by Philip Chiders.
    p. cm.
Includes bibliographical references and index.
ISBN 978-1-63242-498-3
1. Teeth--Diseases. 2. Mouth--Diseases. 3. Dental therapeutics. 4. Oral manifestations of general diseases.
I. Chiders, Philip.
RK307 .E77 2017
617.522--dc23

Foster Academics,
118-35 Queens Blvd., Suite 400,
Forest Hills, NY 11375, USA

ISBN 978-1-63242-498-3 (Hardback)

Printed and bound in the United States of America.

Contents

Preface

This book aims to highlight the current researches and provides a platform to further the scope of innovations in this area. This book is a product of the combined efforts of many researchers and scientists from different parts of the world. The objective of this book is to provide the readers with the latest information in the field.

Dentistry or oral pathology is defined as the branch of medicine that is involved in the examination, diagnosis, prevention and treatment of diseases, disorders and conditions of the oral cavity. This book elucidates the concepts and innovative models around prospective developments with respect to oral pathology and dentistry. It is a valuable compilation of topics, ranging from the basic to the most complex advancements in the field of oral pathology and healthcare. It aims to highlight the importance of dental treatment because it is considered to be as a major public health problem. Students, researchers, dental experts and all associated with oral health care and dentistry will benefit alike from this book.

I would like to express my sincere thanks to the authors for their dedicated efforts in the completion of this book. I acknowledge the efforts of the publisher for providing constant support. Lastly, I would like to thank my family for their support in all academic endeavors.

Editor

An Unusual Erupted Complex Composite Odontoma

Dawasaz Ali Azhar,[1] **Mohammad Zahir Kota,**[2] **and Sherif El-Nagdy**[3]

[1] *Department of Oral Medicine and Radiology, College of Dentistry, King Khalid University, Abha, Saudi Arabia*
[2] *Department of Oral Surgery, College of Dentistry, King Khalid University, Abha, Saudi Arabia*
[3] *Department of Oral Pathology, Faculty of Dentistry, Mansoura University, Dakahliya, Egypt*

Correspondence should be addressed to Dawasaz Ali Azhar; draliazhar@gmail.com

Academic Editors: R. S. Brown, G. Gómez-Moreno, T. Hata, and G. Orsini

Odontomas are malformations of the dental tissues and may interfere with the eruption of the associated tooth. Complex composite odontoma (CO) was described as a distinct entity for the first time by Broca in 1866. This lesion takes place due to the developmental disturbances where the dental components are laid down in a disorganized manner, due to failure of normal morphodifferentiation. Very few cases of erupted complex composite odontomas have been reported in the literature. The case reported here is of an odontoma found in the left mandibular body, associated with an impacted second molar of a 17-year-old Saudi male. Under local anesthesia the odontoma was surgically removed. Histopathological examination confirmed the diagnosis of CO. The impacted second molar which was left in the mandibular body erupted clinically after 6 months. Erupted CO is rarely seen in the mandibular left body. The early diagnosis, followed by a proper treatment at the right time, will result in a favorable prognosis.

1. Introduction

According to the latest classification of the World Health Organization (WHO, 2005), two types of odontomas can be found: complex odontomas and compound odontomas, the latter being twice as common as the former. Odontomas erupting into the oral cavity are rare. The first case was published in 1980, and since then only 17 cases have been reported in the literature. Eight of the 17 cases were complex composite odontomas (COs); the rest were compound odontomas. Pain, swelling, and infection were the most common symptoms, and 13 cases presented an impacted tooth associated with it [1]. COs are found in the mandibular posterior region over impacted teeth which can reach up to several centimeters in size. Radiographically, these lesions manifest as a radiopaque solid mass with occasional nodular elements and are surrounded by a fine radiolucent zone separated from the normal bone by a well-defined cortication line [2].

2. Case Description

A 17-year-old male visited the dental OPD of King Khalid University, Abha, KSA, with a chief complaint of pain in upper left first molar tooth. Routine clinical examination revealed a partially erupted hard mass on the alveolar ridge distal to left mandibular first molar and missing mandibular second molar (Figure 1). Orthopantomograph revealed a unilateral solid single triangular radiopaque structure with apex towards the alveolar ridge (Figure 2). The radiopaque structure was irregular and had a radiolucent zone surrounding it. There was a presence of an impacted second molar with the root apices close to the left lower border of the mandible. Differential diagnoses made based on the clinical and radiological features included complex odontoma, cementoblastoma, ameloblastic fibroodontoma, and Pindborg's tumor. In our case there was a presence of the radiolucent rim around the lesion with the presence of dense radiopacity produced by enamel which helped to distinguish the odontoma. The above lesion was surgically excised under local anesthesia (Figures 3 and 4) and edges of the bones were rounded and the wound was rinsed with saline and sutured with Coated Vicryl 3/0 (Ethicon, Inc., Johnson and Johnson Company, USA). The second molar was left in situ for expected passive eruption. The postoperative course was uneventful. The excised specimen was sent for histopathological examination. The decalcified

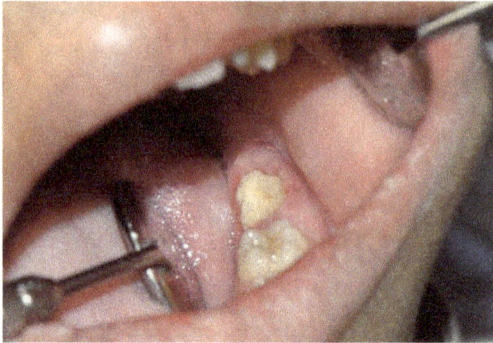

FIGURE 1: Intraoral preoperative photograph.

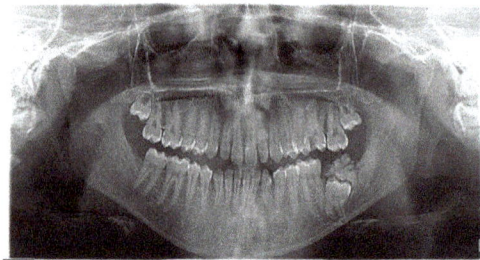

FIGURE 2: Orthopantomograph showing radiopaque structure with impacted mandibular left second molar.

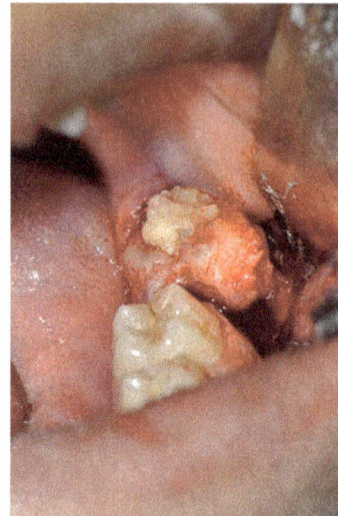

FIGURE 3: Intraoperative photograph showing excision in total.

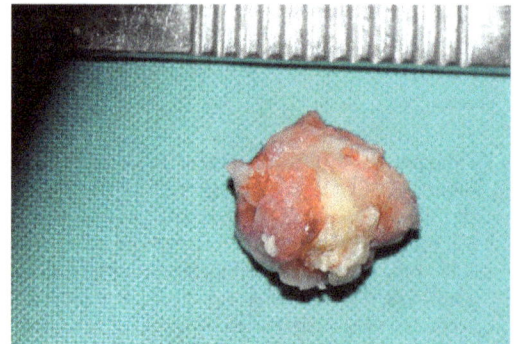

FIGURE 4: Excised specimen.

section showed disorganized dental tissue formed of irregular dentine masses containing multiple hollow circular spaces with pulp tissue and enamel matrix (Figure 5(a)). Other small areas of organized dental tissue resembling normal tooth structure are also seen (Figure 5(b)). Proliferating odontogenic epithelium is also seen in a scanty stroma. The above findings are consistent with complex composite odontoma. At the followup after 6 months it was observed clinically and radiographically (Figures 6 and 7) that the second molar had erupted in its usual position distal to lower left first molar.

3. Discussion

The WHO classification defines CO as follows: "a malformation in which all the dental tissues are represented, individual tissues being mainly well formed but occurring in a more or less disorderly pattern" [2]. The etiology of COs is unknown. Several theories have been proposed, including local trauma, infection, family history, and genetic mutation. It has also been suggested that odontomas are inherited from a mutant gene or interference, possibly postnatally with the genetic control of tooth development [3]. The relative frequency of CO among odontogenic tumors varies between 5% and 30% which means that this lesion is one of the most commonest odontogenic lesion/malformation. The majority of cases (83.9%) occur before the age of 30 with a peak in the second decade of life. The male : female ratio varies between 1.5 : 1 and 1.6 : 1 [4]. It is of interest to note that the majority of odontomas in anterior segment of jaw are

compound composite in type (61%) whereas the majority in posterior segment are CO. Interestingly, both type of odontomas occurred more frequently on the right side of jaw than on the left, such presentation was not seen in our case [5]. Clinically CO is a painless, slow-growing, and expanding lesion that is usually discovered on routine radiographs of the jaw bones, or the failed eruption of a permanent tooth which may lead to the diagnosis of this lesion [3]. The first case of an erupted odontoma was described in 1980 by Rumel et al. The mean patient age was 25–35 years, thus confirming potential presentation of these lesions between the second and third decades of life [6]. The mechanism of odontoma eruption appears to be different from tooth eruption because of the lack of periodontal ligament and root in odontoma. Therefore the force required to move the odontoma is not linked to the contractility of the fibroblasts, as in the case for teeth. Although there is no root formation in odontoma, its increasing size may lead to the sequestration of the overlying bone and hence occlusal movement or eruption. An increase in the size of the odontoma over time produces a force sufficient to cause bone resorption [1].

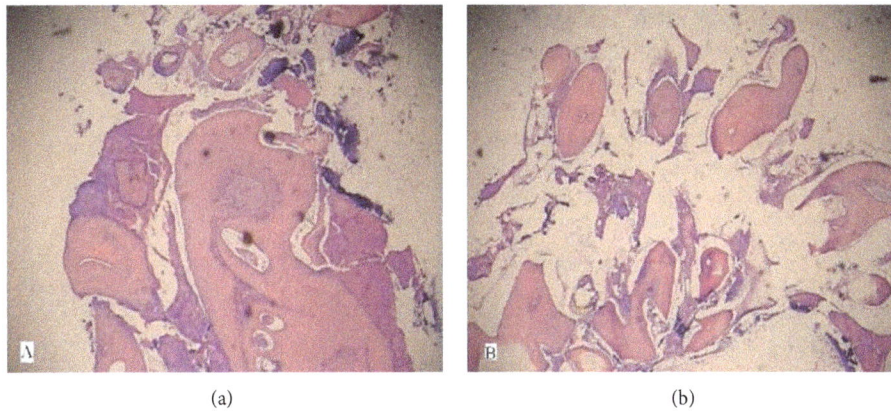

FIGURE 5: H&E stained decalcified section showing (a) disorganized dental tissue formed of irregular dentine masses containing multiple hollow circular spaces with pulp tissue and enamel matrix and (b) small areas of organized dental tissue resembling tooth structure with proliferating odontogenic epithelium seen in a scanty stroma.

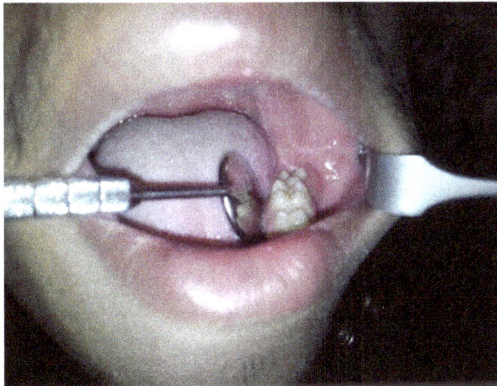

FIGURE 6: Postoperative clinical photograph (6-month followup) showing erupted mandibular left second molar.

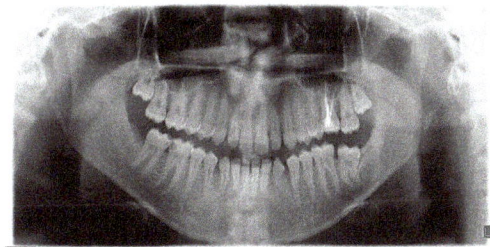

FIGURE 7: Orthopantomograph (6-month followup).

Radiologically, the compound odontoma appears as a collection of tooth-like structures while composite type appears as a calcified mass with a radiodensity similar to tooth structure; both are further surrounded by a narrow radiolucent zone. However there was absence of any corticated border in our case as normally published in previous literature. Unerupted teeth are more commonly associated with compound composite odontoma. However, in our case, presence of unerupted tooth with CO was seen [5]. The lesion appears as a more or less amorphous, solitary mass of calcified material. In some cases, the lesion shows a radiating structure [7].

Rarely odontomas may form peripheral or soft tissue lesions in which they arise outside alveolar bone and may exfoliate or erupt. Such a rare erupted odontoma was present in our case [8].

Microscopically, this lesion consists primarily of a well-delineated, roughly spherical mass of a haphazard conglomerate of mature hard dental tissues. Some examples may include better-ordered, tooth-like structures [9]. Clear spaces and clefts that probably contain mature enamel lost in the process of decalcification are often seen. In some sections at the periphery of the mass, islands of pulp tissue in association with cords and buds of odontogenic epithelium can be found. However, the usual high degree of differentiation of the dental tissues reflects the late stage of morphodifferentiation and maturation of odontogenesis. A thin, fibrous capsule and, in some cases, a cyst wall is seen surrounding the lesion [4].

Conservative surgical enucleation is considered to be the treatment of choice in most cases of CO. During the removal of pathological structures in the mandibular retromolar region in an early age, care should be taken to preserve bone structures on the anterior border of the mandibular ramus, because it might impair jaw development. If needed, a control X-ray should be taken during the surgery. The prognosis is always good since these tumors do not tend to recur [10]. As odontomas are often associated with impacted teeth, the possibility that eruption of the impacted tooth after a presumed obstructive odontoma has been surgically removed is an important issue [11]. In our case, taking into consideration the position of the associated impacted tooth and its presumable path of eruption, it was decided to leave it in situ for passive eruption.

4. Conclusion

Odontomas rarely erupt into the mouth and tend to be associated with impacted teeth. Despite their benign nature, however, their eruption into the oral cavity can give rise to pain, inflammation and infection and different clinical appearance. The treatment of choice is surgical removal of the odontoma, followed by histopathological analysis. In the case of odontomas associated with impacted teeth, the latter should be preserved in situ when a favorable path of eruption exists for facilitating passive eruption of the impacted teeth into the oral cavity.

Conflict of Interests

The authors declare that they have no conflict of interests.

References

[1] G. Serra-Serra, L. Berini-Aytés, and C. Gay-Escoda, "Erupted odontomas: a report of three cases and review of the literature," *Medicina Oral , Patología Oral y Cirugía Bucal*, vol. 14, no. 6, pp. 1–5, 2009.

[2] S. Ora and Ş. Yücetaş, "Compound and complex odontomas," *International Journal of Oral and Maxillofacial Surgery*, vol. 16, no. 5, pp. 596–599, 1987.

[3] G. E. Kaugars, M. E. Miller, and L. M. Abbey, "Odontomas," *Oral Surgery, Oral Medicine, Oral Pathology*, vol. 67, no. 2, pp. 172–176, 1989.

[4] P. Gurdal and T. Seckin, "Odontomas," *Quintessence International*, vol. 2, no. 4, pp. 32–38, 2001.

[5] D. Nisha, K. Rishabh, T. Ashwarya, M. Sukriti, and S. D. Gupta, "An unusual case of erupted composite complex odontoma," *Journal of Dental Sciences and Research*, vol. 2, no. 2, pp. 1–5, 2011.

[6] A. Rumel, A. de Freitas, E. G. Birman, L. A. Tannous, P. T. Chacon, and S. Borkas, "Erupted complex odontoma. Report of a case," *Dentomaxillofacial Radiology*, vol. 9, no. 1, pp. 5–9, 1980.

[7] P. J. Slootweg, "An analysis of the interrelationship of the mixed odontogenic tumors—amelobastic fibroma, ameloblastic fibro-odontoma, and the odontomas," *Oral Surgery Oral Medicine and Oral Pathology*, vol. 51, no. 3, pp. 266–276, 1981.

[8] S. Chandra, A. Bagewadi, V. Keluskar, and K. Sah, "Compound composite odontome erupting into the oral cavity. A rare entity," *Contemporary Clinical Dentistry*, vol. 1, no. 2, pp. 123–126, 2010.

[9] H. P. Philipsen, P. A. Reichart, and F. Prætorius, "Mixed odontogenic tumours and odontomas. Considerations on inter-relationship. Review of the literature and presentation of 134 new cases of odontomas," *European Journal of Cancer B*, vol. 33, no. 2, pp. 86–99, 1997.

[10] S. Dragana, S. Aleksandar, and Č. Snježana, "Complex odontoma associated with an impacted molar," *Serbian Dental Journal*, vol. 54, no. 3, pp. 195–200, 2007.

[11] H. P. Philipsen, W. Thosaporn, P. Reichart, and G. Grundt, "Odontogenic lesions in opercula of permanent molars delayed in eruption," *Journal of Oral Pathology and Medicine*, vol. 21, no. 1, pp. 38–41, 1992.

Sanjad-Sakati Syndrome Dental Management

Hisham Y. El Batawi

Pediatric Dentistry, Sharjah University City, P.O. Box 27272, Sharjah, UAE

Correspondence should be addressed to Hisham Y. El Batawi; helbatawi@sharjah.ac.ae

Academic Editors: I. Anic, A. Epivatianos, and E. F. Wright

Sanjad-Sakati syndrome (SSS) is a rare genetic disorder with autosomal recessive pattern of inheritance characterized by hypoparathyroidism, sever growth failure, mental retardation, susceptibility to chest infection, and dentofacial anomalies. A child with SSS was referred to the dental department seeking dental help for sever dental caries which was attributed to his dietary habits and quality of dental tissues. Full restorative rehabilitation was done under general anesthesia. Two years later, the child presented with recurrent caries affecting uncrowned teeth. High carries recurrence rate was blamed for the nutritional habits endorsed by the parents. Only steel crowned teeth survived such hostile oral environment which suggested shifting of treatment strategy towards full coverage restorations instead of classical cavity preparations and fillings during a second attempt for dental treatment under general anesthesia and for the dental treatment of two cousins of the same child. The author recommends effective health education for parents including the nature of their child's genetic disorder, nutritional needs, and dental health education to improve the life style of such children.

1. Introduction

Sanjad-Sakati syndrome (SSS) is a rare autosomal recessive disorder (OMIM 241410) that is confined to Arab Middle Eastern populations. It is characterized by congenital hypoparathyroidism, hypocalcemia, seizures, hyperphosphatemia, growth retardation, dwarfism, mental retardation, and dysmorphic craniofacial features including microcephaly, deep-seated eyes, depressed nasal bridge, and micrognathia [1].

1.1. Previous Reports

1.1.1. Oman. Al-Ghazali and Dawodu [2], in 1997, reported a case in Oman with the a forementioned features. Computerized tomography (CT) rain scan showed immature myelination suggesting that failure of growth is due to hypothalamic origin.

Thirteen years later, Rafique and Al-Yaarubi [3] claimed the first report of SSS in Omani children where they reported SSS in three siblings (two girls and one boy). The authors highlighted the need for routine DNA counseling for early diagnosis and prevention of associated comorbidities.

1.1.2. Palestine. In 2006, AbuDraz [4] reported two unrelated Palestinian children; both of them had the syndrome's manifestations plus small sized atrial septal defect detected by echocardiogram.

1.1.3. Israel. Platis et al. [5], in 2006, reported one 12-year-old child of Bedouin origin with the syndrome. The child was a product of consanguineous marriage.

1.1.4. Qatar. In 1990, Richardson and Kirk [6] reported eight Qatari children, four boys and four girls, all born to consanguineous parents. Seven of these children had medullary stenosis of long bones.

1.1.5. Saudi Arabia. Sanjad et al., in 1991, reported 12 infants to have the syndrome; eleven of these infants were the product of consanguineous marriages while four has similarly affected siblings.

In this paper, we describe the concerns encountered in dental management of a child with the syndrome and the modifications in treatment plan that had to be done in managing two of his cousins with the same disorder.

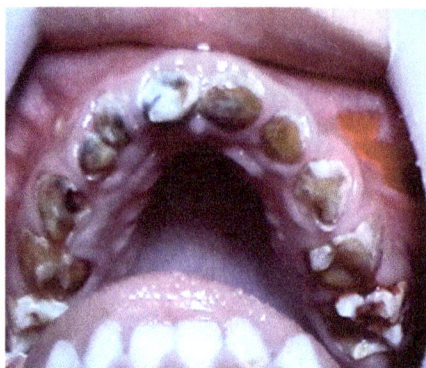

FIGURE 1: Preoperative Sanjad-Sakati intraoral features.

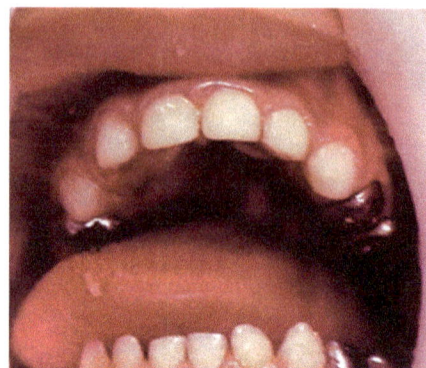

FIGURE 2: Postoperative restorative first attempt.

2. Case Report

A four-year-four-month-old boy belonging to a known tribe in Western Province of Saudi Arabia was referred to the dental department of a private hospital in Jeddah, Saudi Arabia. The child's pediatrician diagnosed the case as Sanjad-Sakati syndrome whose elder brother had the same condition and died at the age of 12 years from severe pneumonia. The child's medical history revealed that he was born at the same hospital with birth weight 1729 grams, occipital-frontal circumference 29 cm, serum calcium 1.5 mm/L, and phosphate 2.6 mmol/L. Walking and speech were delayed as reported in the medical record.

2.1. Pediatric Management. The child had frequent hospitalizations due to recurrent pneumonias. Oral calcium supplements, vitamin D, and Polycose supplement (Abbott Nutrition) were administered in addition to symptomatic anticonvulsive drugs. No growth hormone therapy was administered by pediatrician as it showed no effect on the late older brother.

The child showed typical facial features of short stature, deep sunk eyes, micrognathia, depressed nasal bridge, relatively large ears, and mental retardation. Figure 1 shows an 11-year-old cousin girl of the child with SSS.

2.2. Intraoral Findings. The child presented with sever dental caries and neglected oral hygiene, all upper teeth were badly decayed, and lower molars were also exposed while lower anterior teeth were minimally affected which suggests a nursing bottle pattern of dental caries. High vaulted palate, micrognathia, dental anomaly of extra upper right lateral deciduous incisor, and microdontia were observed in first deciduous molars as well (Figure 2).

2.3. Dental Treatment Plan. Full dental treatment was planned including pulpotomies, steel crowns, restorations, extraction of supernumerary upper right lateral incisor, and parents education regarding nutrition and oral hygiene. Considering the amount of work needed versus the patient's cooperation limits, a decision was made to perform the procedure under general anesthesia.

2.4. Patient Privacy. Informed consents were obtained conforming to the Joint Commission for International Accreditation (JCIA) standards and following the World Medical Association Declaration of Helsinki on Ethical Principles for Medical Research Involving Human Subjects, October 2001.

In a conservative social environment like Saudi Arabia, the author had to get a special consent regarding publication of the three pediatric cases involved in this paper. All parents of the three children permitted publication while only one parent permitted one photograph for publication.

2.5. Anesthesia Management. Preoperative antibiotic prophylaxis was administered for pneumonia concerns. The patient's cooperation level did not allow for intravenous line insertion; accordingly, induction was carried out via facemask with 3% Sevoflurane, Abbott Co., in 100% oxygen. Following insertion of intravenous line, Propofol, Diprivan, AstraZeneca Co., was administered. Nasotracheal intubation was done smoothly with aid of external laryngeal manipulation. During the course of dental procedure, Dexamethasone was given to aid in reducing oral edema. The procedures were done in 130 minutes excluding induction and extubation. During dental management, oxygen saturation was 98-99% and heart rate was 90–125 with the highest reading during dental pulp tissue extirpation. Postoperative recovery was uneventful, and the child was discharged the next day after, pediatric verification that he is fit for discharge.

3. Discussion

Al-Malik, in 2004 [7], reported the oral findings associated with SSS, which included micrognathic mandible and maxilla thin lips, high arched palate, severe dental caries, microdontia, and enamel hypoplasia. In the reported case, all intraoral symptoms reported by Al-Malik were observed with exception of enamel hypoplasia. The parents gave history that the teeth erupted with whitish chalky appearance which turned soon into big cavities and chipping. That statement might be more attributed to the rampant caries resulted from nursing bottle use or early childhood caries than to enamel hypoplasia.

The autosomal recessive pattern of inheritance of hypoparathyroidism resembles that observed in Kenny-Caffey syndrome which is manifested as growth retardation, craniofacial anomalies, small hands and feet, hypocalcaemia, and hypoparathyroidism in addition to radiographic evidence of cortical thickening in long bones; the latter is not reported in SSS. Both syndromes are thought to be allelic as they have been mapped to the same chromosome, share an ancestral haplotype, and both are chaperon diseases caused by a genetic defect in the tubulin [8].

In Arab populations, the deep rooted norm of consanguineous marriage has been widely blamed as a predisposing factor for autosomal recessive diseases such as SSS [9]. The reported case is a product of consanguineous marriage, and two years later, two of the cousins of that child patient were referred to undergo full dental rehabilitation under general anesthesia.

3.1. General Anesthesia. Wasersprung et al. [10], in 2010, reported dental treatment of an SSS child under general anesthesia that went uneventful except for episodes of desaturation (80% SaO_2) that was managed by bronchodilators and ventilation. Al-Malik, in 2004, reported uneventful anesthesia management for an SSS case. In our paper, the child was anesthetized twice with the second time after two years. Both instances went uneventful with no need for intensive care stay. Prophylactic antibiotic coverage was administered to help avoid the risk of chest infection. Tube selection was decided according to the child's weight rather than the child's age.

3.2. Dental Management. Our patient has been subjected to dental treatment under general anesthesia two times with an interval of two years. The aim of the first dental treatment was to restore back all decayed teeth to a nearly normal condition in addition to preventive dental treatment including sealants and fluorides as well. The dental procedures were considered as part of total dental care that included dental health education to the parents regarding nutritional and oral hygiene habits (Figure 3).

After two years, the child appeared with severe recurrent caries in all composite resin filled teeth, with periapical infection related to the upper four incisors. Radiographic examination was not possible due to the patient's limited cooperation and the possible trauma involved during placing the X-ray sensor in such a small oral cavity. All steel crowned teeth were in satisfactory clinical state after the two-year postoperative period.

The parents stated that they failed to quit night bottle feeding and that the child has no muscular strength to chew rough fibrous food. Accordingly, a change of strategy was decided. A second dental rehabilitation under general anesthesia was decided. The second dental management stressed on steel crowns and dental extractions more than restorative procedures, that is, shifting to procedures with more solid prognosis to minimize the child's future dental needs. Further, dental health education concentrated on strict dental hygiene, avoiding night feeding and shifting to

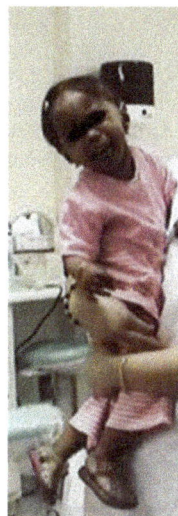

FIGURE 3: A Sanjad-Sakati 11-year-old girl.

healthier semisolid food choices. Strict followup schedule was attempted on monthly bases where dental prophylaxis was performed in each monthly visit.

The same strategy was followed with two cousins of the same child and proved satisfactory on monthly followup bases for two years. Outcome assessment was based on parental satisfaction questionnaire and lack of pain in addition to periodic clinical evaluation. Postoperative body weight monitoring was carried out. No significant postoperative increase in body weight could be observed.

Dental management for SSS children was reported by Al-Malik in 2004 and Waserprung et al. in 2010. No comparisons of fillings versus crowns regarding their longevity were mentioned in both reports. As Waserprung et al. reported anodontia of 12 permanent teeth upon radiographic examination, in our case, X-ray examination was not possible. This does not exclude the possible presence of anodontia in our case which in turn supports our recommendation for the use of steel crowns instead of fillings to prolong the service life of decayed teeth in SSS children.

The use of preformed steel crowns to restore teeth with microdontia has encountered some difficulties especially in lower first primary molar. In our case, we used upper opposite side crowns to restore lower first primary molars due to the smaller mesiodistal width of upper deciduous molars than their corresponding lowers.

Due to the conservative nature of Middle Eastern people in general and Saudi population in particular, the three figures included in this paper were the only photographs approved by the parents for publication. The same cultural habits and traditions may have negative effect on parents preventing genetic counseling which raises concerns regarding proper documentation and reporting of cases as well as incidence studies.

4. Conclusion

The author underlines the importance of premarriage genetic counseling and education related to consanguinity and reproductive health in the Arab world. Constructive teamwork management is a must for successful management of children with Sanjad-Sakati syndrome.

Children with Sanjad-Sakati syndrome lack the growth and development of proper masticatory apparatus which renders them in continuous need for soft and semisolid food. This constitutes a challenge for their restorative dental treatment. This paper recommends the use of steel crowns if possible. Dental treatment should be directed to modalities with unquestionable prognosis and try to prolong the durability of primary molars to improve mastication and dietary habits, thus promoting the child's general health and quality of life.

Dental health education for parents of SSS children regarding nutrition and oral hygiene is of prime importance as well as watchful postoperative followup.

Conflict of Interests

The author declares no conflict of interests neither with the institution where the work has been conducted nor with the manufacturers or suppliers of material and medicaments described in this paper.

References

[1] S. A. Sanjad, N. A. Sakati, Y. K. Abu-Osba, R. Kaddoura, and R. D. G. Milner, "A new syndrome of congenital hypoparathyroidism, severe growth failure, and dysmorphic features," *Archives of Disease in Childhood*, vol. 66, no. 2, pp. 193–196, 1991.

[2] L. I. Al-Ghazali and A. Dawoudu, "The syndrome of hypoparathyroidism, severe growth failure, developmental delay and distinctive faces," *Clinical Dysmorphology*, vol. 6, no. 3, pp. 233–237, 1997.

[3] B. Rafique and S. Al-Yaarubi, "Sanjad Sakati syndrome in omani children," *Oil Market Journal*, vol. 25, no. 3, pp. 227–229, 2010.

[4] A. AbuDraz, "Sanjad Sakati syndrome," *Pakistani Medical Journals*, vol. 2, no. 1, 2006.

[5] C. M. Platis, D. Wasersprung, L. Kachko, I. Tsunzer, and J. Katz, "Anesthesia management for the child with Sanjad-Sakati syndrome," *Paediatric Anaesthesia*, vol. 16, no. 11, pp. 1189–1192, 2006.

[6] R. J. Richardson and J. M. W. Kirk, "Short stature, mental retardation, and hypoparathyroidism: a new syndrome," *Archives of Disease in Childhood*, vol. 65, no. 10, pp. 1113–1117, 1990.

[7] M. I. Al-Malik, "The dentofacial features of Sanjad-Sakati syndrome: a case report," *International Journal of Paediatric Dentistry*, vol. 14, no. 2, pp. 136–140, 2004.

[8] A. S. Teebi, "Hypoparathyroidism, retarded growth and development, and dysmorphism or Sanjad-Sakati syndrome: an Arab disease reminiscent of Kenny-Caffey syndrome," *Journal of Medical Genetics*, vol. 37, no. 2, article 145, 2000.

[9] G. O. Tadmouri, P. Nair, T. Obeid, M. T. Al Ali, N. Al Khaja, and H. A. Hamamy, "Consanguinity and reproductive health among Arabs," *Reproductive Health*, vol. 6, no. 1, article 17, 2009.

[10] D. Wasersprung, C. M. Platis, S. Cohen et al., "Case report: Sanjad—sakati syndrome: dental findings and treatment," *European Archives of Paediatric Dentistry*, vol. 11, no. 3, pp. 151–154, 2010.

3

Mandibular Ameloblastoma in an Elderly Patient

Kokoro Nagata, Kasumi Shimizu, Chu Sato, Hiroshi Morita, Yoshihiro Watanabe, and Toshiro Tagawa

Departments of Oral and Maxillofacial Surgery, and Clinical Sciences, Medical Life Science Mie University Graduate School of Medicine, 2-174 Edobashi, Tsu, Mie 514-8507, Japan

Correspondence should be addressed to Kokoro Nagata; kokoro-m@clin.medic.mie-u.ac.jp

Academic Editors: M. A. Polack and M. O. Sayin

Ameloblastomas frequently occur in relatively young people, but are rarely seen in people aged 80 years or older. We report a case of mandibular ameloblastoma in an elderly patient with a review of the literature. The patient was a 82-year-old man who noticed swelling of the gingiva approximately 2 weeks prior to his initial visit. Computed tomography showed a radiolucent area with little radiopacity. Internal uniformity was observed at the site, with thinning of cortical bone which lacked continuity in some areas. The excision and curettage were performed under general anaesthesia. No recurrence has been observed 14 months after surgery.

1. Introduction

Among odontogenic tumours, ameloblastomas have the highest rate of occurrence after odontomas [1]. They are said to comprise between 10% and 50% of all odontogenic tumours [2–4]. The age group predilection peaks in the 20s and 30s, with the average age being between 30 and 40 years, and the majority of cases occur in the 30 to 60 years age group [1, 2, 5–7]. Based on these figures, ameloblastomas are considered to be fairly rare in the elderly. We present a case of ameloblastoma in the mandible of an 82-year-old man and discuss the occurrence of this tumour in the elderly.

2. Case Presentation

An 82-year-old Japanese man presented with swelling of the gingival in the molar region of the left mandible. Approximately 2 weeks prior to the first visit, the patient noticed swelling of the gingiva, and panoramic X-rays were taken at a dental clinic. The images revealed radiolucent findings at the site, and the patient was referred to our facility for examination. The patient had a moderate physique and was well nourished, but he was taking medication for hypertension.

Intraoral findings showed that the upper and lower jaws were edentulous, with a relatively irregular border from the centre of the mandible to the gingiva of the molar region on the left side. Diffuse swelling and surface ulceration were observed. There was neither tenderness nor numbness of the lips (Figure 1).

Panoramic radiographs revealed a barely perceptible, polycystic radiolucent area with slightly irregular margins in the left molar region of the mandible (Figure 2).

Computed tomography showed a radiolucent area with little radiopacity. Internal uniformity was observed at the site, with thinning of cortical bone which lacked continuity in some areas (Figure 3). After 1 month, a biopsy and a needle aspiration were performed. Five millilitres of yellow-white content was aspirated. The results of bacteriological analysis were negative. Histopathological findings revealed that the squamous epithelium was accompanied by chronic inflammatory cell infiltration. Based on these findings, a diagnosis of benign tumor of the mandible was made, and after 2 months, excision and curettage were performed under general anaesthesia. The lesion partially adhered to the bone, and the surface of the peripheral bone was slightly rough. An inferior alveolar neurovascular bundle was also observed below the tumour, and this was preserved. After excision of the tumor in one piece, curettage was performed and the wound was left open. Seven months after surgery, there has been no recurrence of the tumour, and the patient is currently being monitored as an outpatient.

TABLE 1: Intraosseous ameloblastoma.

Year	Author	Sex	Age	Location	Pathological type	Treatment	Race
1986	Ohyama et al. [8]	M	82	Maxilla	Follicular type	Excision (general anesthesia)	Japanese
1991	Iwata et al. [9]	F	83	Maxilla	Follicular type	Excision (general anesthesia)	Japanese
1998	John et al. [10]	F	80	Maxilla	Plexiform type	Excision (general anesthesia)	Black
1998	Lee et al. [11]	F	83	Mandible	Desmoplastic type	Marginal resection	Asian
2004	Koya et al. [12]	M	81	Mandible	Desmoplastic type	Marginal resection (general anesthesia)	Japanese
2010	This case	M	82	Mandible	Follicular type	Excision and curettage (general anesthesia)	Japanese

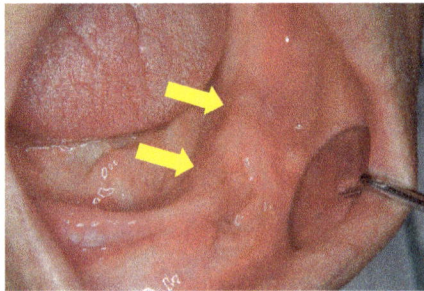

FIGURE 1: Intraoral findings at the first visit. The upper and lower jaws were edentulous, with a relatively irregular border from the centre of the mandible to the gingiva of the molar region on the left side. Diffuse swelling was observed, accompanied by surface ulceration.

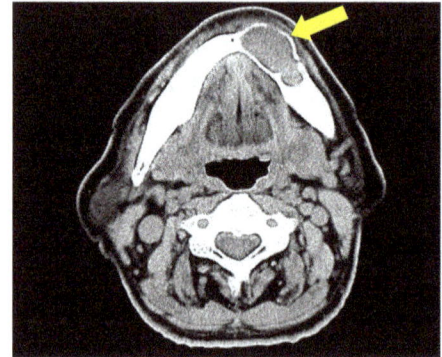

FIGURE 3: Computed tomography view. This shows thinning of peripheral bone was observed, with the bone lacking continuity in some areas.

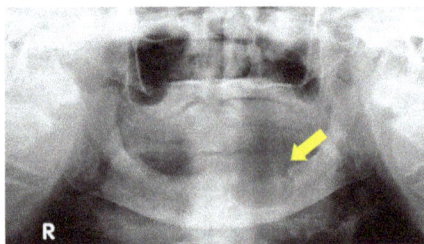

FIGURE 2: Panoramic X-ray view. A polycystic radiolucent area with an irregular margin can be seen in the molar region of the mandible on the left side.

The extracted tumour measured 3 × 2.5 cm and was milky-white in colour, with a slightly rough surface. The transverse section was mostly cystoid, but solid portions were also observed (Figure 4). Histopathological diagnosis was follicular-type ameloblastoma. Haematoxylin-eosin staining revealed alveolar cell hyperplasia with a funicular structure in the fibrosing interstitial tissue, as well as a palisade arrangement (Figure 5).

3. Discussion

Ameloblastomas have a relatively high rate of occurrence and are seen across a wide spectrum of ages [1]. The peak occurrence rate is in the 20s and 30s and reports of these tumours in elderly patients are rare [2, 5–7]. A thorough search by the authors found only 11 reports cases of ameloblastoma

worldwide in patients aged 80 or older between 1977 and 2010. In six of these cases, including the case reported here, the ameloblastoma was located in the centre of the jaw [8–12], and there were three cases each in the maxilla and the mandible. In terms of histological type, three cases were of the follicular type, two were desmoplastic, and one was plexiform (Table 1). The five remaining cases were peripheral ameloblastomas [13–17], two of which occurred in the maxilla, one in the mandible or gingiva, and two in the buccal mucous (Table 2). The ratio of men to women in these 11 cases was 4 : 7, although this may be related to the longer life expectancy of women than men. Of the 11 cases, eight cases were Japanese patients, one was of Asian ethnicity, one was African, and in one case the ethnicity was not noted. Reichart et al. categorised ameloblastoma patients into three ethnicities and found that the mean ages at the time of diagnosis were 28.7, 39.9, and 41.2 years for patients of African, Caucasian and Asian ethnicity, respectively [6]. The fact that the age at occurrence among Asian patients is higher may be because more than 80% of the cases in patients 80 years of age or older occur in Asians.

In reports by Philipsen et al. [18] and Wettan et al. [19], peripheral ameloblastoma comprises 1–10% of all ameloblastoma cases, but in our study of elderly patients, five of the 11 cases studied (45.5%) were peripheral ameloblastomas. According to a 2005 classification by WHO, the mean age of occurrence for intraosseous ameloblastoma is 37 years, while the mean age of patients with peripheral ameloblastomas is 51 years, and 64% of all cases occur between 50 and 70 years of

TABLE 2: Peripheral ameloblastoma.

Year	Author	Sex	Age	Location	Treatment	Race
1977	Frankel et al. [13]	F	92	Maxillary gingiva	Excision (general anesthesia)	Not noted
1988	Takeda et al. [14]	F	89	Mandibular gingiva	Excision and curettage (local anesthesia)	Japanese
1992	Ohuchida et al. [15]	F	81	Maxillary gingiva	Excision (general anesthesia)	Japanese
2007	Yamanishi et al. [16]	M	80	Buccal mucosa	Excision (general anesthesia)	Japanese
2009	Isomura et al. [17]	F	88	Buccal mucosa	Excision (general anesthesia)	Japanese

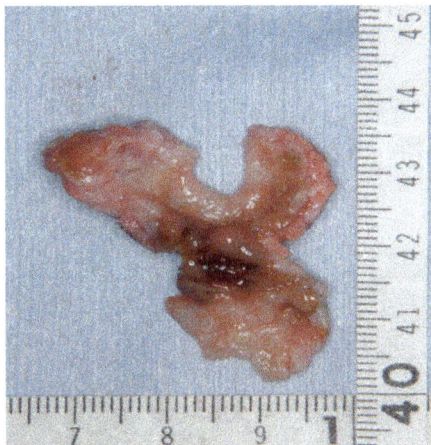

FIGURE 4: The excised tumor. It was milky-white in colour, with a slightly rough surface. The transverse section was largely cystoid, but solid portions were also observed.

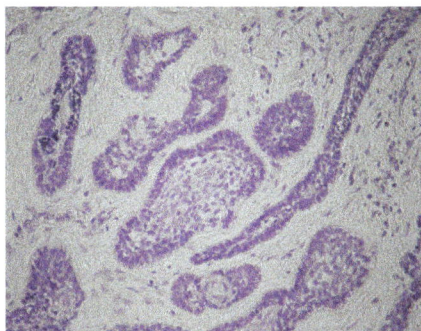

FIGURE 5: Histopathological findings. Alveolar cell hyperplasia with a funicular structure in the fibrosing interstitial tissue was observed, as well as a palisade arrangement (Haematoxylin and eosin staining, ×150).

age [1]. This advanced age may reflect the fact that the age of occurrence is higher for peripheral ameloblastomas. Based on these facts, intraosseous ameloblastomas in elderly patients, as in the case described here, are believed to be relatively rare. Moreover, it is possible that figures for peripheral ameloblastomas include those that occur as a result of alveolar bone being absorbed as a function of ageing, in which case the tumour remains in the soft tissue.

Among reported cases of intraosseous that were diagnosed preoperatively, there have been three cases, including the one described here, in which a benign tumour was suspected [8, 10]: one case of cyst [9], one case in which a clear diagnosis could not be made [11], and one case of malignant tumour [12]. When diagnosing ameloblastomas in elderly patients, there is frequently missing or defective dentition in the affected area, and there are no typical signs such as root absorption. Thus, it is important to differentiate patients with tumours from those with cystic diseases such as residual cysts.

A number of therapies are being investigated for the treatment of ameloblastomas, but in elderly patients, considering their overall physical condition and age, it is necessary to select a minimally invasive surgical approach. Even when the tumour was resected, resection was sometimes performed under local anaesthesia, due to the patient's overall physical condition and the need to preserve the function of the affected area [14] and cases in which the tumour was resected

to the greatest possible extent [9]. In the case described here, after a diagnosis of ameloblastoma was confirmed by intraoperative frozen section diagnosis, the tumour was extracted and curettage was performed. Repeat curettage would generally be performed after 6 months or 1 year, but instead the patient was monitored, due to his advanced age. The authors believe that ongoing, close monitoring will be necessary for this patient.

References

[1] D. G. Gardner, K. Heikinheimo, M. Shear, H. P. Philipsen, and H. Coleman, "Ameloblastomas," in World Health Organization Classification of Tumors. Pathology and Genetics of Head and Neck Tumors, L. Barnes, J. W. Eveson, P. Reichart, and D. Sidransky, Eds., pp. 296–300, IARC Press, Lyon, France, 2005.

[2] M. Takagi, Atlas of Oral Pathology, Bunkodo, Tokyo, Japan, 2004.

[3] T. D. Daley, G. P. Wysocki, and G. A. Pringle, "Relative incidence of odontogenic tumors and oral and jaw cysts in a Canadian population," Oral Surgery, Oral Medicine, Oral Pathology, vol. 77, no. 3, pp. 276–280, 1994.

[4] K. Kasahara, I. Kobayashi, T. Fujiwara et al., "Clinical Study of the odontogenic tumors," Journal of the Japan Stomatological Society, vol. 43, pp. 661–671, 1994.

[5] E. M. Robert and S. Diane, Oral and Maxillofacial Pathology, Quintessence Publishing, Hanover Park, Ill, USA, 2003.

[6] P. A. Reichart, H. P. Philipsen, and S. Sonner, "Ameloblastoma: Biological profile of 3677 cases," European Journal of Cancer B, vol. 31, no. 2, pp. 86–99, 1995.

[7]   D. G. Gardner, "Critique of the 1995 review by Reichart et al. of the biologic profile of 3677 ameloblastomas," *Oral Oncology*, vol. 35, no. 4, pp. 443–449, 1999.

[8]   S. Ohyama, N. Koga, M. Koga et al., "Ameloblastoma of the maxilla: report of a case," *Japanese Journal of Oral and Maxillofacial Surgery*, vol. 32, pp. 434–440, 1986.

[9]   M. Iwata, K. Nishijima, S. Takagi et al., "Ameloblastoma of the maxilla: report of four cases and review of the literature," *Japanese Journal of Oral and Maxillofacial Surgery*, vol. 37, pp. 1826–1834, 1991.

[10] G. John, K. L. Stewart, R. I. Steven, R. B. Julius, and P. S. Marshall, "Plexiform ameloblastoma involving the maxillary antrum," *The New York State Dental Journal*, vol. 64, pp. 34–36, 1998.

[11] C. Y. Lee, J. Lee, K. Hirata, and C. E. Tomich, "Desmoplastic variant of ameloblastoma in an 83-year-ald Asian female: report of a case with literature review," *Hawaii Dental Journal*, vol. 29, no. 3, pp. 12–24, 1998.

[12] E. Koya, M. Mihara, K. Nakashiro, S. Shintani, and H. Hamakawa, "A case of desmoplastic ameloblastoma in an elderly patient," *Japanese Journal of Oral Diagnosis and Oral Medicine*, vol. 17, pp. 58–61, 2004.

[13] K. A. Frankel, J. D. Smith, and L. S. Frankel, "Soft tissue ameloblastom in a 92-year-old woman," *Archives of Otolaryngology*, vol. 103, pp. 499–500, 1977.

[14] Y. Takeda, M. Kuroda, and A. Suzuki, "Ameloblastoma of mucosal origin," *Acta Pathologica Japonica*, vol. 38, no. 8, pp. 1053–1060, 1988.

[15] M. Ohuchida, S. Tanaka, J. Kusukawa, A. Nagata, T. Okina, and T. Kameyama, "A case of peripheral ameloblastoma arising in the maxilla," *Japanese Journal of Oral and Maxillofacial Surgery*, vol. 38, pp. 1437–1438, 1992.

[16] T. Yamanishi, S. Ando, T. Aikawa et al., "A case of extragingival peripheral ameloblasotoma in the buccal mucosa," *Journal of Oral Pathology and Medicine*, vol. 36, no. 3, pp. 184–186, 2007.

[17] E. T. Isomura, S. Ishimoto, T. Yamada, Y. Ono, and M. Kishino, "Case report of extragingival peripheral ameloblastoma in buccal mucosa," *Oral Surgery, Oral Medicine, Oral Pathology, Oral Radiology and Endodontology*, vol. 108, no. 4, pp. 577–579, 2009.

[18] H. P. Philipsen, P. A. Reichart, H. Nikai, T. Takata, and Y. Kudo, "Peripheral ameloblastoma: biological profile based on 160 cases from the literature," *Oral Oncology*, vol. 37, no. 1, pp. 17–27, 2001.

[19] H. L. Wettan, P. A. Patella, and P. D. Freedman, "Peripheral ameloblastoma: review of the literature and report of recurrence as severe dysplasia," *Journal of Oral and Maxillofacial Surgery*, vol. 59, no. 7, pp. 811–815, 2001.

4

Endodontic Treatment of Type II Dens Invaginatus in a Maxillary Lateral Incisor

Dilek Helvacioglu-Yigit and Seda Aydemir

Department of Endodontics, Faculty of Dentistry, University of Kocaeli, 41190 Kocaeli, Turkey

Correspondence should be addressed to Seda Aydemir, aydemirseda@yahoo.com

Academic Editors: A. L. S. Guimaraes and M. A. Polack

Dens invaginatus is a developmental anomaly that results in an enamel-lined cavity intruding into the crown or root before the mineralization phase. It typically affects permanent maxillary lateral incisors, central incisors, and premolars. This paper describes the root canal treatment of Oehlers' type II dens invaginatus in maxillary left lateral incisors. A 16-year-old boy presented to the Faculty of Dentistry, University of Kocaeli, to receive his dental treatments. During the caries removal, the pulp was exposed then anendodontic treatment was initiated. Two canals, one of which represented the invagination, were instrumented, irrigated, and then obturated with a lateral condensation technique.

1. Introduction

Dens invaginatus is a developmental anomaly that results in an enamel-lined cavity intruding into the crown or root before the mineralization phase [1, 2]. The literature suggests several aetiologic factors. These are stimulation and subsequent proliferation and ingrowth of cells of the enamel organ into the dental papilla; retardation of a focal group of cells, with those surrounding continuing to proliferate normally during the dental development; external factors like trauma and infection; and also genetic factors [3, 4]. Three invagination categories were proposed by Oehlers [5] to separate the different types of dens invaginatus by the radiographic appearance of invagination: type I: minimal invagination, enamel lined, confined within the crown of the tooth, and does not extend beyond the level of the external amelocemental junction; type II: enamel lined and extends into the pulp chamber but remains within the root canal with no communication with the periodontal ligament; type III: the invagination penetrates through the root, perforating the apical area and having a second foramen in the apical or periodontal area, but there is no immediate communication with the pulp [2, 4].

The most frequently affected tooth is the maxillary lateral incisor [2, 3, 6]. In a decreasing order of frequency, other teeth that develop this anomaly are the maxillary central incisors, premolars, canines, and molars [2, 6]. The occurrence of this anomaly in mandibular teeth has been reported in a few cases [4, 7]. The clinical appearance of dens invaginatus varies considerably. The crown of affected teeth can have normal morphology or it can also show unusual forms such as a greater buccolingual dimension, peg-shaped form, barrel-shaped form, conical shapes and talon cusps [1, 2, 8]. A deep foramen caecum might be the first clinical sign indicating the presence of an invaginated tooth. As this area is difficult to access and clean, caries can develop with a subsequent pulp necrosis and apical pathosis [2, 6, 9].

2. Case Presentation

A 16-year-old male patient who did not have any problems in his medical history was referred to the Faculty of Dentistry, University of Kocaeli, for his dental treatments. After clinical and radiologic evaluations, we detected caries on the maxillary left lateral incisor which had unusual anatomy (Figures 1(a), 1(b), and 1(c)). The initial periapical radiographic examination revealed that the maxillary left lateral incisor showed an abnormal morphology with an invagination (Oehlers' type II). During the removal of deep dentin caries,

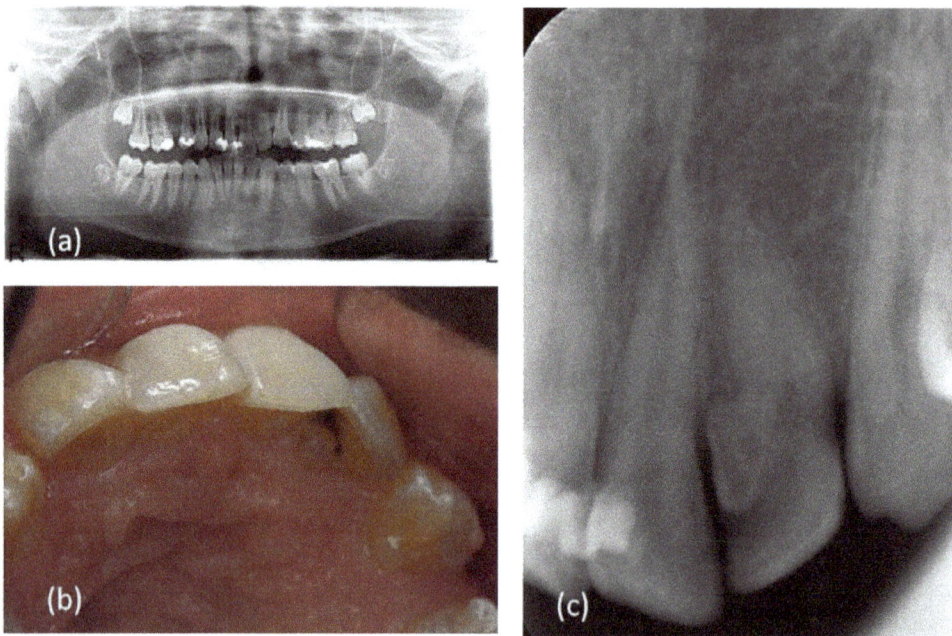

FIGURE 1: (a) Preoperative panoramic radiograph, (b) preoperative photograph: palatinal view, and (c) preoperative radiograph revealing the maxillary left lateral incisor with an unusual anatomy.

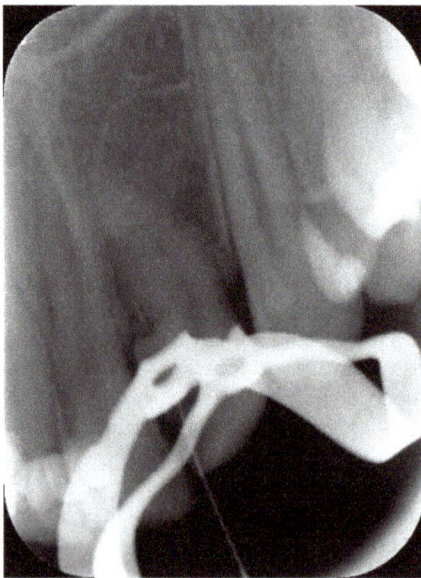

FIGURE 2: Radiograph showing the fusion of the main canal and invagination.

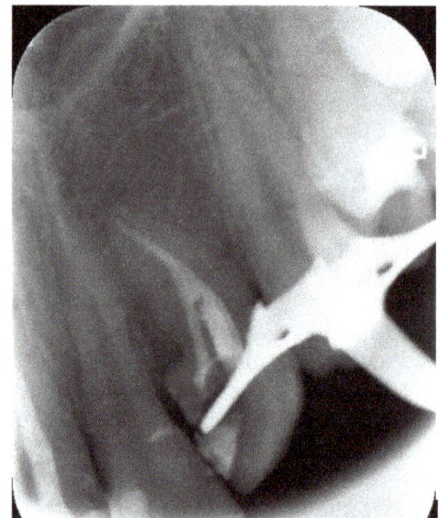

FIGURE 3: Obturation of root canals.

the pulp tissue was exposed. The patient was anesthetised, and rubber dam was placed and stabilised using widgets. The main canal and invaginated canal communicated at the middle of the root. The working length was established by a Raypex 5 apex locator (VDW Endodontic Synergy, Munich, Germany). A radiograph showed the fusion of the main canal and invagination (Figure 2). The root canals were prepared with stainless steel H files (Mani Inc., Tochigi, Japan) using

a step-back technique. The irrigation was copious throughout with a 2.5% sodium hypochlorite solution, and EDTA (MD-ChelCream, META BIOMED, Chungbuk, the Republic of Korea) was used for chelation. The root canals were dried with paper points and (Precise Dental, Zapopan, Mexico) obturated with a lateral condensation technique with a 0.02 tapered gutta-percha (Diadent, Choongchong Buk Do, the Republic of Korea) and an AH plus (Dentsply De Trey GmbH, Konstanz, Germany) root canal sealer (Figure 3). A two-step self-etch adhesive system (Clearfil SE Bond, Kuraray Medical Inc., Japan) was used in order to perform

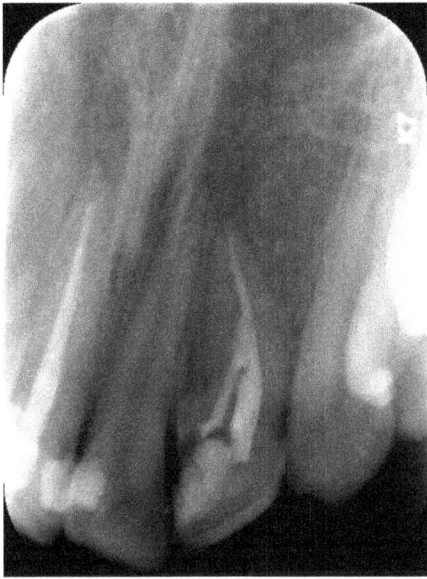

FIGURE 4: Recall radiograph after 6 months.

a restorative treatment. The teeth were restored with a nanofilled resin composite (CLEARFIL MAJESTY Esthetic, Kuraray Medical Inc., Japan). Six months later, the tooth was asymptomatic and all clinical findings were within normal limits (Figure 4).

3. Discussion

Several endodontic treatment options of dens invaginatus have been reported, including nonsurgical, surgical, and combined approaches [4, 8, 10–13]. In this paper, the nonsurgical root canal treatment was sufficient since there was no periapical lesion. There are reports of cases in the literature where the pulp tissues were not involved and only the invaginations were cleaned and treated [14, 15]. However, in most cases, the invagination and the pulp tissues can be connected [3, 15]. Cleaning and shaping procedures of the root canal are difficult because the shape of the canal is deformed by the invagination. Like our case in an Oehlers type II dens invagination, the anomaly does not extend all the way to the apex; therefore, access to the apical third of the root canal is less difficult.

The first difficulty of the cases of dens invaginatus is preparing the access cavity. The root canal debridement of the invagination is difficult, because of the unpredictable shape and narrow access. Stainless steel files using with a chelator such as EDTA and copious irrigation of sodium hypoclorite make the preparation easier allowing thorough debridement of the root canal.

4. Conclusion

Dens invaginatus is a rare malformation of the teeth, showing a broad spectrum of morphologic variations in size and form of the crowns and roots. The complex anatomy of

these anomalies makes treatment procedures harder. Further followup of these cases should not be neglected to evaluate the treatment success.

References

[1] Y. P. Reddy, K. Karpagavinayagam, and C. V. Subbarao, "Management of dens invaginatus diagnosed by spiral computed tomography: a case eport," *Journal of Endodontics*, vol. 34, no. 9, pp. 1138–1142, 2008.

[2] F. V. Vier-Pelisser, A. Pelisser, L. C. Recuero, M. V. So, M. G. Borba, and J. A. Figueiredo, "Use of cone beam computed tomography in the diagnosis, planning and follow up of a type III dens invaginatus case," *International endodontic journal*, vol. 45, pp. 198–208, 2012.

[3] A. Alani and K. Bishop, "Dens invaginatus. Part 1: classification, prevalence and aetiology," *International Endodontic Journal*, vol. 41, no. 12, pp. 1123–1136, 2008.

[4] C. C. Monteiro-Jardel and F. R. F. Alves, "Type III dens invaginatus in a mandibular incisor: a case report of a conventional endodontic treatment," *Oral Surgery, Oral Medicine, Oral Pathology, Oral Radiology and Endodontology*, vol. 111, no. 4, pp. e29–e32, 2011.

[5] F. A. C. Oehlers, "Dens invaginatus (dilated composite odontome). I. Variations of the invagination process and associated anterior crown forms," *Oral Surgery, Oral Medicine, Oral Pathology*, vol. 10, no. 11, pp. 1204–1218, 1957.

[6] S. C. Yeh, Y. T. Lin, and S. Y. Lu, "Dens invaginatus in the maxillary lateral incisor," *Oral Surgery, Oral Medicine, Oral Pathology, Oral Radiology, and Endodontics*, vol. 87, no. 5, pp. 628–631, 1999.

[7] B. Carvalho-Sousa, F. Almeida-Gomes, L. Gominho, and D. Albuquerque, "Endodontic treatment of a periradicular lesion on an invaginated type III mandibular lateral incisor," *Indian Journal of Dental Research*, vol. 20, no. 2, pp. 243–245, 2009.

[8] S. M. G. de Sousa and C. M. Bramante, "Dens invaginatus: treatment choices," *Endodontics and Dental Traumatology*, vol. 14, no. 4, pp. 152–158, 1998.

[9] M. Jung, "Endodontic treatment of dens invaginatus type III with three root canals and open apical foramen," *International Endodontic Journal*, vol. 37, no. 3, pp. 205–213, 2004.

[10] M. Hülsmann, "Dens invaginatus: aetiology, classification, prevalence, diagnosis, and treatment considerations," *International Endodontic Journal*, vol. 30, no. 2, pp. 79–90, 1997.

[11] K. Er, A. Kuştarci, Ü. Özan, and T. Taşdemir, "Nonsurgical endodontic treatment of dens invaginatus in a mandibular premolar with large periradicular lesion: a case report," *Journal of Endodontics*, vol. 33, no. 3, pp. 322–324, 2007.

[12] P. Beltes, "Endodontic treatment in three cases of dens invaginatus," *Journal of Endodontics*, vol. 23, no. 6, pp. 399–402, 1997.

[13] A. M. Chaniotis, G. N. Tzanetakis, E. G. Kontakiotis, and K. I. Tosios, "Combined endodontic and surgical management of a mandibular lateral incisor with a rare type of dens invaginatus," *Journal of Endodontics*, vol. 34, no. 10, pp. 1255–1260, 2008.

[14] T. Tsurumachi, "Endodontic treatment of an invaginated maxillary lateral incisor with a periradicular lesion and a healthy pulp," *International Endodontic Journal*, vol. 37, no. 10, pp. 717–723, 2004.

[15] R. George, A. J. Moule, and L. J. Walsh, "A rare case of dens invaginatus in a mandibular canine," *Australian Endodontic Journal*, vol. 36, no. 2, pp. 83–86, 2010.

5

Complex Composite Odontoma with Characteristic Histology

Sujatha Govindrajan,[1] **J. Muruganandhan,**[1] **Shaik Shamsudeen,**[1] **Nalin Kumar,**[1]
M. Ramasamy,[2] **and Srinivasa Prasad**[3]

[1] *Department of Oral and Maxillofacial Pathology, Sri Venkateswara Dental College and Hospital, Thalambur, Chennai 603103, India*
[2] *Department of Orthodontics, Sri Venkateswara Dental College and Hospital, Thalambur, Chennai 603103, India*
[3] *Department of Oral and Maxillofacial Surgery, Sri Venkateswara Dental College and Hospital, Thalambur, Chennai 603103, India*

Correspondence should be addressed to J. Muruganandhan; drmurugan@outlook.com

Academic Editors: I. El-Hakim and S. R. Watt-Smith

Odontomas are the most commonly occurring odontogenic tumors, which are considered by many to be hamartomas rather than neoplasms. These clinically asymptomatic tumors are classified into complex and compound odontomas. They are usually discovered in radiographs and rarely cause bony expansion or infection. This paper discusses a case report of a complex odontoma exhibiting all the structural features and defects of enamel, dentine, and cementum in succession, with an overview on its etiology.

1. Introduction

Hamartomas of tooth forming tissues are termed as odontoma. They are the most common tumor of epithelial and mesenchymal origin and account for 22% of all odontogenic tumors [1]. This nonaggressive benign tumor contains enamel, dentin, cementum, and pulp either arranged in an orderly manner resembling a rudimentary tooth called compound odontoma or arranged in a haphazard manner called complex odontoma. Complex odontoma is less common when compared to the compound, and they present in ratio of 1 : 2 [2]. Odontomas rarely erupt in the oral cavity. We present a case of a partially erupted odontoma in the right third molar region.

2. Case Report

A 28-year-old male patient reported to a private clinic with a complaint of pain in the right lower posterior tooth region for about one week. On intraoral examination, a partially erupted tooth-like structure was seen. The pain was intermittent and was aggravated on chewing. Radiographic investigation revealed the presence of near-spherical opaque mass resembling calcified tissue measuring about 2 cm in diameter. The radiopaque mass with a density greater than bone and equal or greater than that of tooth was surrounded by a radiolucent rim in all areas except the erupted portion distal to normally erupted second molar (Figure 1).

Removal of the mass was planned under local anaesthesia. Mucoperiosteal flap was raised distal to 47, and the calcified mass was removed. The spherical mass was about 2 cm in diameter with small irregular areas of indentations. The inferior side of the mass showed a hollow invagination giving the appearance of a small cup (Figure 2). The specimen was sent for histopathological examination. A diagnosis of complex odontoma was made clinically.

Ground sections were done on the dissected halves of the hard tissue mass. The ground section showed areas of enamel, dentine, and cementum in succession (Figure 3). The enamel showed uneven thickness and undulating surface. Hypocalcified areas like lamellae, spindles, tufts, and incremental lines were seen (Figures 4 and 5). Some areas showed irregular rod patterns and gnarled enamel (Figure 6).

The dentinoenamel junction was regular and scalloped in some areas. The underlying dentine showed "S" shaped dentinal tubules. Primary and secondary dentine types were observed with clearly visible incremental lines (Figure 7). Hypocalcified areas like interglobular dentine and Tomes' granular layer were also observed (Figures 8 and 9). Dead tracts were also seen (Figure 9). Next to the dentine there

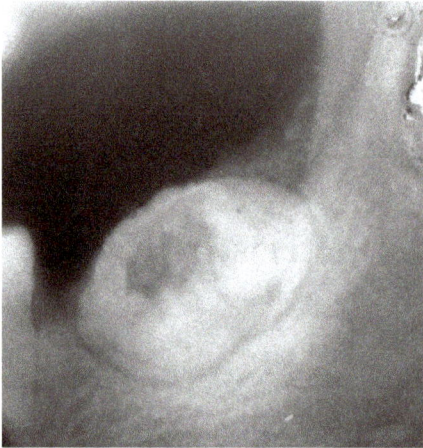

FIGURE 1: Radiographic image of the odontoma.

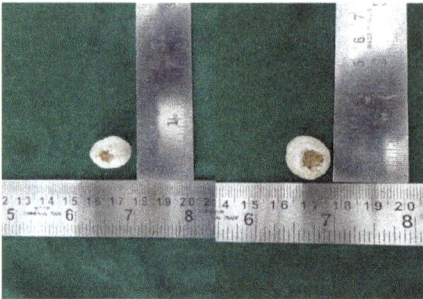

FIGURE 3: Enamel, dentine and cementum in succession (photomicrograph, ground section 10x).

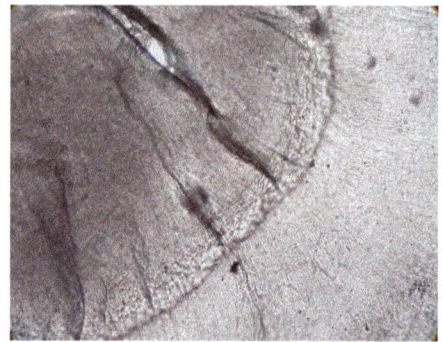

FIGURE 2: Superior and inferior surface of odontoma.

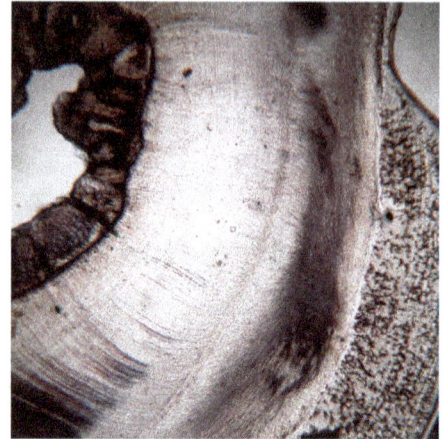

FIGURE 4: Presence of lamellae, spindles and tufts (photomicrograph, ground section 10x).

was a layer of cementum of varying thickness. Both types of cementum were observed. The cellular cementum was more prominent with numerous cementocytes. Each cementocyte had about 8–10 canaliculi, which are branching and oriented away from the dentinal surface (Figure 10).

3. Discussion

Paul Braco in 1867 was the first to coin the term odontoma and defined the term as tumors formed by the overgrowth or transition of complete dental tissue [3]. It is a growth in which both the epithelial and mesenchymal cells exhibit complete differentiation resulting in formation of enamel and dentin by the functional ameloblasts and odontoblasts. These odontogenic cells are usually disorganized, and the enamel, dentine, and pulpal tissue are laid down in an abnormal pattern [4]. Our case represented the presence of functional ameloblast, odontoblast, and cementoblast by formation of these normal hard tissue structures. WHO has classified four tumors which arise from mixed tissue origin giving normal enamel and dentine formation, odontoma being the most common of them [5].

According to WHO, this lesion is "a malformation in which all the dental tissues are represented, individual tissues being mainly formed but occurring in more or less disorderly pattern." When the calcified tissues are simply arranged in an irregular mass bearing no morphological similarity to rudimentary teeth, they are termed complex odontoma. A compound odontoma comprises calcified structures arranged in an orderly pattern that result in many teeth-like structures, but without morphological resemblance to normal tooth [6]. Our case presented as an irregular mass and was classified as a complex odontoma.

The etiology of odontoma is not clear, and various causes like local trauma, infection, hereditary anomalies like Gardner's syndrome, Hermann's syndrome, odontoblastic hyperactivity, and alteration in genetic components responsible for tooth development are also considered [7]. Hitchin suggested that odontomas are inherited (through a mutant gene) due to interference, possibly postnatal, with genetic control of tooth development [8]. Experimental studies in rats suggested the role of trauma in formation of odontomas [9].

Sources of cells for odontomas could be mature ameloblasts, cell rests of Serres, or extraneous odontogenic epithelial cells [1, 10–12]. These cells can be stimulated by either environmental or genetic factors. Genetic factors could be either due to inheritance of abnormal genes or mutation of the responsible genes and interference in the mechanism of genes controlling tooth formation [7].

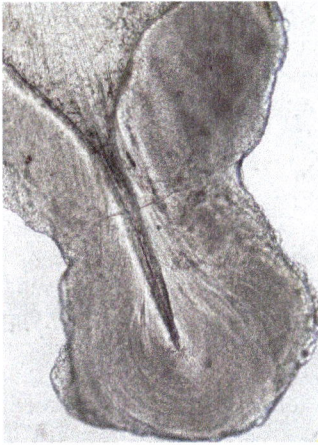

FIGURE 5: Incremental lines of enamel (photomicrograph, ground section 10x).

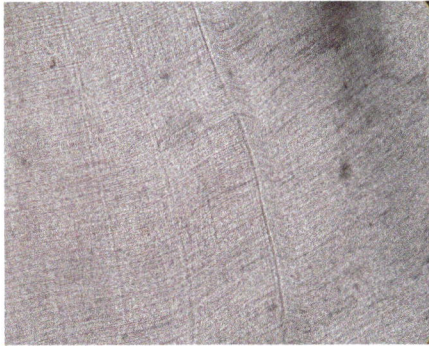

FIGURE 6: Dentinal tubules with incremental lines (photomicrograph, ground section 10x).

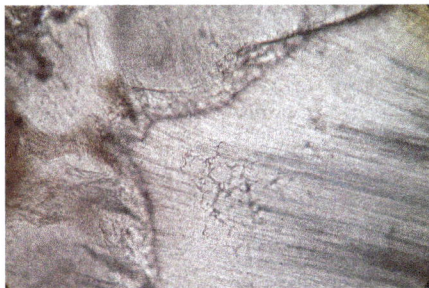

FIGURE 7: Interglobular dentine (photomicrograph, ground section 10x).

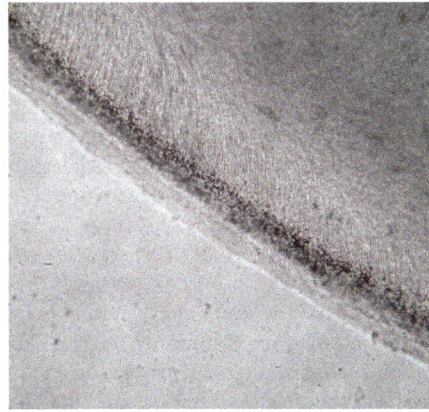

FIGURE 8: Tomes granular layer (photomicrograph, ground section 10x).

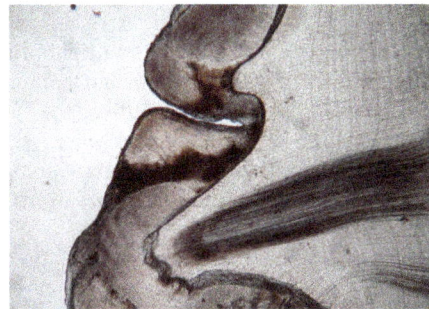

FIGURE 9: Dead tracts and gnarled enamel (photomicrograph, ground section 10x).

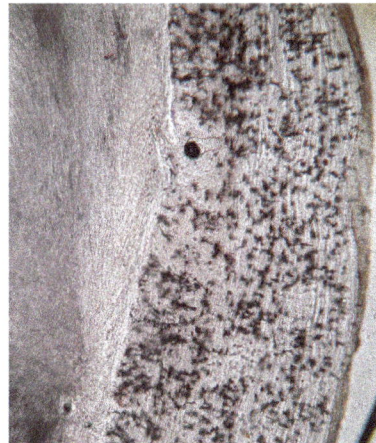

FIGURE 10: Cemetocytes with canaliculi (photomicrograph, ground section 10x).

Environmental factors like trauma, growth pressure, and infection may play a role in the pathogenesis of odontoma. A vertically directed force in the form of trauma which is directed to the permanent tooth bud through the deciduous tooth can lead to morphological changes in the permanent tooth bud leading to formation of odontomas [13]. Studies by Glasstone (1952) and Rushton (1957) have supported the role of trauma in the development of odontoma [8]. Levy states that the stage of development during which the trauma has occurred determines the development of hypoplastic teeth, odontomas, and supernumerary tooth [9]. Presence of odontoma in sites other than tooth bearing regions suggests that trauma could have possibly displaced the developing tooth germ leading to its malformation [14].

Growth pressure due to inadequate space is been quoted as the etiology in some odontomas. This theory by Hitchin states that abnormal pressure from the deciduous roots over the developing tooth germ could lead to the formation of odontomas [8, 15, 16]. Infections can cause the division of tooth germ or interfere with tooth development [7].

Odontomas were discovered at any age but the most prevalent age of detection was the second decade of life with a slight predilection for occurrence in males when compared to females [17]. Compound odontomas are more common in the anterior segment of the jaws (61%), and complex odontomas are more common in the posterior segment (59%), with higher occurrence in the right than in the left side [4]. Compound odontomas are commonly seen in the incisor-cuspid region of maxilla and complex type in the premolar-molar region of mandible [18]. In our case, the patient was a middle aged male patient with the complex odontoma occurring in the right posterior segment of the mandible.

Odontomas are clinically asymptomatic, although occasionally retention of deciduous teeth, noneruption, swelling, pain, tooth displacement, cortical bone expansion, and infection may be noted [19]. Alterations to neighboring teeth such as malpositioning, devitalisation, malformation, aplasia, and retained teeth were observed in 70% of the cases [20]. Odontomas are classified as intraosseous when seen totally embedded in the bone with or without signs of eruption and extraosseous when present in the soft tissues over the tooth bearing bone [21].

Eruption of odontomas is different from a normal tooth as there is lack of periodontal ligament. As there is no root formation, the increasing size of the odontoma leads to sequestration of the overlying bone by causing pressure and eventually occlusal movement and eruption [22]. Bone remodeling is considered as the other possible factor in initiating eruption. Cellular activity in reduced enamel epithelium and dental follicles is required for eruption. Epidermal growth factor β [EGF-β] and transforming growth factor [TGF] are expressed by signals from reduced enamel epithelium, helping in production of colony-stimulating factor by the follicular cells, recruiting osteoclasts to the follicle. Proteases secreted by reduced enamel epithelium also help in breakdown of follicle and produce a path of least resistance [23].

Diagnosis of odontomas is usually by radiographs. A routine intraoral radiograph helps in diagnosing the presence of odontoma and the classification is usually by visualization. A compound odontoma, in a radiograph shows well-organized malformed tooth or tooth-like structures in a radiolucent follicle-like space whereas the complex type shows irregularly shaped radiopacity surrounded by a radiolucent rim. In cases where there are numerous tooth-like structures in a compound odontoma, differentiating the two becomes difficult [7]. If both visual and radiographic images fail to give a definite diagnosis as in some cases, other procedures like histologic examination are used. In our case, though we established a diagnosis of complex odontoma through radiographic and visual examination, we decided to see the histological features through ground section.

Ground section usually reveals the presence of all hard tissues in succession representing enamel, dentine, and cementum. Hypocalcified areas of both enamel and dentine are

seen. In our case, the microscopy showed remarkable features that make for interesting discussion. Treatment of odontomas is usually by conservative surgical removal and preservation of impacted or embedded tooth if present.

4. Conclusion

Odontomas are common odontogenic tumors, which are usually asymptomatic and are diagnosed by routine radiographs. Etiology of this tumor is not clear, and López-Areal in his study has supported the role of injury during childhood for formation of odontomas [24]. In our case, though the patient did not give a clear history of childhood injury, presence of the normal structures in an orderly pattern gives us an opinion that some mild interference during formation of third molar has occurred.

Acknowledgment

The authors thank their lab technician Mrs. M. Elavarasi for helping them prepare this slide.

References

[1] S. N. Bhaskar, "Odontogenic tumors of jaws," in *Synopsis of Oral Pathology*, pp. 292–2303, Mosby, 7th edition, 1986.

[2] D. M. Cohen and I. Bhattacharyya, "Ameloblastic fibroma, ameloblastic fibro-odontoma, and odontoma," *Oral and Maxillofacial Surgery Clinics of North America*, vol. 16, no. 3, pp. 375–384, 2004.

[3] E. Sprawson, "Odontomas," *British Dental Journal*, vol. 62, pp. 177–201, 1937.

[4] G. W. Shafer, M. K. Hine, and B. M. Levy, Eds., *A Text Book of Oral Pathology*, WB Saunders, Philadelphia, Pa, USA, 4th edition, 1983.

[5] J. J. Pindborg, I. R. H. Kramer, and H. Torloni, "Histologic typing of odontogenic tumors, jaw cysts and allied lesions," in *International Histological Classification of Jaw Tumors*, vol. 5, pp. 29–230, World Health Organisation, Geneva, Switzerland, 1970.

[6] I. R. H. Kramer, J. J. Pindborg, and M. Shear, *Histological Typing of Odontogenic Tumors*, WHO International Histological Classification of Tumors, Springer, Berlin, Germany, 2nd edition, 1992.

[7] V. Satish, M. C. Prabhudevi, and R. Sharma, "Odontoma: a brief overview," *International Journal of Clinical Pediatric Dentistry*, vol. 4, pp. 177–185, 2011.

[8] A. D. Hitchin, "The etiology of the calcified composite odontomas," *British Dental Journal*, vol. 130, pp. 475–482, 1971.

[9] B. A. Levy, "Effects of experimental trauma on developing first molar teeth in rats," *Journal of Dental Research*, vol. 47, no. 2, pp. 323–327, 1968.

[10] E. F. Torreti and R. Carrel, "Compound odontoma in a twelve-year-old girl," *ASDC Journal of Dentistry for Children*, vol. 50, no. 5, pp. 376–378, 1983.

[11] O. Fijerskov, "Odontogenesis," in *Histology of the Human Tooth*, I. A. Mjor and O. Fijerskov, Eds., pp. 21–31, Munksgaard, Copenhagen, Denmark, 1st edition, 1979.

[12] R. M. Smith, J. E. Tuner, and A. L. Ribbins, *Atlas of Oral Pathology*, CV Mosby, St Louis, Mo, USA, 1981.

[13] J. O. Andreason, "Injuries to developing teeth," in *Textbook and Color Atlas of Traumatic Injuries to Teeth*, J. O. Andreason and F. M. Andreason, Eds., pp. 457–494, Mosby, Copenhagen, Denmark, 3rd edition, 1993.

[14] A. Shteyer, S. Taicher, and Y. Marmary, "Odontoma in the sub-condylar region," *British Journal of Oral Surgery*, vol. 17, no. 2, pp. 161–165, 1979.

[15] P. Gurdal and T. Seckin, "Odontomas," *Quintessence International*, vol. 4, article 32, 2001.

[16] A. D. Hitchin and W. D. Mchugh, "Three coronal invaginations in a dilated composite odontome," *British Dental Journal*, vol. 97, pp. 90–92, 1954.

[17] M. Vengal, H. Arora, S. Ghosh, and K. M. Pai, "Large erupting complex odontoma: a case report," *Journal of the Canadian Dental Association*, vol. 73, no. 2, pp. 169–172, 2007.

[18] O. P. Kharbanda, C. S. Sambi, and K. Renu, "Odontoma: a case report," *Journal of the Indian Dental Association*, vol. 58, pp. 269–271, 1986.

[19] M. S. Tuzum, "Orofacial pain associated with an infected complex odontoma—case report," *Australian Dental Journal*, vol. 3, pp. 352–354, 1990.

[20] M. Kaneko, M. Fukuda, T. Sano, T. Ohnishi, and Y. Hosokawa, "Microradiographic and microscopic investigation of a rare case of complex odontoma," *Oral Surgery, Oral Medicine, Oral Pathology, Oral Radiology, and Endodontics*, vol. 86, no. 1, pp. 131–134, 1998.

[21] L. Junquera, J. C. de Vicente, P. Roig, S. Olay, and O. Rodríguez-Recio, "Intraosseus odontoma erupted into the oral cavity: an unusual pathology," *Medicina Oral, Patologia Oral y Cirugia Bucal*, vol. 10, no. 3, pp. 248–251, 2005.

[22] A. R. Ten Cate and A. Nanci, "Physiologic tooth movements: eruption and shedding," in *Ten Cate's Oral Histology: Development, Structure and Function*, A. Nanci, Ed., pp. 275–298, Mosby, St. Louis, Mo, USA, 2003.

[23] P. B. Sood, B. Patil, S. Godhi, and D. C. Shetty, "Multiple supernumerary teeth and odontoma in the maxilla: a case report," *Contemporary Clinical Dentistry*, vol. 1, pp. 45–46, 2010.

[24] L. López-Areal, F. Silvestre Donat, and J. Gil Lozano, "Compound odontoma erupting in the mouth: 4-year follow-up of a clinical case," *Journal of Oral Pathology and Medicine*, vol. 21, no. 6, pp. 285–288, 1992.

6

A Rare Case Report of Amlodipine-Induced Gingival Enlargement and Review of Its Pathogenesis

Sanjeev Joshi[1] and Sucheta Bansal[2]

[1] Department of Prosthodontics Including Crown and Bridge & Implantology, Himachal Institute of Dental Sciences,
Paonta Sahib, Himachal Pradesh 173025, India
[2] Department of Oral and Maxillofacial Pathology, Himachal Institute of Dental Sciences, Paonta Sahib,
Himachal Pradesh 173025, India

Correspondence should be addressed to Sanjeev Joshi; sanjeevjoshimds@gmail.com

Academic Editors: P. Lopez Jornet and M. Peñarrocha

Gingival enlargement is a common clinical feature of gingival and periodontal diseases. It is an unwanted side effect of certain systemic drugs given for nondental treatment. It is being reported with three main groups of drugs like calcium channel blockers (CCBs), immunosuppressants, and anticonvulsants. Among calcium channel blockers, nifedipine causes gingival hyperplasia in about 10% of patients, whereas the incidence of amlodipine-, a third generation calcium channel blocker, induced gingival hyperplasia is very limited. There are very few reports of amlodipine-induced gingival enlargement at a dose of 5 mg. We report a case of amlodipine-induced gingival enlargement in a 45-year-old hypertensive patient taking amlodipine at a dose of 5 mg.

1. Introduction

Drug-induced gingival enlargement was first reported in 1939 by Kimball with chronic usage of the antiepileptic drug phenytoin [1]. Currently, more than 20 prescription medications are associated with gingival enlargement [2]. Drugs associated with gingival overgrowth can be broadly categorized into three major groups according to their therapeutic actions, namely, anticonvulsants, immunosuppressants, and calcium channel blockers [3, 4].

Amlodipine is a new dihydropyridine calcium channel blocker that is used in the management of both hypertension and angina. Ellis et al. [5] first reported gingival sequestration of amlodipine and amlodipine-induced gingival overgrowth. Since then, very few cases of amlodipine-induced gingival hyperplasia have been reported in the dental literature although there are numerous reports of nifedipine- (another member of calcium channel blockers) induced gingival overgrowth till date. There are less data on reports of hyperplasia with amlodipine at a dose of 5 mg, even after taking it for more than 6 months [6, 7].

But, in the present case, the gingival hyperplasia occurred at a dose of 5 mg within 6 months of use.

2. Case Report

A 45-year-old male patient came to the department with the chief complaint of loose teeth in upper and lower front jaw regions since 1 year with swollen and bleeding gums. Patient first noted bead like nodular growth over the gums which progressively enlarged to the present size covering almost entire teeth interfering with further cleaning of teeth.

The patient was hypertensive since 1.5 years and was under medication Coronol-AM (atenolol, 50 mg + amlodipine, 5 mg) once daily. He denied the history of any adverse habits.

The patient was moderately built and nourished with no signs of anaemia and jaundice and noncyanosed. His vital signs were within the normal range.

Intraoral examination revealed generalized enlargement of attached gingival extending up to marginal and interdental gingiva. Surface of the gingiva appears lobulated with loss of scalloping (Figure 1). Poor oral hygiene status of patient was assessed by the presence of local irritating factors which surrounded the teeth.

Based on drug history and clinical examination of the patient provisional diagnosis of combined gingival

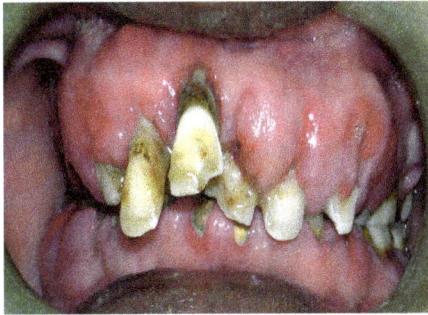

FIGURE 1: Showing generalized amlodipine-induced gingival enlargement.

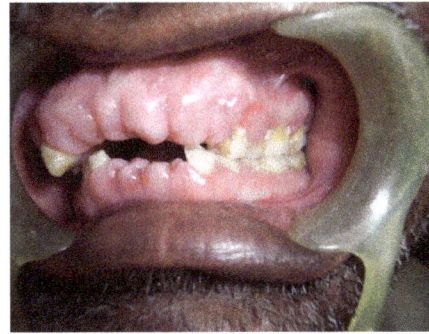

FIGURE 3: Showing response to therapy after 1.5 months.

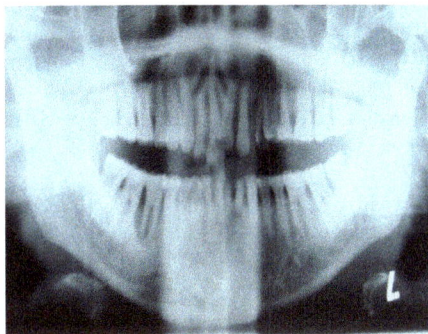

FIGURE 2: Orthopantomography revealed generalized bone loss.

enlargement was made. Complete hemogram of the patient was done, but all the parameters were within the normal range. Orthopantomogram was taken which revealed generalized bone loss (Figure 2).

After this, incisional biopsy was done. Histopathological report revealed few areas of hyperplastic orthokeratinized and parakeratinised stratified squamous epithelium and connective tissue exhibiting mixture of dense and loose fibrous component. Inflammatory cell infiltrate with PMLs and dilated blood capillaries with few areas of calcifications were also evident.

Correlating history, clinical examination, and investigations, final diagnosis of combined gingival enlargement (amlodipine induced and inflammatory) was made. Patient was referred to periodontics department for further treatment. In the preliminary phase, extraction of teeth (11, 21, 22, 23, 31, 32, and 34) with hopeless prognosis was recommended. Planned sessions of scaling and root planning with drug change with the patient's physician consent were performed. Patient was put on tablet Normadate 100 mg twice daily and was evaluated after the period of 1.5 months. There was drastic change in the clinical picture of gingiva with complete loss of inflammatory component (Figure 3).

3. Discussion

Amlodipine is a 3rd generation dihydropyridine calcium antagonist which is structurally similar to nifedipine but pharmacodynamically comparable to it. In patients with

hypertensive heart disease the prevalence of gingival overgrowth associated with amlodipine is lower than that associated with other calcium channel blocking agents including nifedipine [6]. Drug-induced gingival overgrowth usually occurs within the first 3 months of starting drug therapy at a dose of 10 mg/day and begins as an enlargement of the interdental papilla. Although few cases of amlodipine-induced hyperplasia have been reported, the present case is interesting as it occurred with a low dose of amlodipine (5 mg) and appeared on administration for 6 months.

Seymour et al. [8] gave a review on the pathogenesis of drug-induced gingival overgrowth in which they considered it as a multifactorial model, involving an interaction of several factors, which expands on the interaction between drug and metabolite with the gingival fibroblasts. Predisposing factors for these changes are age, genetic predisposition, pharmacokinetic variables, drug-induced alterations in gingival connective tissue homeostasis, histopathology, ultrastructural factors and inflammatory changes, and drug-induced action on growth factors.

The underlying mechanism behind drug-induced gingival hyperplasia involves inflammatory and noninflammatory pathways. The proposed noninflammatory mechanisms include defective collagenase activity due to decreased uptake of folic acid, blockage of aldosterone synthesis in adrenal cortex, and consequent feedback increase in adrenocorticotropic hormone level and upregulation of keratinocyte growth factor. Alternatively, inflammation may develop as a result of direct toxic effects of concentrated drug in crevicular gingival fluid and/or bacterial plagues. This inflammation could lead to the upregulation of several cytokine factors such as transforming growth factor-β1 [9–11].

Many studies have been conducted which showed that amlodipine cannot induce gingival hyperplasia at 5 mg once daily dose even if taken for more than 6 months. It can be caused only at a dose of 10 mg/day [6, 8]. The present case is unique in that even 5 mg/day dose of amlodipine caused gingival hyperplasia after 6 months of use.

The mechanism through which these drugs induce gingival enlargement is still poorly understood. It has been found that phenytoin and calcium channel blockers inhibit the intracellular Ca^{2+} uptake thereby stimulating gingival fibroblasts. Not all the patients receiving the same drug develop gingival enlargement. Possible reason can be that individuals with gingival enlargement have fibroblasts with an abnormal susceptibility to the drug. It has also been proposed that the susceptibility to pharmacologically induced gingival enlargement may be governed by existence of differential proportions of fibroblast subset in each individual which exhibit a fibrogenic response to these medications. It has also been shown that the functional heterogenicity exists in gingival fibroblasts in response to various stimuli [12].

A synergestic enhancement of collagenous protein synthesis by human gingival fibroblasts is found when these cells are exposed simultaneously to calcium channel blockers and elevated levels of interleukin-1β (a proinflammatory cytokine) in inflamed gingival tissues. Interleukin-6 also plays a role in fibrogenic responses of gingiva to these medications. Interleukin-6 targets fibroblasts which trigger the proliferation of fibroblasts and exert the positive regulation on collagen and glycosaminoglycans synthesis. So this cytokine has been proposed to play a pathogenic role in fibrotic gingival enlargement [8].

Clinical relevant doses of cyclosporins trigger gingival fibroblasts to exhibit significant reduced levels of matrix metalloproteinases-1 and -3 secretions which lead to accumulation of extracellular matrix components [13]. There is a strong correlation between the production of inactive collagenase and responding fibroblasts. Because of reduced folic acid uptake, there is limited production of activator protein which converts inactive collagenase to active collagenase. Limited amount of collagenase becomes available [8].

Treatment consists of stopping the offending drug if possible with the patient's physician consent and providing the supplements of folic acid and ascorbic acid. Reduction in the size of the gingival overgrowth has been reported within a week of drug withdrawal and may lead to full resolution [14].

Patients benefit from effective oral hygiene measures, professional tooth cleaning, scaling, and root planning [15]. If gingival enlargement persists after careful consideration of the previously mentioned approaches, these cases need to be treated by surgery, either by gingivectomy or flap surgery. In present case patient was subjected to planned sessions of scaling and root planning with substitute drug Normadate 100 mg twice daily. On evaluating the patient after the period of 1.5 months drastic change in the clinical picture of gingiva with complete loss of inflammatory component was seen.

4. Conclusion

We conclude that the gingival hyperplasia could occur with amlodipine even at a small dose (5 mg). Physicians and dentists should be aware of the etiologic medications that can induce gingival hyperplasia and be able to identify changes in the oral cavity in such patients and to prevent, diagnose, and successfully manage them. It can be treated locally and systemically with combined effort of medical and dental physician. So, cooperative teamwork between the patient, his physician, and the dental health care professional is mandatory to minimize and successfully treat such unwanted side effects of drugs.

References

[1] S. Pradhan and P. Mishra, "Gingival enlargement in antihypertensive medication," *Journal of the Nepal Medical Association*, vol. 48, no. 174, pp. 149–152, 2009.

[2] T. D. Rees and R. A. Levine, "Systemic drugs as a risk factor periodontal disease initiation and progression," *Compendium of Continuing Education in Dentistry*, vol. 16, no. 1, pp. 20–42, 1995.

[3] "Drug associated gingival enlargement," *Journal of Periodontology*, vol. 75, no. 10, pp. 1424–1431, 2004.

[4] P. Garzino-Demo, M. Carbone, M. Carrozzo, R. Broccoletti, and S. Gandolfo, "An increase in gingival volume induced by drugs (phenytoin, cyclosporine and calcium antagonists). A review of the literature," *Minerva Stomatologica*, vol. 47, no. 9, pp. 387–398, 1998.

[5] J. S. Ellis, R. A. Seymour, J. G. Steele, P. Robertson, T. J. Butler, and J. M. Thomason, "Prevalence of gingival overgrowth induced by calcium channel blockers: a community-based study," *Journal of Periodontology*, vol. 70, no. 1, pp. 63–67, 1999.

[6] M. G. Jorgensen, "Prevalence of amlodipine-related gingival hyperplasia," *Journal of Periodontology*, vol. 68, no. 7, pp. 676–678, 1997.

[7] M. G. Triveni, C. Rudrakshi, and D. S. Mehta, "Amlodipine-induced gingival overgrowth," *Journal of Indian Society of Periodontology*, vol. 13, no. 3, pp. 160–163, 2009.

[8] R. A. Seymour, J. M. Thomason, and J. S. Ellis, "The pathogenesis of drug-induced gingival overgrowth," *Journal of Clinical Periodontology*, vol. 23, no. 3, pp. 165–175, 1996.

[9] A. Nyska, M. Shemesh, H. Tal, and D. Dayan, "Gingival hyperplasia induced by calcium channel blockers: mode of action," *Medical Hypotheses*, vol. 43, no. 2, pp. 115–118, 1994.

[10] R. I. Marshall and P. M. Bartold, "A clinical review of drug-induced gingival overgrowths," *Australian Dental Journal*, vol. 44, no. 4, pp. 219–232, 1999.

[11] A. Lafzi, R. M. Z. Farahani, and M. M. Shoja, "Amlodipine-induced gingival hyperplasia," *Medicina Oral, Patología Oral y Cirugía Bucal*, vol. 11, no. 6, pp. E480–E482, 2006.

[12] R. A. Seymour, "Calcium channel blockers and gingival overgrowth," *British Dental Journal*, vol. 170, no. 10, pp. 376–379, 1991.

[13] S. Sonmez, C. Cavdar, C. Gunduz et al., "Do MMP-1 levels of gingival fibroblasts have a role in the gingival overgrowth of cyclosporine-treated patients?" *Transplantation Proceedings*, vol. 40, no. 1, pp. 181–183, 2008.

[14] P. G. Raman, V. N. Mishra, and D. Singh, "Nifedipine induced gingival hyperplasia," *The Journal of the Association of Physicians of India*, vol. 36, no. 3, pp. 231–233, 1988.

[15] M. Mavrogiannis, J. S. Ellis, J. M. Thomason, and R. A. Seymour, "The management of drug-induced gingival overgrowth," *Journal of Clinical Periodontology*, vol. 33, no. 6, pp. 434–439, 2006.

7

Clinical Guidelines and Management of Ankyloglossia with 1-Year Followup

Mayur S. Bhattad, M. S. Baliga, and Ritika Kriplani

Department of Pedodontics and Preventive Dentistry, Sharad Pawar Dental College and Hospital, Sawangi 442001, Wardha, Maharashtra, India

Correspondence should be addressed to Mayur S. Bhattad; mayur_b99@yahoo.co.in

Academic Editors: N. Brezniak, I. El-Hakim, and P. Lopez Jornet

The tongue is an important oral structure that affects speech, position of teeth, periodontal tissue, nutrition, swallowing, nursing, and certain social activities. Ankyloglossia (tongue tie) is a congenital anomaly characterized by an abnormally short, thick lingual frenulum which affects movement of tongue. Though the effect of ankyloglossia in general appears to be a minor condition, but a major difference exists concerning the guidelines for tongue-tie division. There are no accepted practical criteria for the management of such condition, and hence this paper aims at bringing all the compilation in examination, diagnosis, treatment, and management of tongue tie together for better clinical approach.

1. Introduction

The tongue is an important organ that affects speech, position of the teeth, periodontal tissue, nutrition, and swallowing [1]. Most of us think of tongue tie as a situation we find ourselves in when we are too excited to speak. Tongue tie is the nonmedical term for a relatively common physical condition that limits the use of the tongue, which is actually called as ankyloglossia [2].

Before birth, a strong cord of tissue guides the development of oral frenulum which is positioned in the centre of the mouth. After birth, this lingual frenulum continues to guide the position of erupting teeth. As the child grows, it recedes and becomes thin. This frenulum is visible when we look at the mirror under the tongue. In some children, the frenulum is especially tight, or it fails to recede and may cause tongue immobility [2]. Hence ankyloglossia is defined as a developmental anomaly of the tongue characterized by an abnormally short, thick lingual frenum resulting in limitation of tongue movement [3], or in simple terms, tongue tie is present when the lingual frenulum is attached close to the tongue tip, resulting in reduced tongue movement.

Various studies using different diagnostic criteria found a prevalence of ankyloglossia between 4 and 10% [4, 5], and

the incidence of tongue tie varies from 0.2% to 5% depending on the population examined [3]. It is more common in males, with male to female ratio of 2.5 : 1.0 [5]. Ankyloglossia in infants has an incidence rate from 25% to 60%, and its presence can lead to difficulty in breastfeeding ranging from failure to thrive to even refusing the breast [4, 6–8].

Ankyloglossia can also be a part of certain rare syndromes like Smith-Lemli-Opitz syndrome, orofacial digital syndrome, Beckwith Weidman syndrome, Simpson-Golabi-Behmel syndrome, and X-linked cleft palate with autosomal dominant or recessive trait [5, 9–12].

Ankyloglossia in children poses a diagnostic challenge for dentists. Recent reviews have revealed very minimal information about what constitutes an abnormal lingual attachment and what criteria should be used to justify surgical intervention. Hence the purpose of this report is to describe ankyloglossia, its clinical significance, and what guidelines should be followed before planning surgical intervention.

2. Case Reports

Case Number 1. A 12-year-old female patient reported to the Department of Pedodontics and Preventive Dentistry with

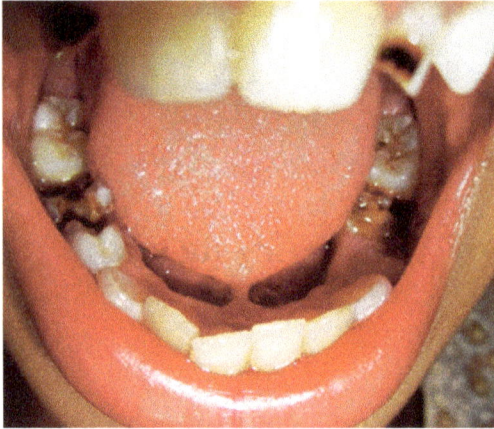

FIGURE 1: Preoperative photograph (Case 1).

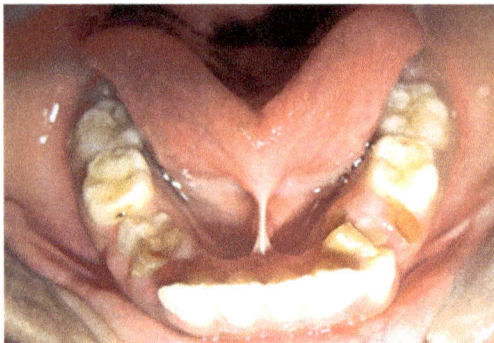

FIGURE 2: Preoperative photograph (Case 2).

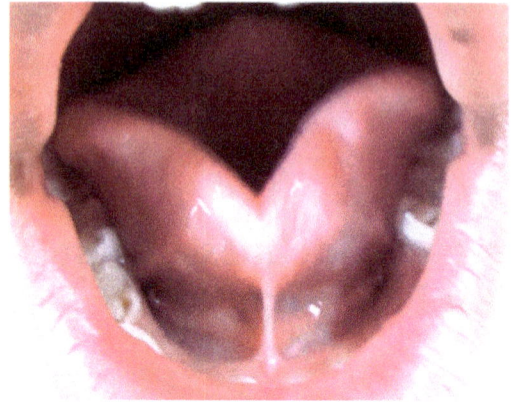

FIGURE 3: Preoperative photograph (Case 3).

TABLE 1: Kotlow's classification.

Type	Movement of the tongue
Clinically acceptable, normal range of free tongue movement	Greater than 16 mm
Class I: Mild ankyloglossia	12 to 16 mm
Class II: Moderate ankyloglossia	8 to 11 mm
Class III: Severe ankyloglossia	3 to 7 mm
Class IV: Complete ankyloglossia	less than 3 mm

the chief complaint of pain in lower right and left posterior region. Oral examination of the patient revealed not only multiple decayed teeth in lower arch but also an ankyloglossia with thick, short frenulum, restricted tongue protrusion, and lifting of the tip of the tongue (Figure 1).

Case Number 2. An 8-year-old male patient reported to the Department of Pedodontics and Preventive Dentistry with the chief complaint of pain in upper right posterior region. After clinical examination, decayed tooth and ankyloglossia with restricted tongue movements were also observed. A bifid or heart shape of the anterior tip of the tongue was seen upon attempted extension (Figure 2).

Case Number 3. An 11-year-old male patient reported to Department of Pedodontics and Preventive Dentistry with the chief complaint of improper speech, and his parents also reported that he was not able to chew solid foods. Clinical examination revealed that patient had ankyloglossia with thick frenum, restricted tongue movements like protrusion, and lifting of the tip of the tongue and a bifid or heart shape of the anterior tip of the tongue, was observed. To assess the extent of limitation of tongue movement, the mouth was carefully inspected under adequate illumination with a tongue depressor (Figure 3).

3. Clinical Assessment

All the 3 cases were assessed clinically by Kotlow's criteria (Table 1) in which normal range of motion of the tongue was assessed [1], Hazelbaker's assessment tool (Table 2) to observe the functional movement and appearance of the tongue [13], and speech analysis to identify and rectify defective speech [3, 14].

Upon diagnosis of an ankyloglossia, the patient's parents were informed about the nature of the lesion, its functional implications, and the variety of surgical approaches. The patient's family and medical history were noncontributory. Patient's height and weight were appropriate for their age. ENT and general physical examination revealed insignificant findings. Hematologic examination of the patients was within normal range. After obtaining informed consent, the following procedures were carried out for correction of lingual frenum.

4. Clinical Management

In the first and second case (cases number 1 and 2), frenum attachment was revised by conventional frenectomy. A topical anesthetic was applied to the underside of the tongue following which block anesthesia was given. After achieving objective symptoms, a suture was passed at the middle of the tongue to control its movements, and two hemostat was used to clamp the frenum: one at the under surface of the tongue and another at the floor of the mouth avoiding salivary gland duct. Incision was placed above and below the hemostats to release the complete frenum. On achieving homeostasis,

TABLE 2: Hazel baker's Assessment tool for appearance and function of the tongue.

Appearance	Function
Appearance of tongue when lifted	Lateralization
2: Round or square	2: Complete
1: Slight cleft in tip apparent	1: Body or tongue but no tongue tip
0: Heart or V-shaped	0: None
Elasticity of frenulum	Lift of tongue
2: Very elastic	2: Tip to mid-mouth
1: Moderately elastic	1: Only edges to mid-mouth
0: Little or no elasticity	0: Tip stays at lower alveolar ridge or rises to mid-mouth only with jaw closure
Length of lingual frenulum when tongue lifted	Extension of tongue
2: >1 cm	2: Tip over lower lip
1: 1 cm	1: Tip over lower gum only 0: Neither of the above, or anterior or mid-tongue humps
0: <1 cm	
Attachment of lingual frenulum to tongue	Spread of anterior tongue
2: Posterior to tip	2: Complete
1: At tip	1: Moderate of partial
0: Notched tip	0: Little or none
Attachment of lingual frenulum to inferior alveolar ridge	Cupping
2: Attached to floor of mouth or well below ridge	2: Entire edge, firm cup
1: Attached just below ridge	1: Side edges only, moderate cup
0: Attached at ridge	0: Poor or no cup
	Peristalsis
	2: Complete, anterior or posterior
	1: Partial, originating posterior to tip
	0: None or reverse

14 = Perfect score, 11 = Acceptable if appearance item score is 10. Frenectomy is necessary if function score is <11 and appearance score is <8.

the area was sutured. The patients were discharged with postoperative instructions.

In the third case (case number 3), frenum was relieved by using diode lasers. A topical anesthetic was applied to the underside of the tongue. Tongue was raised with the thumb and index finger, and the frenum was revised. After achieving homeostasis, patient was discharged with postoperative instructions.

After a week, sutures in all the cases were removed, and case number 3 was referred to speech therapist (Figures 4, 5, and 6). After 1-year followup, all the 3 cases were reassessed again by using the same criterias.

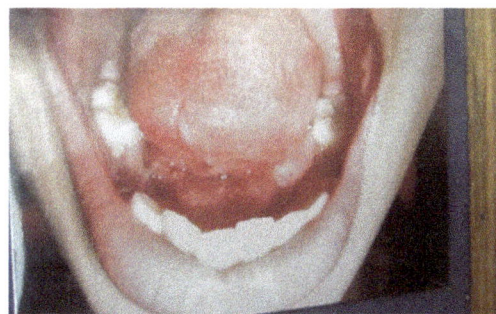

FIGURE 4: Postoperative photograph after 7 days (Case 1).

5. Results

Using the Kotlow's criteria and Hazelbaker's assessment tool, preoperative and postoperative scores were recorded. After 1-year followup, significant improvement in prognosis of symptoms of ankyloglossia was observed (Figures 7, 8, and 9). Free tongue movement increased from 7, 9, and 8 mm to 13, 14, and 15 mm (Table 3), respectively, and functional score of 9, 10, and 10 and appearance score of 6, 6, and 7 were changed to 14, 13, 12, and 9, 9, and 10 (Table 4), respectively. Speech in case number 3 also significantly improved (Table 5).

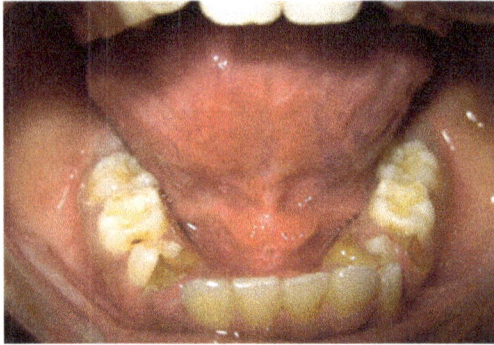

FIGURE 5: Postoperative photograph after 7 days (Case 2).

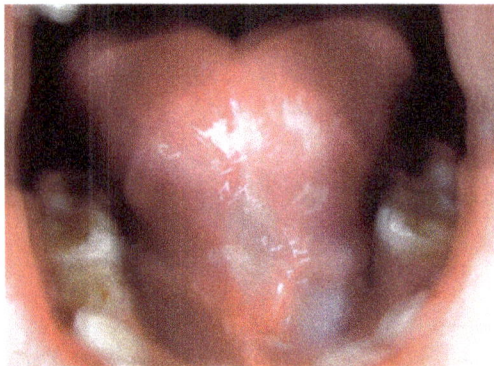

FIGURE 6: Postoperative photograph after 7 days (Case 3).

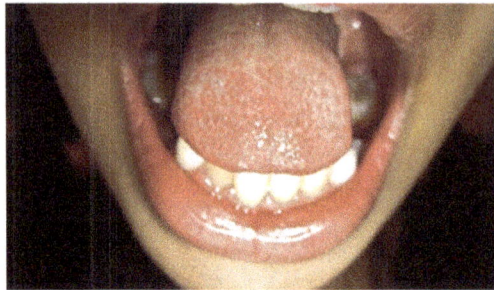

FIGURE 7: Postoperative photograph after 1 year (Case 1).

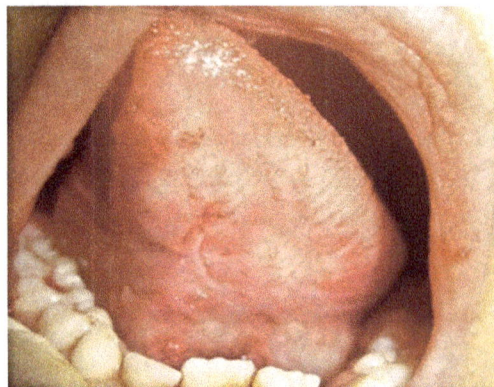

FIGURE 8: Postoperative photograph after 1 year (Case 2).

TABLE 3: Pre-operative and post-operative assessment of free tongue movement in all the 3 cases by using Kotlow's criterias.

Case number	Pre-operative free tongue movement	Diagnosis	Post-operative, free tongue movement	Diagnosis
1	7 mm	Class III	13 mm	Class I
2	9 mm	Class II	14 mm	Class I
3	8 mm	Class II	15 mm	Class I

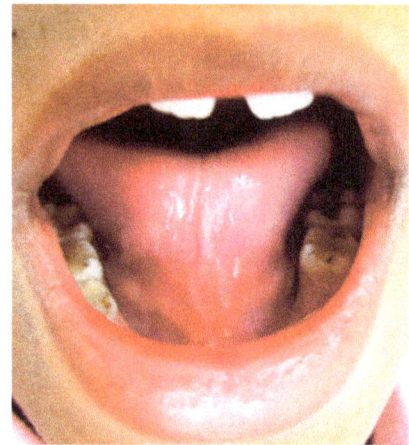

FIGURE 9: Postoperative photograph after 1 year (Case 3).

6. Discussion

Anatomical definition of ankyloglossia consists of descriptions as well as absolute measurements. Descriptions include the attachment of the frenulum to the tongue, the attachment of the frenulum to the inferior alveolar ridge, the elasticity of the lingual frenulum, and the appearance of the tongue when lifted. Absolute measurements include the length of the lingual frenulum when the tongue is lifted as well as the free tongue length [15].

According to Wallace, functional definition includes it as a condition in which the tip of the tongue cannot be protruded beyond the lower incisor teeth because of a short frenulum. On the other hand, tongue movement is more complex than simple protrusion, and as a result functional assessments criteria have included tongue lateralization, tongue lift, tongue spread, tongue cupping, and tongue snap back [15].

Ankyloglossia can be divided into partial or complete ankyloglossia. The academy of Breastfeeding Medicine Protocol defines partial ankyloglossia as the presence of a sublingual frenulum which changes the appearance and/or function of the infant's tongue because of its decreased length, lack of elasticity or attachment too distal beneath the tongue or too close to or onto the gingival ridge. Complete ankyloglossia is a condition in which there is extensive fusion of the tongue to the floor of the mouth which is extremely rare [16].

TABLE 4: Pre-operative and post-operative assessment of functional and appearance score of all the 3 cases by using Hazel-Baker's assessment tool.

Case number	Pre-operative function score	Pre-operative appearance score	Post-operative function score	Post-operative appearance score
1	9	6	14	9
2	10	6	13	9
3	10	7	12	10

TABLE 5: Pre-operative and post-operative assessment of speech in all the 3 cases.

Case number	Pre-operative associated problem	Post-operative associated problem
1	No speech abnormality	—
2	No speech abnormality	—
3	Defective speech	Improvement of speech

7. Consequences of Not Treating the Tongue Tie

Appearance of the tongue could be abnormal in some individuals. Improper chewing and swallowing of food could increase the gastric distress and bloating, and snoring and bed wetting at sleep are common among tongue tied children. It also affects children who want to participate in routine play which involves tongue movements, gestures, and speech. Dental caries could occur due to food debris not being removed by the tongue's action of sweeping the teeth and spreading of saliva. Malocclusion like open bite due to thrust created by being tongue tied, spreading of lower incisors with periodontitis, and tooth mobility due to long-term tongue thrust are associated problems. It also affects self-esteem because it has been noted clinically that occasionally an older child or adult will be self-conscious or embarrassed about their tongue tie that they may be teased by their classmates for their anomaly. In infant feeding problem may be experienced due to latching on to the nipple which may compress the nipple against the gum resulting in nipple pain in mothers, and due to this the mothers may often try to shift the baby to a bottle [3, 16–18].

8. Clinical Guidelines for Management of Ankyloglossia

There is a wide difference of opinion regarding its clinical significance and optimal management. In many children, ankyloglossia is asymptomatic, and the condition may resolve spontaneously, or affected children may learn to compensate adequately for their decreased lingual mobility. Some children, however, benefit from surgical intervention of their tongue tie. Parents should be educated about the possible long-term effects of tongue tie, so that they may make an informed choice regarding possible therapy.

For effective management proper clinical guidelines are mandatory. In ankyloglossia, the most important factor to be considered is the normal range of motion of the tongue which should be determined by using Kotlow's criteria [1] in which classification ranges from class I to class IV. The tip of the tongue should able to protrude outside the mouth without clefting and should be able to sweep the upper and lower lips easily, without straining. When the tongue is retruded, it should not blanch the tissue lingual to the anterior teeth and should not put excessive forces on the mandibular anterior teeth. The lingual frenum should not create a diastema between the mandibular central incisor, and the frenum should not prevent an infant from attaching to the mother's nipple during nursing.

The functional movement and appearance of the tongue could be determined by using Hazelbakers assessment tool [15]. In this tool, scores are given to each movement of the tongue and appearance of the tongue. If the functional and appearance score is below 11 and 8, then surgical invention should be considered.

Patients should be asked to pronounce certain words which start from "I," "th," "s," "d," and "t" to check the accuracy of the word pronunciations. If a defective speech is observed, after postoperative wound healing, referral to a speech therapist is mandatory for speech modification. Postoperative tongue muscle exercises like licking the upper lip, touching hard palate with the tip of tongue, and side-to-side movements should be explained to the patient for enhanced tongue movements.

9. Conclusion

Tongue tie affects a considerable number of infants and children. It is perhaps interesting that such a simple condition can cause such controversy and diversity of opinions. However, it is important that accurate information and guidance is given to parents with regard to the indications and potential benefits of tongue-tie revision, and that appropriate provisions are in place for those infants and children who require revision. These case reports offer guidelines which can be used by general and pediatric dentists for diagnosis and treatment of a tongue restriction resulting from ankyloglossia.

References

[1] L. A. Kotlow, "Ankyloglossia (tongue-tie): a diagnostic and treatment quandary," *Quintessence International*, vol. 30, no. 4, pp. 259–262, 1999.

[2] Entnet.org [Internet] American Association of otolaryngologist: head and neck surgery: fact sheet, 2012, http://entnet.org/HealthInformation/Ankyloglossia.cfm.

[3] H. E. Darshan and P. M. Pavithra, "Tongue tie: from confusion to clarity-a review," *International Journal of Dental Clinics*, vol. 3, pp. 48–51, 2011.

[4] L. M. Segal, R. Stephenson, M. Dawes, and P. Feldman, "Prevalence, diagnosis, and treatment of ankyloglossia: methodologic review," *Canadian Family Physician*, vol. 53, no. 6, pp. 1027–1033, 2007.

[5] M. Saeid, Y. Mobin, R. Reza, A. P. Ali, and G. Mohsen, "Familial ankyloglossia (tongue-tie): a case report," *Acta Medica Iranica*, vol. 48, no. 2, pp. 123–124, 2010.

[6] A. H. Messner, M. L. Lalakea, J. Macmahon, E. Bair, and A. Janelle, "Ankyloglossia: incidence and associated feeding difficulties," *Archives of Otolaryngology*, vol. 126, no. 1, pp. 36–39, 2000.

[7] J. L. Ballard, C. E. Auer, and J. C. Khoury, "Ankyloglossia: assessment, incidence, and effect of frenuloplasty on the breastfeeding dyad," *Pediatrics*, vol. 110, no. 5, p. e63, 2002.

[8] P. Tait, "Nipple pain in breastfeeding women: causes, treatment, and prevention strategies," *Journal of Midwifery and Women's Health*, vol. 45, no. 3, pp. 212–215, 2000.

[9] P. Meinecke, W. Blunck, and A. Rodewald, "Smith-Lemli-Opitz syndrome," *American Journal of Medical Genetics*, vol. 28, no. 3, pp. 735–739, 1987.

[10] G. Neri, F. Gurrieri, G. Zanni, and A. Lin, "Clinical and molecular aspects of the Simpson Golabi Behmel syndrome," *American Journal of Medical Genetics*, vol. 79, pp. 279–283, 1998.

[11] C. Braybrook, K. Doudney, A. C. B. Marçano et al., "The T-box transcription factor gene TBX22 is mutated in X-linked cleft palate and ankyloglossia," *Nature Genetics*, vol. 29, no. 2, pp. 179–183, 2001.

[12] P. N. Kantaputra, M. Paramee, A. Kaewkhampa et al., "Cleft lip with cleft palate, ankyloglossia, and hypodontia are associated with TBX22 mutations," *Journal of Dental Research*, vol. 90, no. 4, pp. 450–455, 2011.

[13] A. K. Hazelbaker, *The assessment tool for lingual frenulum function (ATLFF): use in a lactation consultant private practice [thesis]*, Pacific Oaks College, Pasadena, Calif, USA, 1993.

[14] N. Ketty and P. A. Sciullo, "Ankyloglossia with psychological implications," *ASDC Journal of Dentistry for Children*, vol. 41, no. 1, pp. 43–46, 1974.

[15] R. V. Johnson, "Tongue-tie—exploding the myths," *Infant*, vol. 2, pp. 96–99, 2006.

[16] J. Ballard, C. Chantry, and C. R. Howard, "Guidelines for the evaluation and management of neonatal ankyloglossia and its complications in the breastfeeding dyad," Academy of Breastfeeding Medicine, 2004, http://www.bfmed.org/Media/Files/Protocols/ankyloglossia.pdf.

[17] A. Tuli and A. Singh, "Monopolar diathermy used for correction of ankyloglossia," *Journal of Indian Society of Pedodontics and Preventive Dentistry*, vol. 28, no. 2, pp. 130–133, 2010.

[18] A. Kupietzky and E. Botzer, "Ankyloglossia in the infant and young child: clinical suggestions for diagnosis and management," *Pediatric Dentistry*, vol. 27, no. 1, pp. 40–46, 2005.

8

Treatment of the Atrophic Upper Jaw: Rehabilitation of Two Complex Cases

Andrea Enrico Borgonovo,[1] **Andrea Marchetti,**[1] **Virna Vavassori,**[1] **Rachele Censi,**[2] **Ramon Boninsegna,**[3] **and Dino Re**[1]

[1] Istituto Stomatologico Italiano, Department of Oral Rehabilitation, School of Oral Surgery, University of Milan,
via Pace, 21, 20122 Milan, Italy
[2] Department of Implantology and Periodontology III, Istituto Stomatologico Italiano, Milan, Italy
[3] Department of Clinical and Experimental Sciences, University of Brescia, Italy

Correspondence should be addressed to Virna Vavassori; virna.vavassori@hotmail.it

Academic Editors: S. S. de Rossi and R. Sorrentino

In reconstructive surgery, the fresh frozen homologous bone (FFB) represents a valid alternative to the autologous bone, because FFB allows bone regeneration thanks to its osteoinductive and osteoconductive properties. The purpose of this work is to describe the surgical-implant-prosthetic treatment of two complex cases using FFB. In particular, fresh frozen homologous bone grafts were used to correct the severe atrophy of the maxilla, and, then, once the graft integration was obtained, implant therapy was performed and implants placed in native bone were immediately loaded.

1. Introduction

The implant-prosthetic rehabilitation is a current practice in clinic dentistry and is characterized by safe and predictable results in the long term [1]. However, in order to obtain the success of implant therapy, in the preliminary stages it is essential to assess and classify the amount of available bone. In fact, this evaluation is fundamental for the correct implant placement, according to the principles of modern prosthetically driven implant placement [2].

Several classifications have been proposed to assess the amount of available bone. In the Lekholm and Zarb [3] classification (1985), the jaw bone shape is classified on a five degree scale. Cawood and Howell [4] (1988) proposed another classification that differentiates the atrophies according to an analysis of three-dimensional alveolar ridges. The presence of unfavorable crestal anatomy, which may result from different situations such as atrophy, periodontal disease, iatrogenic or congenital defects, trauma, or oncological resection, is not an absolute contraindication to dental implant placement. In fact, with the advances and evolution occurring in implant dentistry, new surgical techniques have been developed and refined in order to allow the correction of bone defects and the implant-prosthetic management of compromised sites.

One of the most common procedures for the correction of bone defects involves autologous (or autogenous) bone grafting (bone is harvested from the patient's own body). Autologous bone is typically harvested from intraoral sources [5] as the chin, the mandibular ramous, the tuber maxilla or from extraoral sources as the iliac crest, the fibula, and even parts of the skull [6]. Other graft materials, which are used in clinical practice, are the xenograft bone substitutes, derived from a species other than human, such as bovine, the allograft bone, like autogenous bone which is derived from humans, and at last, the artificial bone, such as bioglass, hydroxyapatite, or calcium phosphate [2]. For the reconstruction of extended bone defects, autologous or homologous bone grafts are preferred, in form of blocks, in order to restore the correct vertical and/or horizontal dimensions.

Only recently, the homologous bone has been introduced in the reconstructive surgery and maxillofacial surgery, although it has been used for many years in orthopedics for complex surgical operations with clinical results consolidated in the long term [7, 8]. The homologous bone is obtained from a living donor (usually from patients undergoing total hip replacement) or from cadavers [9]. In the latter case, the harvesting is made within 12/24 hours of death, in a sterile environment. The parts that are collected are then sent to the Tissue Bank to be subjected to serological tests, tests to detect antibodies and antigens and blood culture. Once completed these exams, the bone is processed and depending on the type of preparation, three distinct physical forms can be distinguished.

   (i) "Fresch frozen" (FFB)—the processing of the fresh frozen homologous bone does not provide decalcification nor irradiation. The FFB is initially disinfected with a polichemotherapic disinfection solution (72 hours at −4°C), then washed with saline solution, divided into blocks, packed in double sterile pouch, and preserved at −80°C in a tank [10];

   (ii) lyophilized homologous bone (FDB)—the bone tissue is ground into particles of 500 microns–5 mm, delipidated with pure ethanol, dehydrated, and frozen;

   (iii) demineralized and lyophilized homologous bone (DFDB)—in addition to the processes for freeze-drying, the bone is subjected to a further step that provides for the immersion in citric acid for 6–16 hours in order to demineralize the resulting particles.

Each of these types of homologous bone has precise indications, management, and contraindications [11, 12].

In implant surgery, the standard protocol for the management of complex cases in which bone grafting is performed, includes healing times of not less than 5-6 months for graft integration [13]. After this period and after verifying the success of the reconstructive therapy, dental implants can be placed in the grafted sites. The implant techniques, as described by Brånemark [14], require a submerged healing of endosseous implants placed in regenerated bone for a period of about 6 months and 3-4 months for implants placed in native bone [15]. At the end of this period, it is possible to functionalize the implants with temporary restorations. Although the protocol proposed by the Swedish school is still valid, the research has been directed towards the study of new protocols that present a shorter healing phase in order to reduce the duration of overall rehabilitation. In particular, considering the immediate loading techniques for dental implants [16, 17], several clinical studies [18, 19] showed that the immediate loading protocols can be applied with predictable results for implants placed in native bone, and excellent results were obtained also for implants placed in areas reconstructed with bone grafts but only in certain selected cases.

In this paper, the surgical-implant-prosthetic treatment of three complex cases is described. In particular, fresh frozen homologous bone grafts were used to correct the severe atrophy of the maxilla, and, then, once the graft integration was obtained, implant therapy was performed and implants placed in native bone were immediately loaded.

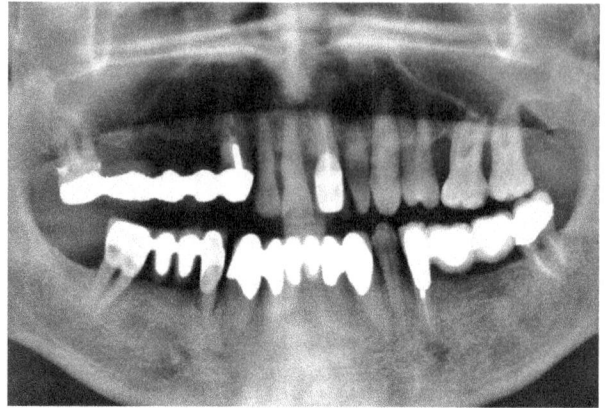

FIGURE 1: Case 1: Initial panoramic radiograph (OPT).

2. Case Series

Case 1. The patient A. M., 56 years old, male came to our attention presenting, in the upper jaw, edentulous multiple sites, mobility of the remaining teeth, periodontal disease, and severe atrophy of the maxillary edentulous alveolar ridge. The patient clearly required that the prosthetic rehabilitation be exclusively fixed and did not accept provisional phases with removable dentures. Based on the clinical examination and the evaluation of radiographs (panoramic radiograph (Figure 1) and computed tomography of the maxilla with DentalScan reconstructions), it was decided to treat the atrophic upper jaw with a combined sinus lift procedure and local ridge augmentation using bone grafts in the areas from 1.4 to 1.6, performed under general anesthesia. In addition, it was decided to conserve not compromised teeth until the bone grafts were integrated in order to proceed, in a second phase, with implant placement and immediate loading.

The patient was adequately informed about the use of FFB grafts and the subsequent implant-prosthetic treatment plan. The preoperative phase included blood tests, an interview with the anesthesiologist for the general anesthesia, the signature of the informed consent form for the surgery, the test to determine the patient's blood group, and the signature of a specific informed consent form for the bone graft from the Tissue Bank. Once the preliminary phase was completed, the tissue specimen was then booked at the reference Tissue Bank, and in particular, a specimen harvested from the iliac crest was required.

Initially, the avulsion of the element 16 was performed and after 40 days, the reconstructive surgery was programmed. On the day of surgery, a sealed container with the graft preserved under controlled temperature was delivered. Once freed from its outer packaging, the specimen was still wrapped in a sealed double sterile bag. It was then transferred to the operating room, where the double bag was opened in a sterile environment and the tissue specimen was defrozen in an abundant solution of saline and rifampicin at a temperature of 37°C for one hour, in compliance with the instructions provided by the reference Bank. Once the specimen had been defrozen, it was debrided to remove nonbony tissue,

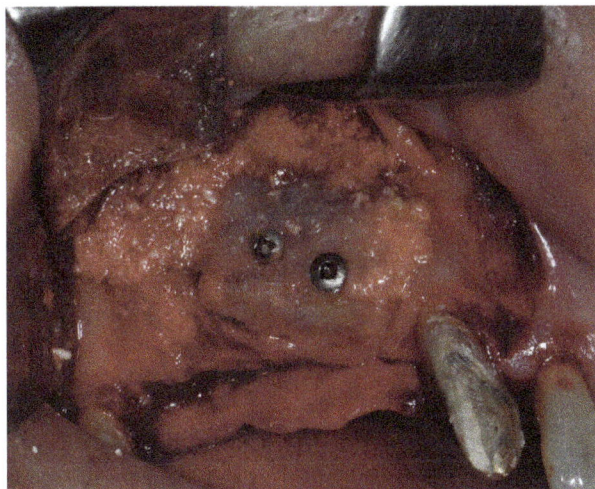

FIGURE 2: The atrophic upper jaw is treated with a combined sinus lift procedure and local ridge augmentation using fresh frozen homologous grafts.

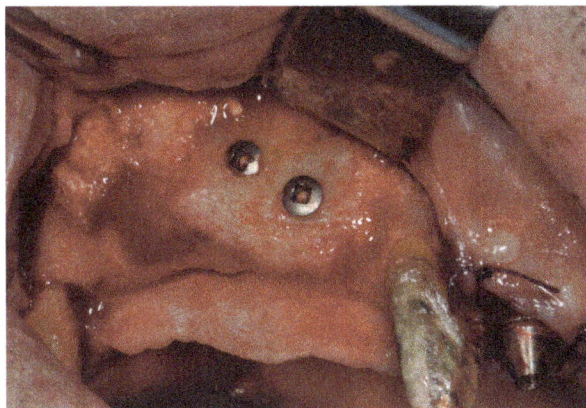

FIGURE 3: The surgical site is reopened.

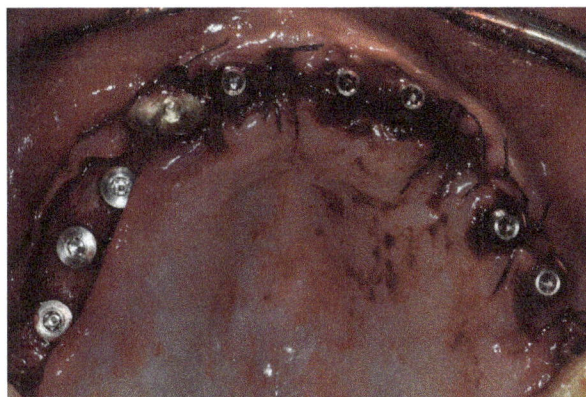

FIGURE 4: Implant placement.

cut into blocks and contoured or morcellized, based on the treatment plan. The bone deficit was corrected by means of a major sinus lift and an onlay graft using a precontoured allogenic cancellous bone (FFB) block harvested from an iliac crest. The graft was then fixated with osteosynthesis screws. The subantral cavity and the gaps between the graft and the alveolar bone were then filled with allogeneic bone (FFB) chips (Figure 2). The whole thing, including the screws, were then covered with the same morcellized bone, which was maintained in situ by means of resorbable collagen membranes. The wound was closed by sutures after releasing and passivating the flaps. At the clinical controls conducted in the weeks following the surgery and at radiographic examination (OPT) performed 1 month after the surgical procedure, there was no evidence of any complications. Three months later, the avulsions of the elements 12, 11, 21, 22, 24, and 26 were performed, whereas the elements 17, 13, 23, and 27 were maintained in situ and rehabilitated temporarily with a reinforced resin bridge in order to control the vertical dimension, the occlusion and the mandibular movements. At five months, the surgical site was reopened (Figure 3) and the fixation screws were removed. The bone tissue appeared vital and well integrated; no bone resorption was revealed.

Eight endosseous dental implants (BlueSky, Bredent, Senden, Germany) were inserted at the level of areas 1.6, 1.4, 1.5, 1.2, 2.1, 2.2, 2.4, and 2.5 using a customized surgical template (Figure 4). The dental implants, placed in regenerated bone in the areas 1.6, 1.4, 1.5, were left submerged and loaded at 6 months. Considering the dental implants placed in the incisal region and those located in the areas 2.4 and 2.5, the resulting torque insertion was greater than 35 N/cm. For this reason, immediate loading was performed, and a provisional screw-retained implant prosthesis was fixed on dental implants (Figure 5). Six months after implant placement, a definitive metal ceramic prosthetic rehabilitation was performed (Figures 6, 7, and 8).

Case 2. The patient M. P., 60 years old, female required the rehabilitation of the upper jaw because only the incisive teeth were present in the arch. In the posterior regions, the alveolar bone was particularly resorbed (Figure 9). Firstly, the sinus lift procedure and the local ridge augmentation were performed using fresh frozen bone harvested from iliac crest (Figure 10). When the bone graft was well integrated (Figure 11), 6 implants were placed in the posterior areas (NobelReplace, Nobel Biocare, Gothenburg, Sweden) (Figure 12). Five months after implant insertion, the implant sites were reopened, and contextually, the incisive teeth were extracted and postextractive implants were placed in regions 1.1 and 2.1 (Figures 13 and 14). All implants were restored with a Toronto bridge (Figure 15).

3. Discussion

When programming a correct treatment plan, the preliminary stages, involving clinical and radiographic examinations, represent the key to determine which treatment strategy should be taken. In particular, the analysis of data acquired by CT with or without the aid of diagnostic and surgical masks, the diagnostic wax-up and the three-dimensional models allow to accurately assess if the quality

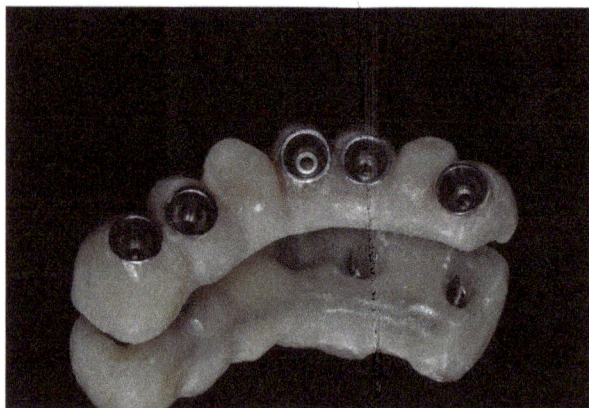

FIGURE 5: Provisional prosthesis.

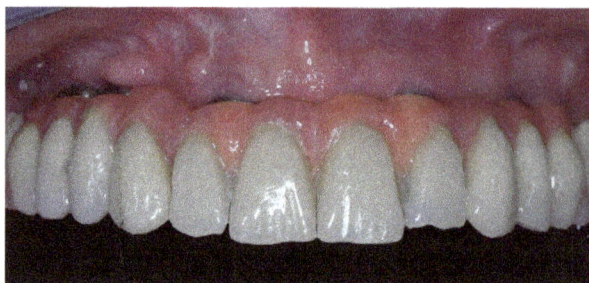

FIGURE 7: Final screw-retained implant prosthesis.

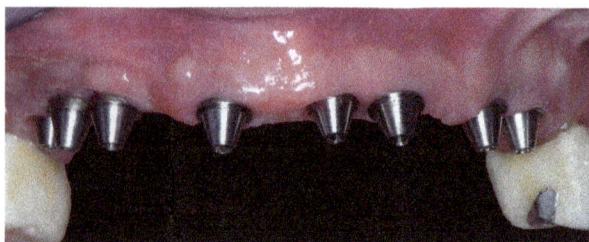

FIGURE 6: Clinical view. It is possible to appreciate the optimal soft tissue health.

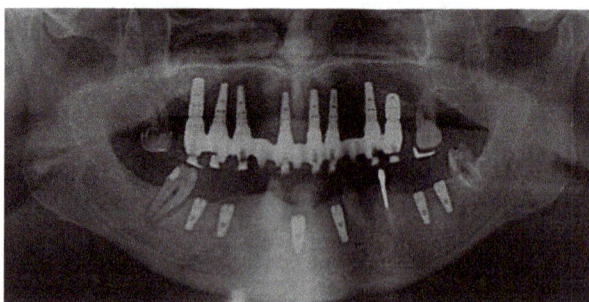

FIGURE 8: Radiographic followup.

and quantity of bone are appropriate for achieving high primary dental implant stability, or if simultaneous regenerative techniques are required, or if the implants should be placed after bone reconstructive surgery. In this regard, Buser et al. [20] introduced a classification that relates the bone defect with the possibility of positioning the implants. This classification distinguishes bone defects in 4 classes:

(i) Class 1: bone volume is ideal both in thickness and height for the correct implant positioning;

(ii) Class 2: moderate horizontal bone resorption does not permit a correct implant axis orientation;

(iii) Class 3: transversal bone resorption. The bone quantity is not sufficient for implant placement, and, for this reason, it is essential to regenerate the bone around fenestrations and dehiscences. In this case, the regenerative techniques are performed in association with implant insertion;

(iv) Class 4: insufficient bone thickness that requires preliminary regenerative techniques and, in a second phase, the performance of implant therapy.

However, when programming a treatment plan, it is important to evaluate the quantitative assessment of bone and to define the implant size and the functional and aesthetic goals of implant rehabilitation. Clinical practice has shown how, in certain cases, it is possible to obviate the preimplant reconstructive surgery using for example, the "short-implants" which have a good behavior in the short

and long term as confirmed by the literature [21]. In other cases, however, even in the presence of a sufficient amount of bone for implant insertion, there is no possibility of ensuring the aesthetic and/or functional success of the treatment plan if reconstructive techniques are not performed. In fact, as demonstrated by Dietrich et al. [22] in a 10-year study of 2017 implants, the percentage of implant success is significantly influenced by the thickness of the vestibular bone wall during implant placement. The implant sites that originally had more than 1 mm of vestibular bone wall present a success rate of 96.6% at 5-year followup, while for those implants which originally present less than 1 mm of thickness on the vestibular side, the success rate was 89, 3%. Therefore, the three-dimensional presence of bone around the implants significantly influences the success rates and, if not adequate, determines an aesthetic and/or functional failure of implant rehabilitation. Anyway, nowadays the surgical techniques of preimplant bone reconstruction are highly predictable and are indicated in the presence of vertical and horizontal bone defects.

The autologous bone tissue is considered the gold standard in preimplant bone reconstruction [23]. In fact it ensures the complete absence of adverse immune reaction because the bone is harvested from the patient's own body. In addition, the autologous bone is both osteoconductive, because it provides mechanical support to the vessels and to the cellular elements that will colonize the site of grafting, and osteoinductive because it stimulates osteogenesis [24]. Moreover, since it contains mature cellular elements, the autologous bone has a partial capacity of osteogenesis. However, the autologous bone tissue also presents disadvantages [25, 26]. In fact, the autologous bone graft is indicated in

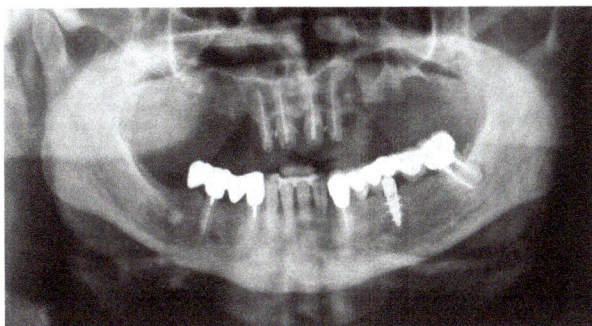

FIGURE 9: Case 2: initial OPT.

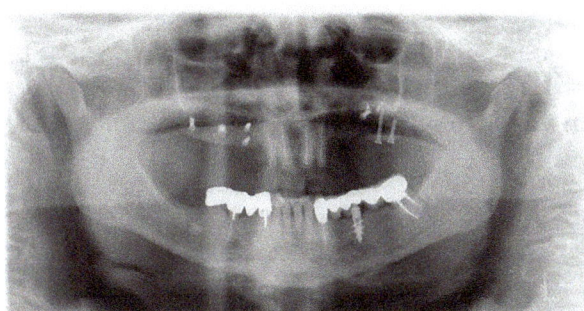

FIGURE 11: The radiographic image shows that bone grafts are well integrated.

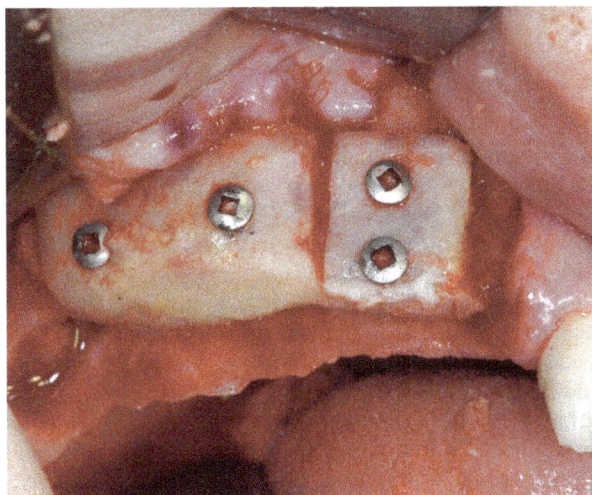

FIGURE 10: The patient is treated with sinus lift procedure and local ridge augmentation using fresh frozen bone.

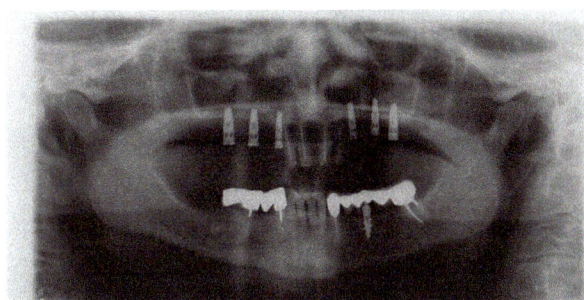

FIGURE 12: Panoramic radiograph after implant placement.

partially edentulous patients because the ridge defects are less severe and more localized, necessitating a smaller quantity of bone. In contrast, an extraoral donor site is often required for bone augmentation where ridge resorption is extreme and extensive. Extraoral bone donor sites provide additional procedural requirements, increased procedure time, and high morbidity and can result in intra- and postoperative complications such as infections of donor or recipient sites.

Considering these issues relative to autologous bone graft, research has been directed towards the study of bone substitutes of various origin (homologous, heterologous, and synthetic). In particular, the homologous fresh frozen (FFB) bone graft has osteoconductive properties and can act as a scaffold by providing structural support during the bone replacement phase. When performed correctly, freezing does not affect the BMPs contained in the bone, so its osteoinductive properties are left unchanged [10, 27]. In consideration of the doubts on the possible interaction between incompatible blood groups and the risk of viral transmission, it must be considered that the assessment of general allogeneic bone donor fitness is more selective than for organ donors and it is based on the collection of in-depth information on the potential donor's medical/social/sexual history, accompanied

by a set of instrumental examinations to protect the recipient from transmissible disease [28]. The risk of transmission of viral diseases is now extremely low as PCR serological tests are performed on the donor and then repeated on the tissue during the preparation steps [9]. However, even if the risk of infections is practically absent, the patient should be informed. In addition, the patient must also be informed that he can start donating blood again after control test 90 days after the allogeneic grafting procedure, and the patient can donate all organs with the exception of bone. The use of homologous FFB grafts has some advantages including

(i) osteoconductive and osteoinductive qualities,

(ii) reduction of postoperative discomfort for the patient due to the lack of donor site,

(iii) availability of graft in suitable quantity and quality,

(iv) limited costs, and

(v) reduction of operating time because the grafts are prepared on stereolithographic models in a preliminary phase.

The macroscopic clinical results showed in all the clinical cases a successful bone regeneration that allowed the reestablishment of the morphology and bone volume of the alveolar process. Moreover, after five months from graft placement, during the second surgical phase, bone showed a good blood support that indicates the process of bone turnover with new bone formation. The bone regeneration obtained by the FFB graft integration has also been confirmed

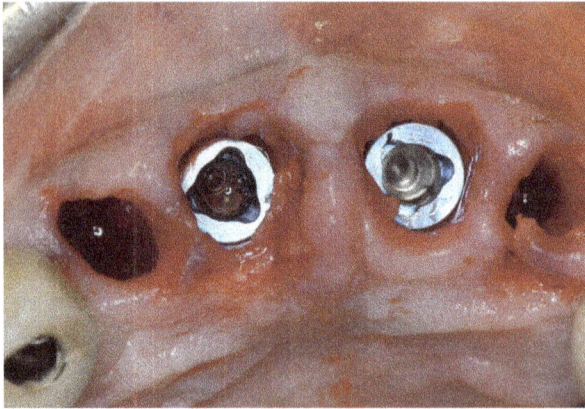

FIGURE 13: Two postextractive implants are inserted in the incisal area.

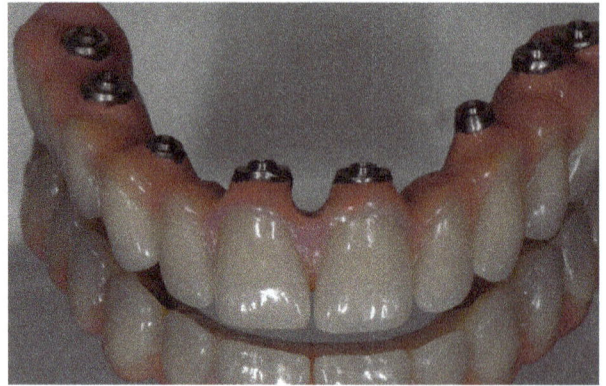

FIGURE 15: Toronto dental bridge.

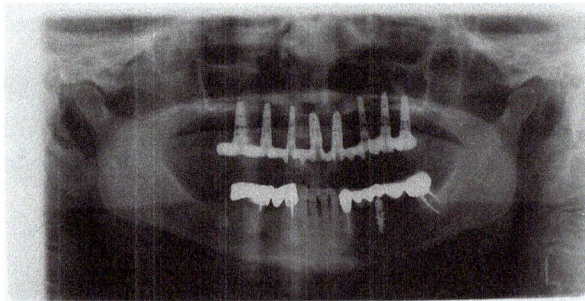

FIGURE 14: Final X-ray picture.

by several studies that have used homologous FFB bone for reconstructive preimplant surgery. In the clinical cases reported, during implant insertion, a good quality bone was noticed and all implants showed a good primary stability with insertion torque of 35 N/cm. In the literature, studies that refer to the success and survival rates of titanium dental implants placed in regenerated bone using FFB grafts are rather limited. One of the first studies was published in 1992 by Perrott [29] who used FFB graft of iliac crest to rehabilitate, in 8 patients, severe bone atrophy of the jaw. After completing the prosthetic rehabilitation, one implant failed to integrate with regenerated bone, and consequently, the survival rate that resulted was equal to 95.8%. In 2009, Franco [30] evaluated the survival and success rated of implants with narrow diameter (NDI) placed, in regenerated bone with FFB grafts. In this study, 91 ND implants were placed and there were only five failures during a mean observation period of 25 months. The implant survival rate was 95.7%, confirming the results obtained also by Perrott.

In another study by the same group of authors [9], implants placed in regenerated jaws with FFB grafts were considered. In particular, 21 patients were treated with 28 onlay FFB grafts, and afterwards, 63 titanium dental implants were inserted. During a mean period of 20 months, 2 implants were lost and the survival rate amounted to 96.8%. The studies relating to the implant position in regenerated

bone with FFB grafts, even if limited, report encouraging results, similar to those in which the dental implants are positioned in regenerated bone with autologous bone tissue.

For implants placed in native bone and immediately loaded, the osseointegration of all implants was obtained without any complication in the short and long term. The implant-prosthetic techniques of immediate loading are consolidated surgical procedures and are supported by numerous studies. In the literature, in fact, several experimental and histological studies conducted on animal and human models are reported, and these works show that immediate-loaded implants provide promising results compared to delayed-loaded implants. In the clinical cases where the immediate loading is indicated, the immediate implant functionalization allows to obtain a significant reduction of costs and operating time for the patients, and, in particular, if the treatment plan is complex, immediate loading permits a quick restoration of function and esthetics.

4. Conclusion

In reconstructive surgery, fresh frozen homologous bone (FFB) allows bone regeneration with its replacement by new bone formation thanks to FFB osteoinductive and osteoconductive properties. In addition, compared to autologous bone, the homologous bone tissue is available in unlimited quantities, allows the reduction of the operating time, and does not have all the disadvantages of the intra- or extraoral surgical site donor.

Therefore, the fresh frozen homologous bone represents a valid alternative to the autologous bone, even for the reconstructions of atrophic jaws. The literature has, in fact, shown that survival rates for implants placed in homologous and autologous bone are comparable with survival rates of over 95% for implants placed in sites regenerated using FFB.

Conflict of Interests

The authors declare that there is no conflict of interests.

References

[1] Å. Leonhardt, K. Gröndahl, C. Bergström, and U. Lekholm, "Long-term follow-up of osseointegrated titanium implants using clinical, radiographic and microbiological parameters," *Clinical Oral Implants Research*, vol. 13, no. 2, pp. 127–132, 2002.

[2] E. D'Aloja, E. Santi, G. Aprili, and M. Franchini, "Fresh frozen homologous bone in oral surgery: case reports," *Cell and Tissue Banking*, vol. 9, no. 1, pp. 41–46, 2008.

[3] U. Lekholm and G. A. Zarb, "Patient selection and preparation," in *Tissue-Integrated Prosthesis: Osseointegration in Clinical Dentistry*, P. I. Branemark, G. A. Zarb, and T. Albrektsson, Eds., pp. 199–209, Quintessence, Chicago, Ill, USA, 1985.

[4] J. I. Cawood and R. A. Howell, "A classification of the edentulous jaws," *International Journal of Oral and Maxillofacial Surgery*, vol. 17, no. 4, pp. 232–236, 1988.

[5] J. A. Leonetti and R. Koup, "Localized maxillary ridge augmentation with a block allograft for dental implant placement: case reports," *Implant Dentistry*, vol. 12, no. 3, pp. 217–226, 2003.

[6] P. S. Petrungaro and S. Amar, "Localized ridge augmentation with allogenic block grafts prior to implant placement: case reports and histologic evaluations," *Implant Dentistry*, vol. 14, no. 2, pp. 139–148, 2005.

[7] S. N. Khan, F. P. Cammisa Jr., H. S. Sandhu, A. D. Diwan, F. P. Girardi, and J. M. Lane, "The biology of bone grafting," *The Journal of the American Academy of Orthopaedic Surgeons*, vol. 13, no. 1, pp. 77–86, 2005.

[8] H. Burchardt, "The biology of bone graft repair," *Clinical Orthopaedics and Related Research*, vol. 174, pp. 28–42, 1983.

[9] F. Carinci, G. Brunelli, I. Zollino et al., "Mandibles grafted with fresh-frozen bone: an evaluation of implant outcome," *Implant Dentistry*, vol. 18, no. 1, pp. 86–95, 2009.

[10] L. G. de Macedo, N. L. de Macedo, and A. do Socorro Ferreira Monteiro, "Fresh-frozen human bone graft for repair of defect after adenomatoid odontogenic tumour removal," *Cell and Tissue Banking*, vol. 10, no. 3, pp. 221–226, 2009.

[11] K. Gajiwala and A. Lobo Gajiwala, "Use of banked tissue in plastic surgery," *Cell and Tissue Banking*, vol. 4, no. 2–4, pp. 141–146, 2003.

[12] E. S. Kalter and T. M. By, "Tissue banking programmes in Europe," *British Medical Bulletin*, vol. 53, no. 4, pp. 798–816, 1997.

[13] A. H. Reddi, S. Weintroub, and N. Muthukumaram, "Biological principles of bone induction," *The Orthopedic Clinics of North America*, vol. 18, no. 2, pp. 207–212, 1987.

[14] P. I. Brånemark, B. O. Hansson, R. Adell et al., "Osseointegrated implants in the treatment of the edentulous jaw. Experience from a 10-year period," *Scandinavian Journal of Plastic and Reconstructive Surgery*, vol. 16, pp. 1–132, 1977.

[15] L. Cordaro, D. Sarzi Amadè, and M. Cordaro, "Clinical results of alveolar ridge augmentation with mandibular block bone grafts in partially edentulous patients prior to implant placement," *Clinical Oral Implants Research*, vol. 13, no. 1, pp. 103–111, 2002.

[16] K. Vandamme, I. Naert, L. Geris, J. Vander Sloten, R. Puers, and J. Duyck, "The effect of micro-motion on the tissue response around immediately loaded roughened titanium implants in the rabbit," *European Journal of Oral Sciences*, vol. 115, no. 1, pp. 21–29, 2007.

[17] S. B. Goodman, Y. Song, A. Doshi, and P. Aspenberg, "Cessation of strain facilitates bone formation in the micromotion chamber implanted in the rabbit tibia," *Biomaterials*, vol. 15, no. 11, pp. 889–893, 1994.

[18] S. Isaksson and P. Alberius, "Maxillary alveolar ridge augmentation with onlay bone-grafts and immediate endosseous implants," *Journal of Cranio-Maxillofacial Surgery*, vol. 20, no. 1, pp. 2–7, 1992.

[19] M. G. Donovan, N. C. Dickerson, L. J. Hanson, and R. B. Gustafson, "Maxillary and mandibular reconstruction using calvarial bone grafts and Branemark implants: a preliminary report," *Journal of Oral and Maxillofacial Surgery*, vol. 52, no. 6, pp. 588–594, 1994.

[20] D. Buser, K. Dula, U. Belser, H. P. Hirt, and H. Berthold, "Localized ridge augmentation using guided bone regeneration. 1. Surgical procedure in the maxilla," *The International Journal of Periodontics & Restorative Dentistry*, vol. 13, no. 1, pp. 29–45, 1993.

[21] F. Pieri, N. N. Aldini, M. Fini, C. Marchetti, and G. Corinaldesi, "Rehabilitation of the atrophic posterior maxilla using short implants or sinus augmentation with simultaneous standard-length implant placement: a 3-year randomized clinical trial," *Clinical Implant Dentistry and Related Research*, 2012.

[22] U. Dietrich, R. Lippold, T. Dirmeier, N. Behneke, and W. Wagner, "Statistische Ergebnisse zur Implantatprognose am Beispiel von 2017 IMZ-Implantaten unterschiedlicher Indikationen der letzten 13 Jahre," *Zeitschrift für Zahnärztliche Implantologie*, vol. 9, pp. 9–18, 1993.

[23] J. A. Leonetti and R. Koup, "Localized maxillary ridge augmentation with a block allograft for dental implant placement: case reports," *Implant Dentistry*, vol. 12, no. 3, pp. 217–226, 2003.

[24] H. Burchardt, "The biology of bone graft repair," *Clinical Orthopaedics and Related Research*, vol. 174, pp. 28–42, 1983.

[25] P. S. Petrungaro and S. Amar, "Localized ridge augmentation with allogenic block grafts prior to implant placement: case reports and histologic evaluations," *Implant Dentistry*, vol. 14, no. 2, pp. 139–148, 2005.

[26] M. Franco, A. Viscioni, L. Rigo, R. Guidi, G. Brunelli, and F. Carinci, "Iliac crest fresh frozen homografts used in pre-prosthetic surgery: a retrospective study," *Cell and Tissue Banking*, vol. 10, no. 3, pp. 227–233, 2009.

[27] S. N. Khan, F. P. Cammisa Jr., H. S. Sandhu, A. D. Diwan, F. P. Girardi, and J. M. Lane, "The biology of bone grafting," *The Journal of the American Academy of Orthopaedic Surgeons*, vol. 13, no. 1, pp. 77–86, 2005.

[28] E. D'Aloja, E. Santi, G. Aprili, and M. Franchini, "Fresh frozen homologous bone in oral surgery: case reports," *Cell and Tissue Banking*, vol. 9, no. 1, pp. 41–46, 2008.

[29] D. H. Perrott, R. A. Smith, and L. B. Kaban, "The use of fresh frozen allogeneic bone for maxillary and mandibular reconstruction," *International Journal of Oral and Maxillofacial Surgery*, vol. 21, no. 5, pp. 260–265, 1992.

[30] M. Franco, A. Viscioni, L. Rigo et al., "Clinical outcome of narrow diameter implants inserted into allografts," *Journal of Applied Oral Science*, vol. 17, no. 4, pp. 301–306, 2009.

9

Trismus Pseudocamptodactyly Syndrome:
A Sporadic Cause of Trismus

Prathima Sreenivasan,[1] Faizal C. Peedikayil,[2] Sumal V. Raj,[3] and Manasa Anand Meundi[4]

[1] *Department of Oral Medicine and Radiology, Kannur Dental College, Anjarakkandy, Kannur, Kerala 670612, India*
[2] *Department of Pedodontics, Kannur Dental College, Anjarakkandy, Kannur, Kerala 670612, India*
[3] *Department of Oral Medicine and Diagnostic Radiology, Sri Sankara Dental College, Akathumuri, Varkala, Kerala 695318, India*
[4] *Department of Oral Medicine and Radiology, Dayananda Sagar College of Dental Sciences, Shavige Malleshwara Hills,*
   Kumaraswamy Layout, Bangalore 560078, India

Correspondence should be addressed to Prathima Sreenivasan; prathimasumal@gmail.com

Academic Editors: C. Ledesma-Montes, G. Spagnuolo, and E. F. Wright

Trismus pseudocamptodactyly syndrome is a very rare autosomal dominant inherited disorder characterized by the inability to completely open the mouth (trismus) and the presence of abnormally short tendon units causing the fingers to curve (camptodactyly). Early diagnosis and management of this condition is important to prevent facial deformities in the patient. Reporting such a case is important as case reports are one of the sources of data for calculating the prevalence of rare diseases. Here, we report a case of trismus pseudocamptodactyly syndrome in an eight-year-old boy with a brief review of the literature.

1. Introduction

Trismus pseudocamptodactyly syndrome (TPS) is a rare autosomal dominant disorder with sporadic incidence [1]. This condition was first reported by Hecht and Beale in 1969 [2] and was named the trismus pseudocamptodactyly syndrome (TPS). It is a type of Distal Arthrogryposis (arthro means joint; grypos means curved). They are a group of autosomal dominant disorders that mainly involve the distal parts of the limbs and also affect the temporomandibular joint leading to congenital deformities. They are characterized by congenital contracture of two or more different areas without a primary neurological or muscular disease [1, 3]. Ten different arthrogryposes have been described till date [1, 3, 4] (Table 1). Diagnostic criteria have been formulated for the diagnosis of each type of distal arthrogryposis. For the upper limb, major diagnostic criteria include campto-dactyly or pseudocamptodactyly (limited passive proximal interphalangeal joint extension with hyperextension of the wrist), hypoplastic and/or absent flexion creases, overriding fingers, and ulnar deviation at the wrist [1, 4]. For the lower limb, major diagnostic criteria are talipes equinovarus,

calcaneovalgus deformities, vertical talus, and/or metatarsus varus. To be considered affected, an individual must exhibit two or more of these major criteria. When a first-degree family member (a parent or a sibling) meets these diagnostic criteria, a person with at least one major diagnostic criterion is considered affected [1, 3, 4]. In the revised and extended classification scheme of distal arthrogryposis, Bamshad et al. classified TPS as distal arthrogryposis type 7 (DA7) [4]. The major diagnostic criteria are trismus and pseudocamp-todactyly [3, 4]. The features of distal arthrogryposis type 7 (DA7) are limited excursion of the mandible, shortened muscle tendon units of the hands (consequently, flexion deformity of the fingers that occurs with wrist extension, camptodactyly), and foot deformities related to shortened muscle legs thereby preventing normal growth and develop-ment [1, 2, 4].

2. Case Report

An eight-year-old boy was reported with a complaint of difficulty in opening the mouth. History revealed that the patient noticed gradual reduction in mouth opening for the

TABLE 1: Classification of distal arthrogryposes.

Syndrome	New label	OMIM number
Distal arthrogryposis type 1	DA1	108120
Distal arthrogryposis type 2A Freeman Sheldon syndrome	DA2A	193700
Distal arthrogryposis type 2B Sheldon Hall syndrome	DA2B	601680
Distal arthrogryposis type 3 Gordon syndrome	DA3	114300
Distal arthrogryposis type 4 Scoliosis	DA4	609128
Distal arthrogryposis type 5 Ophthalmoplegia, ptosis	DA5	108145
Distal arthrogryposis type 6 Sensorineuronal hearing loss	DA6	108200
Distal arthrogryposis type 7 Trismus pseudocamptodactyly	DA7	158300
Distal arthrogryposis type 8 Autosomal dominant pterygium syndrome	DA8	178110
Distal arthrogryposis type 9 Congenital contractural arachnodactyly	DA9	121050
Distal Arthrogryposis type 10 Congenital Planar contractures	DA10	187370

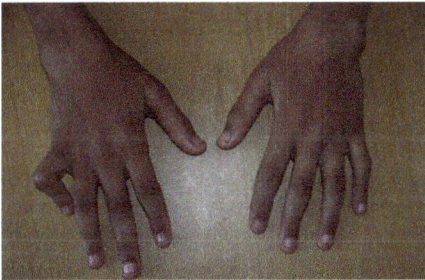

FIGURE 2: Photograph of feet showing contracture of all the toes and valgus deformity of the feet.

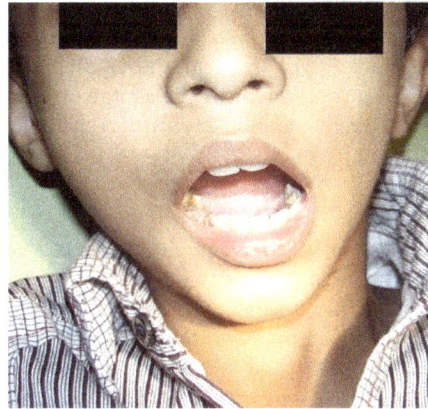

FIGURE 3: Decreased mouth opening with deviation towards left side.

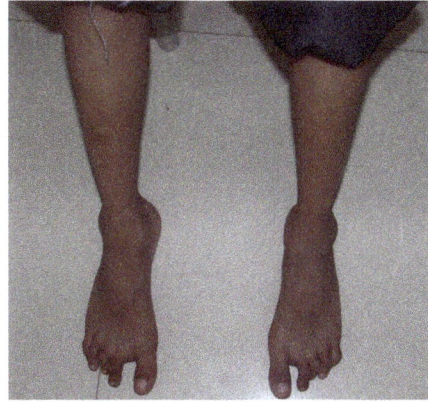

FIGURE 1: Photograph of hand showing camptodactyly-curved little finger.

last one year. Mouth opening had decreased rapidly in the last one month. Family history revealed that his parents had a consanguineous marriage. Mother had pregnancy induced hypertension in the antenatal period due to which a caesarian section was performed. Child was delivered preterm at seven months of gestation, and birth weight was 1.4 kg. Contractures of fingers, knees, and toes were noted at birth. Delay in achieving milestones both motor and speech was obvious. Patchy hair loss and rampant caries were noticed for the last two years. The boy underwent surgical release of the knee contractures at the age of four after which walking was achieved. The contractures in the leg have improved since then. History revealed that his sibling was also a preterm child and died at the fourth day after delivery.

On examination, the patient had normal height and weight. On central nervous system (CNS) examination Memory, intelligence and affect were normal. Hypertonia of both lower limbs with brisk reflexes was noted. Upper limbs showed mild rigidity with normal reflexes. Camptodactyly was present (Figure 1). Contractures of all the toes with valgus deformity were also noted (Figure 2). Hypopigmented macules were noted on the back, buttocks, and both arms. Alopecia areata was also noted.

Malar hypoplasia and retrognathic mandible were present. Mouth opening was 20 mm. Deflection to the left during mouth opening was noted (Figure 3). On intraoral examination, caries involving all the deciduous posterior teeth were noted.

2.1. Radiographic Investigations. Altered shape and flattening of the left condyle was notable in the coronal sectional CT (Figure 4).

2.2. Blood and Biochemistry Parameters Were within Normal Limits. The diagnosis of trismus pseudocamptodactyly syndrome/distal arthrogryposis type 7 was made based on the history of presence of congenital contractures, clinical findings of trismus, camptodactyly, valgus deformities of the feet, and correlating radiographic features of hand and the left condyle.

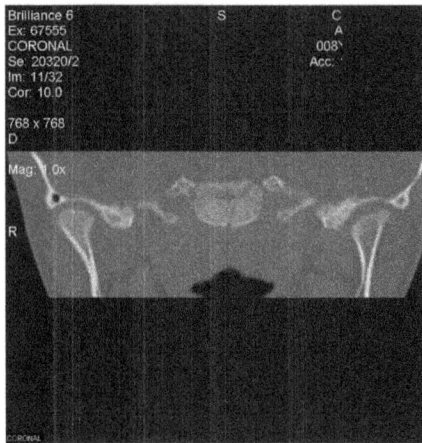

FIGURE 4: Coronal sectional CT showing flattening of the left condyle.

His parents were counseled regarding the temperomandibular joint (TMJ) problem and advised to undergo surgery at the earliest to remove the contracture, relieve the trismus, and prevent mandibular growth retardation.

3. Discussion

Trismus pseudocamptodactyly syndrome is a rare autosomal disorder with sporadic incidence. The disease has variable expressivity, and the severities of clinical features vary widely. Other than trismus and camptodactyly, additionally reported features include shortened hamstring muscles and short stature. No single feature, including either trismus or pseudocamptodactyly, is present in all affected individuals [3, 4]. It does not present uniformly in all patients making it difficult to diagnose. Fibrosis of the muscles of the TMJ, thickening and shortening of periarticular capsular and ligamentous tissues, coronoid hyperplasia [5–7], and condylar deformities with reduced joint space [8–11] have been cited as reasons for contracture in the muscles. Fibrosis of the muscles of TMJ and condylar deformities could be the reason for trismus in our patient.

Genetic studies have proven that it is caused by a single missense mutation in MYH8 that is predicted to cause an arginine-to-glutamine substitution in perinatal myosin. It is inherited in an autosomal dominant pattern [12]. The diagnosis is essentially clinical, and genetic analysis can be used only as an adjunct [4].

The sustained contracture in the masticatory muscles leads to trismus, difficulties in speech, mastication, and mandibular growth retardation. Early diagnosis and detection of TMJ related changes are important in the management of the condition. Though the condition was diagnosed early, the TMJ findings were not detected initially in our patient. The contracture of the masticatory muscles resulted in trismus and functional difficulties which could have been avoided if he had been assessed for TMJ involvement in the initial stages.

Surgical management is the treatment of choice [5–11]. Our patient was also advised surgical release of contracture in the masseter muscle and correction of condylar deformities to improve mouth opening and prevent further mandibular growth retardation.

4. Conclusion

Only a few cases of this condition have been reported in the literature till now. Improved knowledge will allow increased recognition and diagnosis, help in establishing prognosis, provide family counseling, and facilitate treatment. Early detection and appropriate intervention can prevent serious growth retardation and facial deformities. All children diagnosed with distal arthrogryposis should undergo periodic oral and maxillofacial assessment to rule out TMJ involvement. DA7/TPS should be included as a differential diagnosis for long standing trismus in children and adults.

References

[1] M. Bamshad, A. E. van Heest, and D. Pleasure, "Arthrogryposis: a review and update," Journal of Bone and Joint Surgery A, vol. 91, supplement 4, pp. 40–46, 2009.

[2] F. Hecht and R. K. Beale, "Inability to open the mouth fully: an autosomal dominant phenotype with facultative camptodactyly and short stature," Birth Defects Original Article Series, vol. 5, no. 3, pp. 96–98, 1969.

[3] http://omim.org/entry/158300.

[4] M. Bamshad, L. B. Jorde, and J. C. Carey, "A revised and extended classification of the distal arthrogryposes," American Journal of Medical Genetics, vol. 65, no. 4, pp. 277–281, 1996.

[5] R. K. Beals, "The distal arthrogryposes: a new classification of peripheral contractures," Clinical Orthopaedics and Related Research, no. 435, pp. 203–210, 2005.

[6] G. Gasparini, R. Boniello, A. Moro, G. Zampino, and S. Pelo, "Trismus-pseudocamptodactyly syndrome: case report ten years after," European Journal of Paediatric Dentistry, vol. 9, no. 4, pp. 199–203, 2008.

[7] R. Carlos, E. Contreras, and J. Cabrera, "Trismus-pseudocamptodactyly syndrome (Hecht-Beals' syndrome): case report and literature review," Oral Diseases, vol. 11, no. 3, pp. 186–189, 2005.

[8] S. Pelo, F. Boghi, A. Moro, R. Boniello, and R. Mosca, "Trismuspseudocamptodactyly syndrome: a case report," European Journal of Paediatric Dentistry, vol. 4, no. 1, pp. 33–36, 2003.

[9] J. S. Kargel, V. M. Dimas, and P. Chang, "Orthognathic surgery for management of Arthrogryposis Multiplex Congenita: case report and review of the literature," Canadian Journal of Plastic Surgery, vol. 15, no. 1, pp. 53–55, 2007.

[10] S. C. Karras and L. M. Wolford, "Trismus-pseudocampylodactyly syndrome: report of a case," Journal of Oral and Maxillofacial Surgery, vol. 53, no. 1, pp. 80–64, 1995.

[11] P. Hodgson, S. Weinberg, and C. Consky, "Arthrogryposis multiplex congenita of the temporomandibular joint," Oral Surgery Oral Medicine and Oral Pathology, vol. 65, no. 3, pp. 289–291, 1988.

[12] R. M. Toydemir, H. Chen, and V. K. Proud, "Trismus-pseudocamptodactyly syndrome is caused by recurrent mutation of MYH8," American Journal of Medical Genetics A, vol. 140, no. 22, pp. 2387–2393, 2006.

10

Autotransplantation of a Supernumerary Tooth to Replace a Misaligned Incisor with Abnormal Dimensions and Morphology: 2-Year Follow-Up

R. Ebru Tirali,[1] Cagla Sar,[2] Ufuk Ates,[3] Metin Kizilkaya,[4] and S. Burcak Cehreli[1]

[1] Department of Pediatric Dentistry, Faculty of Dentistry, Baskent University, 11. Sokak No. 26, Bahcelievler, 06490 Ankara, Turkey
[2] Department of Orthodontics, Faculty of Dentistry, Baskent University, Ankara, Turkey
[3] Department of Oral and Maxillofacial Surgery, Faculty of Dentistry, Baskent University, Ankara, Turkey
[4] Private Practice, 34100 Istanbul, Turkey

Correspondence should be addressed to R. Ebru Tirali; ebru_aktepe@hotmail.com

Academic Editors: A. Celebić, Y.-K. Chen, C. Evans, C. S. Farah, and C. Landes

Autotransplantation is a viable treatment option to restore esthetics and function impaired by abnormally shaped teeth when a suitable donors tooth is available. This paper describes the autotransplantation and 2-year follow-up of a supernumerary maxillary incisor as a replacement to a misaligned maxillary incisor with abnormal crown morphology and size. The supernumerary incisor was immediately autotransplanted into the extraction site of the large incisor and was stabilized with a bonded semirigid splint for 2 weeks. Fixed orthodontic therapy was initiated 3 months after autotransplantation. Ideal alignment of the incisors was accomplished after 6 months along with radiographic evidence of apical closure and osseous/periodontal regeneration. In autogenous tooth transplantation, a successful clinical outcome can be achieved if the cases are selected and treated properly.

1. Introduction

Autotransplantation (autogenous tooth transplantation) refers to the repositioning of autogenous teeth in another tooth extraction site or a surgically prepared recipient site to replace teeth that are congenitally missing or have poor prognosis [1, 2]. Traumatic injuries affecting anterior teeth which require prosthodontic or orthodontic treatment may also be treated by autotransplantation [1–4]. Finally, autotransplantation can be utilized to replace teeth with shape/size anomalies using donor teeth of normal size and/or morphology [5].

The success of autotransplantation can be influenced by a number of factors, which include patient age, developmental stage of the transplanted tooth, type of tooth transplanted, surgical technique employed, and extra alveolar time span before the tooth is transplanted [1–4]. Root resorption and loss of attachment are the major complications of autogenous tooth transplants. Contraindications for autotransplantation include cardiac anomalies, poor oral hygiene, and poor self-motivation [3].

Autotransplanted teeth result in the maintenance and regeneration of alveolar bone, and the procedure can be performed in growing patients. The aim of this paper is to present the autotransplantation, orthodontic treatment, and 2-year follow-up of a supernumerary incisor as a replacement to a large, fused central incisor.

2. Case Presentation

A healthy, 10-year-old boy was admitted to pediatric dentistry clinic for the management of crowding associated with a large tooth present in the upper jaw. On intraoral examination, the patient's chief complaint was confirmed by the presence of a misaligned maxillary right central incisor. The tooth had a talon cusp-like enamel projection on the labial aspect of the crown and had a large mesiodistal dimension. Owing to the

(a)

(b)

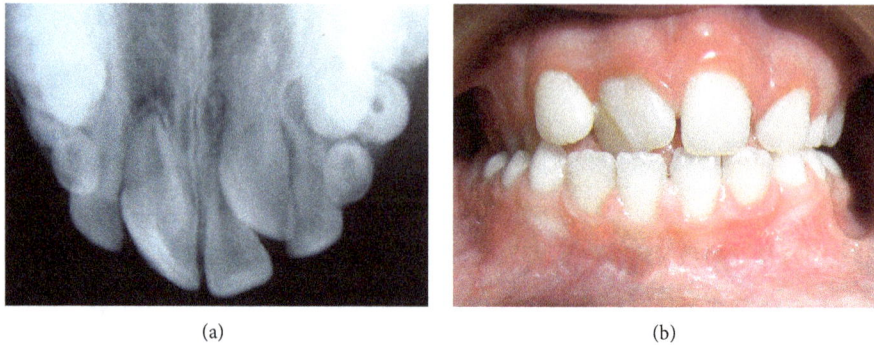

FIGURE 1: (a) Occlusal radiograph of the patient, demonstrating the large incisor and the unerupted supernumerary incisor. (b) Close-up view of the tooth, showing abnormal crown dimensions and morphology.

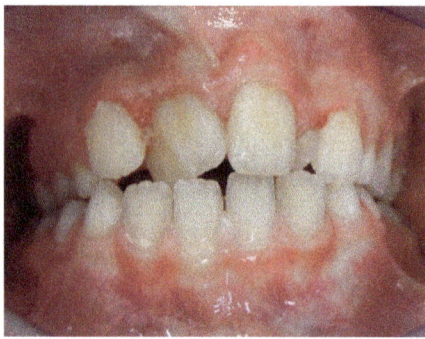

FIGURE 2: View of the supernumerary incisor (arrow), which erupted 4 months after the initial examination.

patient's gagging reflex, a proper radiographic examination of the incisor could not be made. However, the occlusal and periapical radiographs were highly suggestive of a large pulp chamber, and even of the possibility of a fused tooth. The occlusal radiograph also indicated an unerupted supernumerary incisor located on the contralateral side between the central and lateral incisors. The supernumerary incisor had a well-shaped crown and showed advanced root formation with incomplete apical closure (Figure 1).

Among possible treatment options, esthetic reduction of the crown in both the proximal and labial aspects was considered unfavorable due to the presence of a large pulp chamber. Extraction of the tooth and consequent orthodontic correction were also discarded as a treatment alternative, since orthodontic movement of the supernumerary tooth over the midline could result in resorption of the alveolar bone. Finally, the use of the contralateral supernumerary incisor as a replacement for the existing large incisor was considered the best treatment option, since both the radiographic crown dimensions and presence of the immature apex favored the possibility for autotransplantation. The patient and his parents were informed about the treatment options and their possible outcomes. The patient showed up four months later, approving the treatment plan of autotransplantation. During the time, the supernumerary incisor erupted into the crowded maxillary arch in a rotated fashion

(Figure 2). Extraction of the large incisor and autotransplantation of the supernumerary tooth were made one week later under local anesthesia (Figure 3). Stabilization of the autotransplanted incisor was provided by use of a semirigid splint made of 0.9 mm fisherman spring, bonded with acid-etch composite resin. The gingival tissue on the mesial and distal aspects of the tooth crown were sutured to accelerate healing. The patient was prescribed 20 mg/kg amoxicillin two times a day and a chlorhexidine gluconate mouthrinse for 1 week along with strict hygiene instructions. The splint was removed at the end of the second week, and the mobility was observed to be within normal limits. The radiographic followup demonstrated initiation of periradicular healing in the absence of clinical symptoms and pathologic mobility (Figure 4). Orthodontic treatment was initiated 3 months after autotransplantation and the transplanted tooth had an acceptable gingival contour, showed normal mobility, and responded to thermal and electrical pulp tests at the beginning of fixed orthodontic treatment (Figure 5). Clinical and radiographic followup at 2 years demonstrated apical closure, advanced regeneration of the periapical tissues, and reestablishment of the periodontal space along with slight calcific metamorphosis of the root canal space (Figure 6).

3. Discussion

Esthetic management of anterior teeth with abnormal crown dimensions and/or morphology may be quite challenging. As seen herein, the large coronal pulp space may limit the chance of successful reduction of the crown dimensions without possible endodontic complications. In such cases, autotransplantation appears to be a viable treatment option to restore esthetics and function, especially when a suitable donor tooth is available [1–5]. In young individuals, successful tooth transplantation also facilitates dentofacial development, mastication, and speech along with maintenance of the attached gingiva with a natural shape and level [1–4].

High long-term success rates of autotransplantation have been reported in the dental literature [6–8]. The age of the patient, the type, and development stage of the donor tooth are important factors that affect the success of autotransplantation [6, 8]. Further, a healthy periodontal membrane

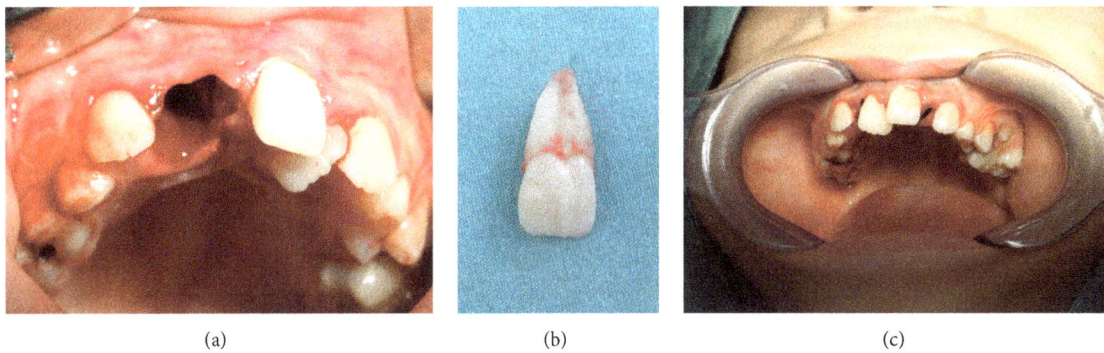

(a)   (b)   (c)

FIGURE 3: (a) View of the extraction socket of the large incisor; (b) the extracted incisor, demonstrating large crown and root dimensions and morphological appearance of a fused tooth; (c) view of the supernumerary incisor, immediately after implantation into the recipient site.

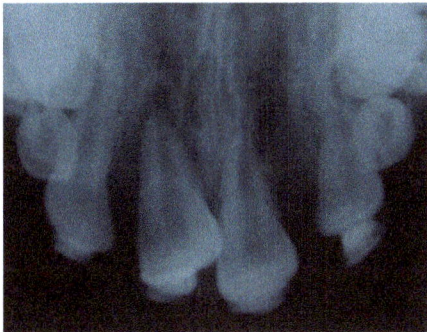

FIGURE 4: Radiographic view of the autotransplanted incisor at the 3rd week.

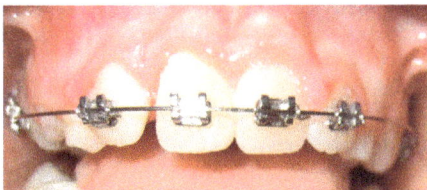

FIGURE 5: View of the incisors during fixed orthodontic treatment.

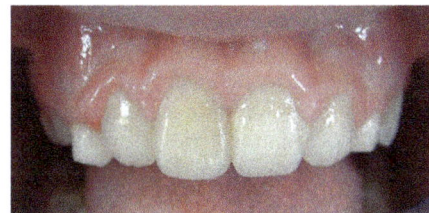

(a)

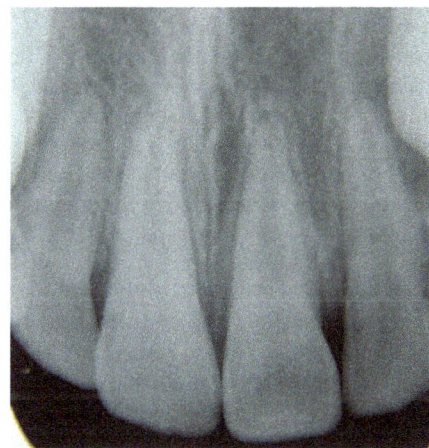

(b)

FIGURE 6: Clinical and radiographic view of the maxillary incisor at 2 years.

should be present on the transplanted tooth and the root morphology of the tooth to be transplanted should be simple. In addition, infection should be absent in the recipient site, and during surgery, the extraoral period should be short and trauma should be minimized [9–11].

As observed in the present case, calcific metamorphosis of the pulp is a common finding in transplanted teeth [5, 12–14]. No endodontic treatment was made since the pulp was vital and asymptomatic. According to Andreasen and Hjorting-Hansen [12], endodontic treatment of such teeth should be started only when a tooth becomes symptomatic or when bone lesions develop. Autotransplanted teeth have been shown to serve without pulpal complications for many years.

The presence of intact and viable periodontal ligament cells on the root surface of the donor tooth is the most critical factor that determines the prognosis of an autotransplanted tooth [1, 3, 11, 15]. Extended extraoral time of the donor tooth significantly affects the viability of the periodontal ligament cells, which leads to unfavorable results such as inflammation or root resorption [4]. In the present case, the supernumerary (donor) incisor was extracted after the fused incisor in order to minimize the extraoral dry time. The autotransplantation was performed immediately thereafter, without immersing the tooth in any kind of transport/storage media.

Along with rapid and atraumatic surgical technique, adequate recipient site affects the prognosis as well [15, 16].

Unlike other organ transplants, tooth transplants require dimensional compatibility between the transplanted tooth and the recipient site [17]. Optimal contact with the recipient site can improve the level of nutrition and the blood supply to the periodontal ligament cells, which can increase the success rate of autotransplantation [3, 18, 19]. In the absence of adequate buccolingual width to accommodate the donor tooth, resorption of the alveolar ridge may occur [18, 19]. In the present case, the buccolingual dimension of the donor tooth was compatible with the width of the transplantation socket, but the mesiodistal size of the donor tooth was considerably smaller. Thus, in order to maximize adaptability, the donor tooth was placed in a rotated fashion and gingival tissue on the mesial and distal aspects of the tooth crown were sutured to optimize postoperative healing. This procedure proved out to be effective, as evidenced by the final clinical and radiographic outcome.

Various techniques have been described to stabilize transplanted teeth, including loose fixation with sutures, ligatures, orthodontic brackets, acid-etch composite and wire splints, and ligature wires or orthodontic appliances [20–22]. The reported duration of splinting varies between 1 week [18, 19] and 4–6 weeks [23, 24]. In selected cases, splinting may not even be necessary [6]. It has been shown that prolonged and rigid fixation has significant negative influence on the success of tooth transplantation [25–27]. Thus, a short-term (2-week) semi-rigid splint was used in the present case.

Transplantation of teeth with immature roots offers high success rates due to the chance of revascularization as well as unimpeded development of the donor tooth and adjacent alveolar bone growth [5, 12, 16, 18]. Transplanted teeth with incomplete root formation possess a 96% rate of pulpal revascularization, while those with complete root formation show considerably lower chances (i.e., about 15%) of pulp regeneration [22, 28]. In the present case, the donor tooth showed advanced root formation, with incomplete apical closure. Since pulpal vitality was maintained after transplantation, no endodontic intervention was performed.

Transplanted teeth can be submitted to orthodontic treatment 3 to 6 months after transplantation [6, 10, 18, 29, 30]. According to Hamamoto et al. [31], orthodontic treatment can be initiated after regeneration of the periodontal space and subsequent radiographic confirmation of the lamina dura. In the present case, tooth alignment was accomplished with a short-term orthodontic intervention which was initiated approximately 4 months following autotransplantation. During the first month of orthodontic treatment, the amount of the force was minimized by leaving the autotransplanted tooth outside of the archwire.

The outcome of autotransplantation can be considered successful if there is no progressive root resorption, the adjacent periodontal tissues adjacent are normal and the crown-to-root ratio is less than 1 [7, 22]. In the present case, the success of autotransplantation also complied with the modified criteria of Chamberlin and Goerig [32]. Accordingly, the tooth was fixed in its socket without discomfort; the patient was chewing satisfactorily and without discomfort; the tooth was not mobile; no pathological condition was seen on the radiograph; the lamina dura appeared normal on the radiographs; and the depths of the sulcus, gingival contour, and gingival colour were normal. In addition, the crown to-root-ratio was less than 1. At the follow-up appointments, no pulpal or periodontal complications were observed.

4. Conclusion

In the presence of a well-shaped supplementary tooth, autotransplantation may be considered as a viable treatment option for replacement of large, misaligned teeth, which impair both esthetics and function. The procedure is cost-effective, one-stage surgery can be used and orthodontic movement is possible. Hence, autotransplantation can be considered as a successful and atraumatic treatment option in growing patients, especially when compared with treatment alternatives such as interim removable prostheses.

References

[1] R. A. Mendes and G. Rocha, "Mandibular third molar auto-transplantation: literature review with clinical cases," *Journal of the Canadian Dental Association*, vol. 70, no. 11, pp. 761–766, 2004.

[2] J. R. Natiella, J. E. Armitage, and G. W. Greene, "The replantation and transplantation of teeth. A review," *Oral Surgery, Oral Medicine, Oral Pathology*, vol. 29, no. 3, pp. 397–419, 1970.

[3] S. Thomas, S. R. Turner, and J. R. Sandy, "Autotransplantation of teeth: is there a role?" *British journal of orthodontics*, vol. 25, no. 4, pp. 275–282, 1998.

[4] M. Tsukiboshi, *Autotransplantation of Teeth*, Quintessence, Chicago, Ill, USA, 2001.

[5] T. Demir, U. Ates, B. Cehreli, and Z. C. Cehreli, "Autotransplantation of a supernumerary incisor as a replacement for fused tooth: 24-month follow-up," *Oral Surgery, Oral Medicine, Oral Pathology, Oral Radiology and Endodontology*, vol. 106, no. 4, pp. e1–e6, 2008.

[6] M. Akkocaoglu and O. Kasaboglu, "Success rate of autotransplanted teeth without stabilisation by splints: a long-term clinical and radiological follow-up," *British Journal of Oral and Maxillofacial Surgery*, vol. 43, no. 1, pp. 31–35, 2005.

[7] E. M. Czochrowska, A. Stenvik, B. Bjercke, and B. U. Zachrisson, "Outcome of tooth transplantation: survival and success rates 17-41 years posttreatment," *American Journal of Orthodontics and Dentofacial Orthopedics*, vol. 121, no. 2, pp. 110–119, 2002.

[8] G. Mensink and R. Van Merkesteyn, "Autotransplantation of premolars," *British Dental Journal*, vol. 208, no. 3, pp. 109–111, 2010.

[9] A. S. Cohen, T. C. Shen, and M. A. Pogrel, "Transplanting teeth successfully: autografts and allografts that work," *The Journal of the American Dental Association*, vol. 126, no. 4, pp. 481–500, 1995.

[10] J. W. F. H. Frenken, J. A. Baart, and A. Jovanovic, "Autotransplantation of premolars: a retrospective study," *International Journal of Oral and Maxillofacial Surgery*, vol. 27, no. 3, pp. 181–185, 1998.

[11] G. M. Raghoebar and A. Vissink, "Results of intentional replantation of molars," *Journal of Oral and Maxillofacial Surgery*, vol. 57, no. 3, pp. 240–244, 1999.

[12] J. O. Andreasen and E. Hjorting-Hansen, "Replantation of teeth. I. Radiographic and clinical study of 110 human teeth replanted

after accidental loss," *Acta Odontologica Scandinavica*, vol. 24, no. 3, pp. 263–286, 1966.

[13] S. Y. Cho and C. K. Lee, "Autotransplantation of a supplemental premolar: a case report," *Journal of the Canadian Dental Association*, vol. 73, no. 5, pp. 425–429, 2007.

[14] R. Kallu, F. Vinckier, C. Politis, S. Mwalili, and G. Willems, "Tooth transplantations: a descriptive retrospective study," *International Journal of Oral and Maxillofacial Surgery*, vol. 34, no. 7, pp. 745–755, 2006.

[15] J. O. Andreasen, "Autotransplantation of molars," in *Atlas of Replantation and Transplantation of Teeth*, WB Saunders, Philadelphia, Pa, USA, 1992.

[16] S. Kvint, R. Lindsten, A. Magnusson, P. Nilsson, and K. Bjerklin, "Autotransplantation of teeth in 215 patients a follow-up study," *Angle Orthodontist*, vol. 80, no. 3, pp. 446–451, 2010.

[17] T. Tsurumachi and Y. Kakehashi, "Autotransplantation of a maxillary third molar to replace a maxillary premolar with vertical root fracture," *International Endodontic Journal*, vol. 40, no. 12, pp. 970–978, 2007.

[18] P. C. Gault and R. Warocquier-Clerout, "Tooth autotransplantation with double periodontal ligament stimulation to replace periodontally compromised teeth," *Journal of Periodontology*, vol. 73, no. 5, pp. 575–583, 2002.

[19] G. Nethander, "Periodontal conditions of teeth autogenously transplanted by a two-stage technique," *Journal of Periodontal Research*, vol. 29, no. 4, pp. 250–258, 1994.

[20] J. O. Andreasen, H. U. Paulsen, Z. Yu, and O. Schwartz, "A long-term study of 370 autotransplanted premolars. Part III. Periodontal healing subsequent to transplantation," *European Journal of Orthodontics*, vol. 12, no. 1, pp. 25–37, 1990.

[21] T. Lundberg and S. Isaksson, "A clinical follow-up study of 278 autotransplanted teeth," *British Journal of Oral and Maxillofacial Surgery*, vol. 34, no. 2, pp. 181–185, 1996.

[22] K. A. M. Marcusson and E. K. Lilja-Karlander, "Autotransplantation of premolars and molars in patients with tooth aplasia," *Journal of Dentistry*, vol. 24, no. 5, pp. 355–358, 1996.

[23] L. Kristerson, "Autotransplantation of human premolars. A clinical and radiographic study of 100 teeth," *International Journal of Oral Surgery*, vol. 14, no. 2, pp. 200–213, 1985.

[24] A. Nordenram, "Autotransplantation of teeth. A clinical investigation," *The British Journal of Oral Surgery*, vol. 7, no. 3, pp. 188–195, 1970.

[25] J. O. Andreasen, "The effect of splinting upon periodontal healing after replantation of permanent incisors in monkeys," *Acta Odontologica Scandinavica*, vol. 33, no. 6, pp. 313–323, 1975.

[26] O. Bauss, R. Schilke, C. Fenske, W. Engelke, and S. Kiliaridis, "Autotransplantation of immature third molars: influence of different splinting methods and fixation periods," *Dental Traumatology*, vol. 18, no. 6, pp. 322–328, 2002.

[27] C. E. Nasjleti, W. A. Castelli, and R. G. Caffesse, "The effects of different splinting times on replantation of teeth in monkeys," *Oral Surgery, Oral Medicine, Oral Pathology*, vol. 53, no. 6, pp. 557–566, 1982.

[28] J. O. Andreasen, H. U. Paulsen, Z. Yu, T. Bayer, and O. Schwartz, "A long-term study of 370 autotransplanted premolars. Part II. Tooth survival and pulp healing subsequent to transplantation," *European Journal of Orthodontics*, vol. 12, no. 1, pp. 14–24, 1990.

[29] O. Bauss, R. Schwestka-Polly, and S. Kiliaridis, "Influence of orthodontic derotation and extrusion on pulpal and periodontal condition of autotransplanted immature third molars," *American Journal of Orthodontics and Dentofacial Orthopedics*, vol. 125, no. 4, pp. 488–496, 2004.

[30] L. Lagerström and L. Kristerson, "Influence of orthodontic treatment on root development of autotransplanted premolars," *American Journal of Orthodontics*, vol. 89, no. 2, pp. 146–150, 1986.

[31] N. Hamamoto, Y. Hamamoto, and T. Kobayashi, "Tooth autotransplantation into the bone-grafted alveolar cleft: report of two cases with histologic findings," *Journal of Oral and Maxillofacial Surgery*, vol. 56, no. 12, pp. 1451–1456, 1998.

[32] J. H. Chamberlin and A. C. Goerig, "Rationale for treatment and management of avulsed teeth," *The Journal of the American Dental Association*, vol. 101, no. 3, pp. 571–475, 1980.

11

Unusual Root Canal Morphology of the Maxillary Second Molar

Neslihan Şımşek, Ali Keleş, and Elçin Tekın Bulut

Department of Endodontics, Faculty of Dentistry, Inonu University, 44280 Malatya, Turkey

Correspondence should be addressed to Neslihan Şımşek; neslihan.akdemir@inonu.edu.tr

Academic Editors: Y.-K. Chen, W. El-Badrawy, T. Kubota, P. Lopez Jornet, M. A. Polack, and U. Zilberman

Introduction. This clinical case report presents the successful endodontic treatment of a maxillary second molar that has a mandibular molar-like anatomy with no palatal root and with each of its roots containing two separate root canals. Cone-beam computed tomography (CBCT) was used to confirm this unusual anatomy. *Methods.* A 34-year-old male patient was referred to the Department of Endodontics at Inonu University's Faculty of Dentistry because of severe pain in his right maxillary second molar. Clinical and radiographic examinations identified unusual roots and root canals anatomy, and CBCT was planned in order to understand the nature of these variations. Cleaning and shaping procedures were performed using the crown down technique with Sybron Endo (Glendora, CA, USA) rotary instruments, and endodontic treatment was completed with gutta-percha cones and AH Plus resin sealers using the cold lateral compaction technique. *Conclusions.* The maxillary second molar exhibits aberrations and variations in terms of the numbers and configurations of its roots and root canals, and CBCT can be a useful imaging technique in endodontics.

1. Introduction

It is known that thorough cleaning and shaping, in apical limits and dimensions, and obturation of all pulp spaces using an inert filling material are essential for root canal therapy. To perform successful endodontic treatment, it is important to have a clear understanding of the root canal system and its variations. The clinician who prepares the canal should expect, and be well equipped for, variations in the numbers of roots and root canal systems, in order to prevent undesirable consequences, including failure [1].

Most studies [2–6] of the morphology of the maxillary second molar have shown that the most frequently encountered type, known as standard morphology, has three roots: one mesiobuccal, one distobuccal, and one palatal. Each of these has a single canal. According to some studies [5–7], the presence of a second mesiobuccal canal is the most common variation found in the maxillary second molar. However, there are also case reports that present maxillary second molars with variations in the numbers of roots and root canals that they have. Benenati [8] presented a maxillary

second molar with two palatal canals, and Deveaux [9] reported a maxillary second molar with two palatal roots. In another case report, Alani [10] described the endodontic treatment of four-rooted maxillary second molars that occur bilaterally. Fahid and Taintor [11] and Zmener and Peirano [12] also reported maxillary molars with three buccal roots, and Kottoor et al. [13] described a CBCT study that found a maxillary second molar with both five roots and five canals.

This clinical case report presents a successful endodontic treatment of a maxillary second molar that has mandibular molar-like anatomy with no palatal root and with each of its roots containing two separate root canals.

2. Case Report

A 34-year-old male patient was referred to the Department of Endodontics at Inonu University's Faculty of Dentistry because of severe pain in his right maxillary second molar. The patient's medical history was unremarkable. Clinical examination revealed that the tooth had a deep composite

(a)

(b)

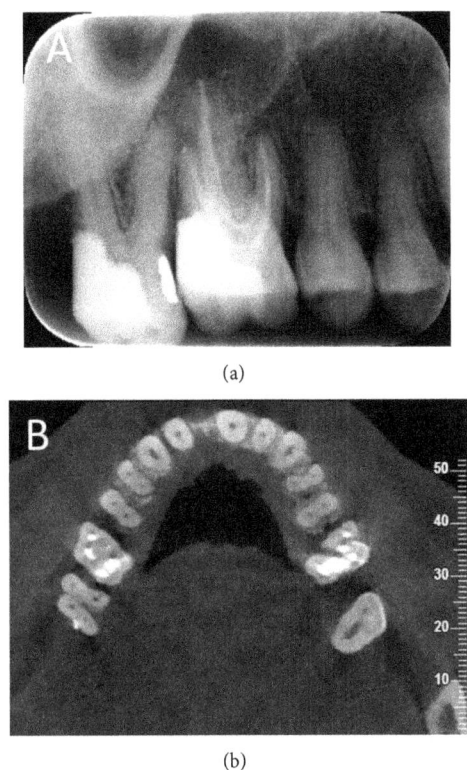

Figure 1: (a) Preoperative radiography showed that the tooth had two roots and no periapical radiolucency. (b) CBCT image revealed the absence of palatal root and two roots with two canals each.

restoration and was not tender to palpation or percussion. The vitality tests were painful for both hot and cold stimulants, and electric pulp test was reduced. A preoperative radiograph showed no periapical radiolucency, and the periapical tissues were normal. Because radiographic examination revealed an unusual formation of the roots and root canals of the involved tooth, cone-beam computed tomography (CBCT-NewTom 5G, QR, Verona, Italy) was planned to acquire a better understanding of the nature of these variations. Informed consent was obtained from the patient. CBCT helped to verify the morphology of the roots and root canals. CBCT image demonstrated that the maxillary second molar tooth has two roots which were located mesially and distally, and each root has two canals (Figure 1). Based on the clinical examination and the patient's complaints, a diagnosis of irreversible pulpitis was established and endodontic treatment was planned.

The tooth was anesthetized, and a rubber dam was put into place to isolate it. Preparation of the access cavity was also completed successfully. After a thorough inspection of the pulp chamber floor had confirmed the location of four root canal orifices, two of which were located mesially and two distally, these root canals were examined with no.10 K-type files (Mani Inc.). The working length was determined by Root ZX mini apex locator (J. Morita, Kyoto, Japan). To facilitate access to the root canals, coronal enlargement was prepared

by using Gates Glidden burs (Mani, Inc., Tochigi, Japan) nos. 1, 2. Cleaning and shaping procedures were performed using twisted file (SybronEndo, Orange, CA) rotary instruments, according to the manufacturer's recommendations. The root canals were irrigated with 2.5% sodium hypochlorite between each of the instrumentations, and 17% EDTA (ethylenediamine tetraacetic acid) solution was used for the final irrigation. After the root canals had been dried, calcium hydroxide was applied as an intracanal medicament, a sterile cotton pellet was placed into the pulp chamber, and Cavit (ESPE, Seefeld, Germany) was used to seal the access cavity. A week later, the patient was asymptomatic. All root canals were obturated with gutta-percha cones and AH Plus (Dentsply De Trey GmbH, Konstanz, Germany) resin sealer, using the cold lateral compaction technique and a final periapical radiograph was taken to confirm the filling of the root canals (Figure 2). After one year, the clinical and radiographic followup revealed that the patient was asymptomatic and the periapical tissues and restored tooth were healthy (Figure 3).

3. Discussion

This case reports on a distinct formation of the roots and root canals of a maxillary second molar. Unlike some cases [9, 14, 15], which reported the presence of extra palatal roots in maxillary second molars, our case reveals the absence of a palatal root. In addition, in our report the roots of the maxillary second molar are positioned mesially and distally, and each has two root canals. In 1989, Libfeld and Rotstein [2] evaluated 1200 teeth in two groups: the first group included 1000 teeth and the second had 200. The study showed that 6% of the teeth in group one had two roots and 12% of those in group two had two roots with two canals. In addition, Peikoff et al. [4], who conducted a study of 520 completed endodontic treatments for maxillary second molars in 1996, described two separate roots, a buccal and a palatal, with one canal in each root as variant 4, with a percentage of 6.9%. A study by Lee et al. [7] also reported that, out of 205 maxillary second molars, 5.8% had two separate roots, with the variations of root canal anatomy frequently found in the buccal roots. Another recent study by Kim et al. [16] used CBCT to analyze the morphology of maxillary first and second molars in a Korean population and found the incidence of two separate roots in 821 maxillary second molars to be 9.8%.

In this paper, the positions of the maxillary second molar's four root canal orifices were observed to be located mesiobuccally, mesiopalatally, distobuccally, and distopalatally, on the pulp chamber floor. Another recent study by Versiani et al. [17], who evaluated the root and root canal morphology of four-rooted maxillary second molars with micro-CT, described a new classification system, based on the configuration of the root canal orifices and their relationship to the pulp chamber floor, in maxillary second molars. Based on this classification system, our study categorized the involved maxillary second molar as type B (trapezoid shaped).

Conventional radiographic images force clinicians to visualize 3D structures based on 2D images, and the need to superimpose adjacent anatomic structures on each other

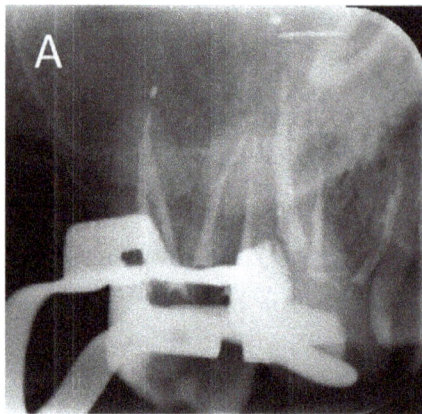

(a)

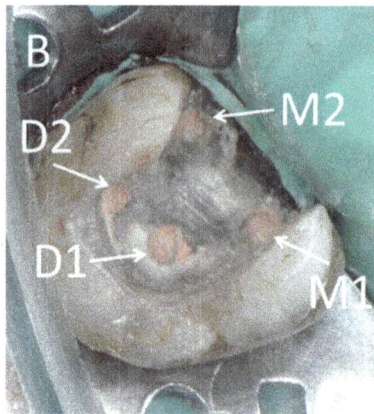

(b)

FIGURE 2: (a) Postoperative periapical radiograph taken immediately after completion of the root canal treatment. (b) The location of four root canal orifices after root canal filling.

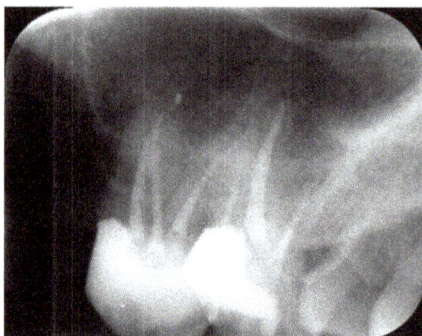

FIGURE 3: A 1-year follow-up periapical radiograph.

for radiographs prevents clinicians from gathering clear, understandable images. CBCT imaging technology, however, with its 3D images eliminates the disadvantages of conventional radiographs [18]. In our case, even though periapical radiographs of the involved tooth revealed variations in root canal anatomy, they did not provide clear information about the nature of this variation. Using CBCT allowed us to acquire

a better understanding of the variation and, therefore, to perform successful endodontic treatment.

4. Conclusions

The maxillary second molar exhibits aberrations and variations in terms of the numbers and configurations of its roots and root canals. Also, the complexity of the root canal system, especially in multirooted teeth, increases with the presence of such variations. CBCT can be a useful imaging technique in endodontics for providing a clear understanding of root canal morphology, especially when there are variations.

Conflict of Interests

The authors declare that they have no conflict of interests.

References

[1] F. J. Vertucci, "Root canal morphology and its relationship to endodontic procedures," *Endodontic Topics*, vol. 10, no. 1, pp. 3–29, 2005.

[2] H. Libfeld and I. Rotstein, "Incidence of four-rooted maxillary second molars: literature review and radiographic survey of 1,200 teeth," *Journal of Endodontics*, vol. 15, no. 3, pp. 129–131, 1989.

[3] P. Neelakantan, C. Subbarao, R. Ahuja, C. V. Subbarao, and J. L. Gutmann, "Cone-beam computed tomography study of root and canal morphology of maxillary first and second molars in an Indian population," *Journal of Endodontics*, vol. 36, no. 10, pp. 1622–1627, 2010.

[4] M. D. Peikoff, W. H. Christie, and H. M. Fogel, "The maxillary second molar: variations in the number of roots and canals," *International Endodontic Journal*, vol. 29, no. 6, pp. 365–369, 1996.

[5] J. D. Pecora, J. B. Woelfel, M. D. Sousa-Neto et al., "Morphologic study of the maxillary molars—part II: internal anatomy," *Brazilian Dental Journal*, vol. 3, no. 1, pp. 53–57, 1992.

[6] A. M. Alavi, A. Opasanon, Y. L. Ng, and K. Gulabivala, "Root and canal morphology of Thai maxillary molars," *International Endodontic Journal*, vol. 35, no. 5, pp. 478–485, 2002.

[7] J. H. Lee, K. D. Kim, J. K. Lee et al., "Mesiobuccal root canal anatomy of Korean maxillary first and second molars by cone-beam computed tomography," *Oral Surgery, Oral Medicine, Oral Pathology, Oral Radiology and Endodontology*, vol. 111, no. 6, pp. 785–791, 2011.

[8] F. W. Benenati, "Maxillary second molar with two palatal canals and a palatogingival groove," *Journal of Endodontics*, vol. 11, no. 7, pp. 308–310, 1985.

[9] E. Deveaux, "Maxillary second molar with two palatal roots," *Journal of Endodontics*, vol. 25, no. 8, pp. 571–573, 1999.

[10] A. H. Alani, "Endodontic treatment of bilaterally occurring 4-rooted maxillary second molars: case report," *Journal of the Canadian Dental Association*, vol. 69, no. 11, pp. 733–735, 2003.

[11] A. Fahid and J. F. Taintor, "Maxillary second molar with three buccal roots," *Journal of Endodontics*, vol. 14, no. 4, pp. 181–183, 1988.

[12] O. Zmener and A. Peirano, "Endodontic therapy in a maxillary second molar with three buccal roots," *Journal of Endodontics*, vol. 24, no. 5, pp. 376–377, 1998.

[13] J. Kottoor, S. Hemamalathi, R. Sudha, and N. Velmurugan, "Maxillary second molar with 5 roots and 5 canals evaluated using cone beam computerized tomography: a case report," *Oral Surgery, Oral Medicine, Oral Pathology, Oral Radiology and Endodontology*, vol. 109, no. 2, pp. e162–e165, 2010.

[14] O. I. A. Ulusoy and G. Görgül, "Endodontic treatment of a maxillary second molar with 2 palatal roots: a case report," *Oral Surgery, Oral Medicine, Oral Pathology, Oral Radiology and Endodontology*, vol. 104, no. 4, pp. e95–e97, 2007.

[15] S. J. Shin, J. W. Park, J. K. Lee, and S. W. Hwang, "Unusual root canal anatomy in maxillary second molars: two case reports," *Oral Surgery, Oral Medicine, Oral Pathology, Oral Radiology and Endodontology*, vol. 104, no. 6, pp. e61–e65, 2007.

[16] Y. Kim, S. J. Lee, and J. Woo, "Morphology of maxillary first and second molars analyzed by cone-beam computed tomography in a korean population: variations in the number of roots and canals and the incidence of fusion," *Journal of Endodontics*, vol. 38, no. 8, pp. 1063–1068, 2012.

[17] M. A. Versiani, J. D. Pecora, and M. D. Sousa-Neto, "Root and root canal morphology of four-rooted maxillary second molars: a micro-computed tomography study," *Journal of Endodontics*, vol. 38, no. 7, pp. 977–982, 2012.

[18] T. P. Cotton, T. M. Geisler, D. T. Hoden, S. A. Schwartz, and W. G. Schindler, "Endodontic applications of cone-beam volumetric tomography," *Journal of Endodontics*, vol. 33, no. 9, pp. 1121–1132, 2007.

12

Basal Cell Ameloblastoma of Mandible

Hemant Shakya,[1] Vikram Khare,[1] Nilesh Pardhe,[2] Ena Mathur,[1] and Mansi Chouhan[1]

[1] *Department of Oral Medicine and Radiology, Mahatma Gandhi Dental College & Hospital, Jaipur 302022, Rajasthan, India*
[2] *Department of Oral & Maxillofacial Pathology, Mahatma Gandhi Dental College & Hospital, Jaipur 302022, Rajasthan, India*

Correspondence should be addressed to Hemant Shakya; shakyamds@gmail.com

Academic Editors: J. C. de la Macorra and M. A. Polack

Ameloblastoma is a slow-growing benign neoplasm that has a strong tendency to local invasion and that can grow to be quite large without metastasizing. Rare examples of distant metastasis of an ameloblastoma in lungs or regional lymph nodes do exist. It has an aggressive and recurrent course and is rarely metastatic. Radiographically it shares common features with other lesions such as the giant cell tumor, aneurysmal bone cyst, and renal cell carcinoma metastasis; a definitive diagnosis can only be made with histopathology. Basal cell ameloblastoma is believed to be the rarest histologic subtype in which the tumor is composed of more primitive cells and has even fewer features of peripheral palisading. Till date, only few cases of basal cell ameloblastoma have been reported in the literature. Considering the rarity of the lesion, we report here an interesting and unique case of basal cell ameloblastoma of the mandible occurring in a very old patient.

1. Introduction

Ameloblastomas are benign locally aggressive, polymorphic neoplasms of proliferating odontogenic epithelial origin, arising from cell rests of enamel organ, either remnants of dental lamina or remnants of Hertwig's sheaths, the epithelial rest of Malassez, the developing enamel organ, basal cell epithelium of the jaws, heterotropic epithelium in the other parts of the body especially the pituitary gland and epithelium of the odontogenic cyst particularly the dentigerous cyst, and the odontomas [1]. Ameloblastomas constitute approximately 1% of all cysts and tumors of the jaws. The occurrence in the mandible is five times higher than in the maxilla. In the literature, the average age of occurrences is 38.9 years [2].

The incidence, clinical and radiological features, behavior, and histopathology of ameloblastomas have been extensively reviewed in numerous publications. They occur in three different clinicoradiographic situations, which deserve separate consideration because of different therapeutic considerations and prognosis [3].

These are

(1) conventional solid or multicystic (about 86% of all cases),

(2) unicystic (about 13% of all cases),

(3) peripheral (extraosseous) (about 1% of all cases).

Several histopathologic patterns of ameloblastomas are commonly described and include the follicular, plexiform, acanthomatous, granular cell, and basal cell patterns. There appears to be rather general agreement that these variations in histopathology patterns do not have any significant bearing on prognosis except unicystic ameloblastoma because of the less aggressive behavior and favorable prognosis [4].

Basal cell variant of ameloblastoma is the least common type. These lesions are composed of nests of uniform baseloid cells and histopathologically very similar to basal cell carcinoma of skin. No stellate reticulum is present in the centre portion of the nest. The peripheral cells around the nest tend to be cuboidal rather than columnar [3].

Though very little information appears in the literature either due to insufficient number of cases reported or due to variations in the clinical or radiological criteria, the pathologist may sometimes fail to differentiate it from intraoral basal cell carcinoma [4].

The purpose of this paper is to present a case of the rarest variant of ameloblastoma (basal cell ameloblastoma) that has

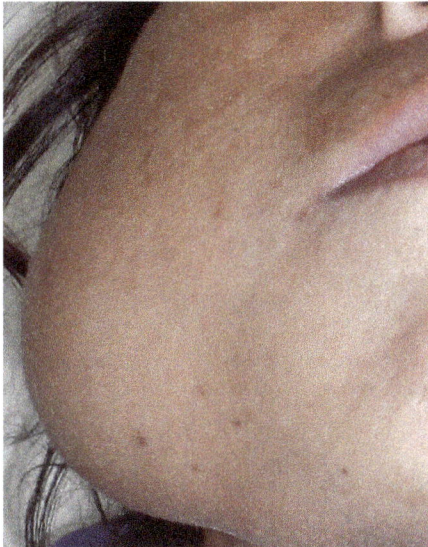

FIGURE 1: Frontal view of the patient showing extraoral swelling in the right lower mandibular region.

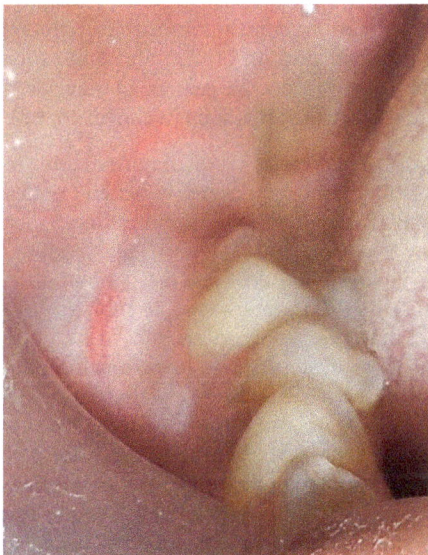

FIGURE 2: Intraoral view of the patient showing obliteration of the right lower buccal vestibule.

occurred in the 6th decade of the age and to provide a brief review of the literature.

2. Case Report

A 50-year-old female patient visited the department of oral medicine and radiology, with a chief complaint of the pain and swelling over the right lower third of the face for 6 months. Extraorally swelling (Figure 1) was oval in shape, size 7 cm × 6 cm and extended anteriorly from the right corner of the oral cavity to posterior border of ramus of mandible. Superiorly from right tragus of ear to 1 cm below

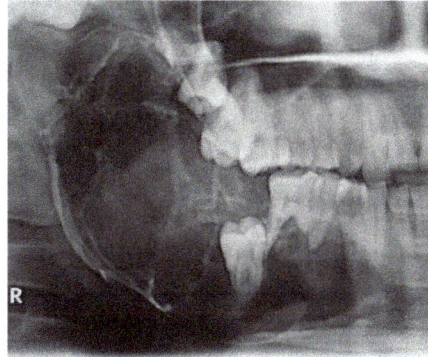

FIGURE 3: OPG of the female patient showing multilocular radiolucent lesion & root resorption of 46.

to the lower border of mandible. Intraoral examination (Figure 2) revealed obliteration of the right lower buccal vestibule. The overlying skin of lesion was normal in color without any sinus and drainage, and there was no local rise in the temperature. The patient had poor oral hygiene and numbness of the lower lip on right side. On the basis of history and clinical examination the provisional diagnosis was given as odontogenic tumur and differential diagnosis was given as odontogenic cyst and bone tumur.

The details of the procedure were explained to the patient and a written informed consent was obtained. The patient was subjected to routine hematological and radiological examination. Radiographically in orthopentomogram (Figure 3) lesion was multilocular and extended mesially from canine to condylar and coronoid region. The panoramic view revealed expansion of lower border of mandible & anterior border of ramus with perforation. Root resorption of 46 was in favour of ameloblastoma. Expansion of lower border of mandible is evident in lateral cephalogram (Figure 4). CT scan (Figure 5) revealed bicortical expansion with perforation.

Incisional biopsy was taken from the site of lesion which shows features of basal cell ameloblastoma. Then the patient was refered to the department of oral and maxillofacial surgery where she underwent hemimandibulectomy and reconstruction was done with a 2.5 mm reconstruction plate; bony reconstruction was not considered due to the advanced age of the patient.

In the histopathology (Figure 6) report, a completely resected lesion showed islands of uniform baseloid cells in a mature fibrous connective tissue stroma. Peripheral cells are columnar & showed reversal of polarity. The cells were stained deeply basophilic and nearly equivalent in staining intensity. In some island, the central portion is completely replaced by baseloid cells and some island shows scanty stellate reticulum like areas. Baseloid cells are hyperchromatic and there is no palisading of nuclei. Healing was uneventful and she was discharged after 7 days.

3. Discussion

Ameloblastomas begin as unilocular lesions and evolve into multilocular lesions, according to the fact that the mean age

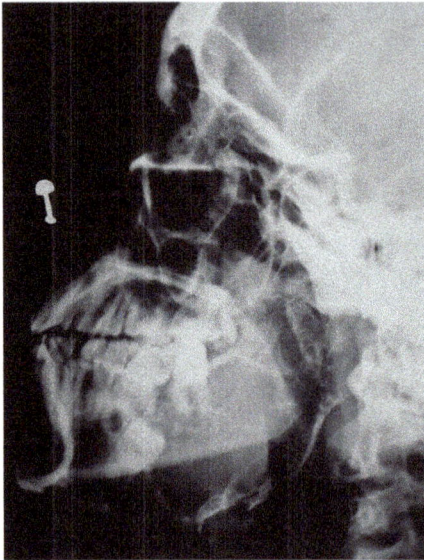

FIGURE 4: Lateral cephalogram of the patient showing expansion of the lower border of mandible.

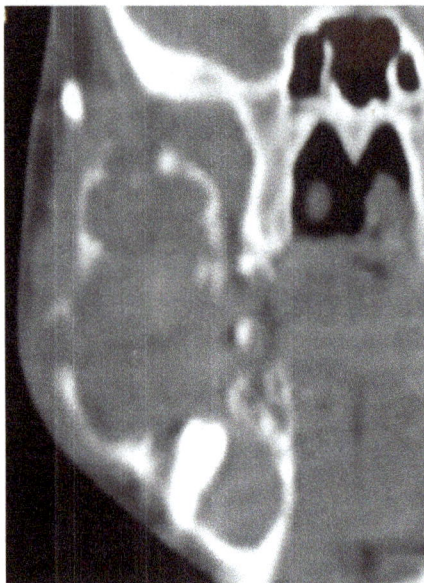

FIGURE 5: CT scan of the patient showing bicortical expansion with perforation.

of patient with unilocular lesion is 26 years, whereas it is 38 years for multilocular ameloblastomas. Radiographically it may appear unilocular or multilocular with soap bubble or honeycomb appearance; buccal and lingual expansion of the cortex invariably accompanies ameloblastoma. Thinned and intact cortex shows egg shell appearance [5].

Worth divided the ameloblastoma into four radiological manifestation categories.

(1) First, resembling a dentigerous cyst without septa, mostly in ramus region. Most frequently anterior wall of ramus lost.

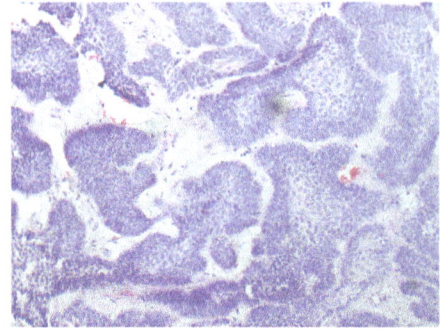

FIGURE 6: Photomicrograph shows island of uniform baseloid cells in a mature fibrous connective tissue stroma.

(2) Second, most common, cystic appearing cavity with distinctive septa (caricature of spider). Perforation in anterior surface of ramus & superior border of the body of mandible. Characteristically, angle of mandible is preserved. The inferior aspect may be ballooned out with a significant smooth downward convexity.

(3) Third, less common multilocular cystic appearance in posterior portion of mandible and ramus. Significant downward enlargement of inferior border of mandible, which maintains a convex lower border.

(4) Fourth, solid varity in which normal bone is replaced by honeycomb appearance in which cavities are relatively small and fairly uniform in size.

The basal cell ameloblastoma is a rare variant of ameloblastoma, which shows a remarkable resemblance to the basal cell carcinoma and published cases of intraoral basal cell carcinoma most likely are basal cell ameloblastoma; only few cases of basal cell subtypes were available for valid statistical analysis. Basal cell ameloblastoma tends to grow in an island-like pattern. The characteristic color gradation in other ameloblastoma is often difficult to appreciate in basal cell type, because baseloid appearing cell rather then stellate reticulum-like appearing cell occupies the center portion of the tumor island. The baseloid cells stain deeply basophilic and equivalent in staining intensity with peripheral layer of cells [6].

The typical cellular morphology and nuclear orientation of peripheral cells are altered. They tend to be low columnar to cuboidal and often do not show reverse nuclear polarity with subnuclear vacuole formation, but hyperchromatism and palisading of nuclei are maintained.

The similarity in the histopathology of this tumor to basal cell carcinoma might point toward the aggressiveness of this lesion. The recurrence rates of basal cell ameloblastoma have not been reported due to the limitation in the number of cases. Basal cell variant like the one reported in the paper needs an appropriate diagnosis based not only on clinical and radiological principles but also on sound histopathologic analysis. Long-term followup is necessary to establish the recurrence rate.

References

[1] Hennry M. Cherrick, "Odontogenic tumors of the jaw," in *Oral and Maxillofacial Surgery*, Daniel M. Laskin, Ed., pp. 626–636, AITBS, New Delhi, India, 2009.

[2] I. A. Small and C. A. Waldron, "Ameloblastoma of the Jaws," *Journal of Oral and Maxillofacial Surgeryand Pathology*, vol. 8, pp. 281–297, 1995.

[3] B. W. Neville, D. D. Damn, C. M. Allen, and J. K. Bouqout, Eds., *Oral and Maxillofacial Pathology*, WB Saunders, Philadelphia, Pa, USA, 2nd edition, 2002.

[4] H. Desai, R. Sood, R. Shah, J. Cawda, and H. Pandya, "Desmoplastic ameloblastoma: report of a unique case and review of literature," *Indian Journal of Dental Research*, vol. 17, no. 1, pp. 45–49, 2006.

[5] R. P. Langland, O. E. Langland, and C. J. Nortje, *Diagnostic Imaging of the Jaw*, Williams & Wilkins, Philadelphia, Pa, USA, 1st edition, 1995.

[6] H. P. Kessler, "Intraosseous ameloblastoma," *Oral and Maxillofacial Surgery Clinics of North America*, vol. 16, no. 3, pp. 309–322, 2004.

13

Clinical and Imaging Findings of True Hemifacial Hyperplasia

Bansari A. Bhuta,[1] **Archana Yadav,**[1] **Rajiv S. Desai,**[1] **Shivani P. Bansal,**[1]
Vipul V. Chemburkar,[2] **and Prashant V. Dev**[2]

[1] *Department of Oral Pathology, Nair Hospital Dental College, Dr. A. L. Nair Road, Mumbai, Maharashtra 400 008, India*
[2] *Department of Radiology, Topiwala National Medical College & B. Y. L. Nair Hospital, Mumbai 400008, India*

Correspondence should be addressed to Rajiv S. Desai; nansrd@hotmail.com

Academic Editors: M. Darling, A. C. B. Delbem, G. Spagnuolo, and K. H. Zawawi

Congenital hemifacial hyperplasia is a rare developmental disorder of unknown etiology, characterized by a marked unilateral facial asymmetry. It involves the hard (bones and teeth) and soft tissues of the face. We report an interesting case of true hemifacial hyperplasia in a 25-year-old male highlighting the clinical and computed tomography imaging findings.

1. Introduction

Congenital hemihyperplasia is a rare developmental disorder characterized by unilateral overgrowth of one or more body parts resulting in marked asymmetry. This phenomenon was first described by Meckel [1] in 1822 and first reported by Kottmeier and Wagner [2] in 1839. Rowe [3] in 1962 classified hemihypertrophy into (1) complex hemihypertrophy, involving the entire half of the body, (2) simple hemihypertrophy affecting one or both limbs, and (3) hemifacial hypertrophy. Depending on involvement of soft tissues, teeth, and bones, he further classified hemifacial hypertrophy into (a) true hemifacial hypertrophy and (b) partial hemifacial hypertrophy. True hemifacial hypertrophy exhibits unilateral enlargement of all tissues, teeth, bones, and soft tissues, characterized by viscerocranial enlargement, bounded by frontal bone superiorly (sparing the eye), inferior border of the mandible inferiorly, midline medially, and ear including the pinna laterally. In partial hemifacial hypertrophy not all structures are enlarged to the same degree or limited to one structure. We prefer to use the term congenital hemifacial hyperplasia although it is usually referred to as hemifacial hypertrophy. The term hyperplasia is more precise histologically, as all tissues show an increase in the number of cells rather than an increase in cell size [4]. The asymmetry usually remains constant with the end of adolescence, and as the skeletal maturation occurs the condition stabilizes thereafter.

We report an interesting case of true hemifacial hyperplasia (THFH) in a 25-year-old male, discussing clinical features, imaging findings, and differential diagnosis in detail to supplement the current literature.

2. Case Report

A 25-year-old male reported to our department for opinion regarding a massive, asymptomatic enlargement of the right half of the face since childhood (Figure 1). The asymmetry had increased with age and ceased to grow after 18 years of age. Family history was unavailable since he was an orphan. Medical examination did not reveal any other health issues. The patient had deferred treatment until now due to the lack of financial resources. Extraoral examination revealed a massive and diffuse enlargement of the right side of the face. The enlargement extended from the midline to the preauricular region, superiorly to the frontal bone and inferiorly to the inferior border of mandible. The nose and chin were deviated towards the left side of the face, with the facial midline describing a gentle arc from nasion to gnathion instead of the usual vertical straight line. The right corner of the mouth was drooped and lips were larger on the right side. The skin of the involved right side of the face was coarser than the unaffected left side. The right pinna was larger than that of the left side. There was monstrous enlargement of the soft tissue over the zygoma, the infraorbital region and the symphyseal region.

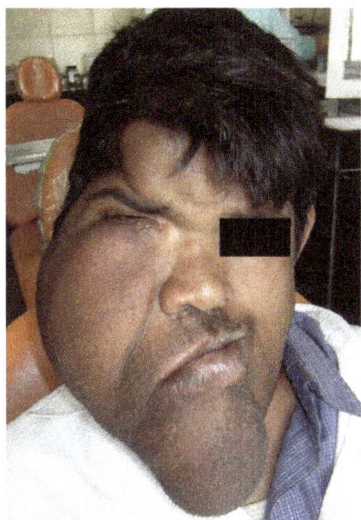

FIGURE 1: Unilateral enlargement of right side of the face. Note the asymmetry of the forehead, cheeks, nose, lips, chin, and the closed eye.

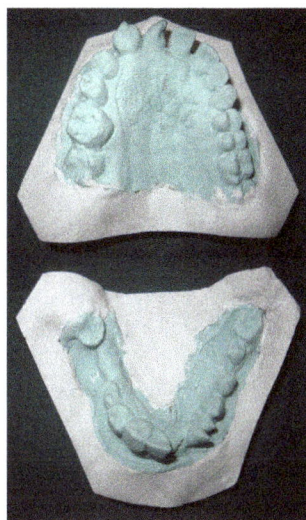

FIGURE 2: Occlusal view of the maxillary and mandibular dental casts showing macrodontia of the right side, midline shift to the left, along with granular surface of the right palatal mucosa.

The enlarged soft tissue mass on the right side of the face caused closure of the right eye, compromising the patient's vision. There appeared to be an excessive increase in size of the right side of the mandible, maxilla, zygoma, and frontal bone, as compared to the contralateral side. On palpation a nontender, soft tissue swelling over the right parietal bone was noticed. No temporomandibular joint disorder or dysfunction was detected. No discrepancy in range of mandibular motion was noted.

Intraoral examination disclosed an obvious alveolar enlargement of the right maxillary and mandibular quadrants as compared to the left quadrants (Figure 2). The surface of the gingival tissue and palate on the right side was granular in appearance. Right half of the tongue showed an obvious enlargement to the midline with polypoid excrescences representing enlargement of the fungiform papillae (Figure 3). The right buccal mucosa was thickened and hung in pendulous folds (Figure 4). A distinct tooth size discrepancy was observed between right and left side. Detailed coronal dimensions of the teeth were measured on the casts with vernier calipers, which revealed major variations in size between the teeth of the affected side compared to the uninvolved side. Right permanent maxillary canine, first premolar, second premolar, first molar, and second molar were larger cervicoincisally, mesiodistally, and labiolingually than those of the left side (Table 1). Similarly, right permanent mandibular lateral incisor, canine, first premolar, and second premolar were larger cervicoincisally, mesiodistally, and labiolingually than those of the left side (Table 2). The above mentioned right maxillary and mandibular teeth were considerably enlarged than their contralateral counterparts. The right permanent maxillary canine, first premolar, second premolar, first molar, and second molar demonstrated 224%, 100%, 63%, 110%, and 75% increase in volume, respectively, than their contralateral counterparts, while the right permanent mandibular lateral

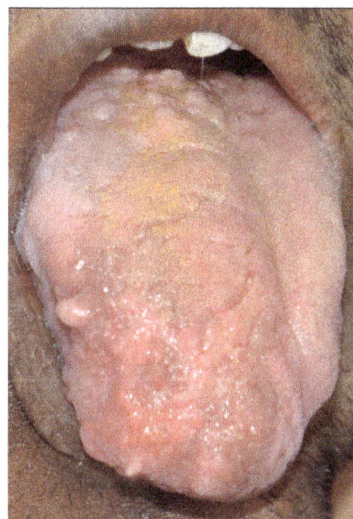

FIGURE 3: Intraoral photograph showing enlargement of right side of the tongue with enlarged papillae.

incisor, canine, first premolar, and second premolar demonstrated 337%, 150%, 116%, and 57.14% increase in volume, respectively, than their contralateral counterparts. The maxillary and mandibular midline was shifted to the left. A generalised crossbite was present due to a prognathic mandible (Figure 5). The occlusal plane on the right side was canted downwards.

The panoramic radiograph showed enlarged right body of the mandible with the widening of the right inferior alveolar canal (Figure 6). PA Skull showed enlargement of right half of mandible, maxilla, and zygoma (Figure 7). Soft tissue enlargement was seen on the right side of the face and also encircling the symphysis.

TABLE 1: Comparison of crown sizes of the maxillary teeth.

| Dimension (mm) | Maxillary arch | | | | | | | | | |
| | Canine | | 1st premolar | | 2nd premolar | | 1st molar | | 2nd molar | |
	L	R	L	R	L	R	L	R	L	R
Cervicoincisal	11	17	9	12	9	10	9	12	9	11
Mesiodistal	7	11	8	9	7	8	11	13	10	13
Labiolingual	6	8	6	8	7	9	9	12	10	11
Total surface volume (cu. mm)	462	1496	432	864	441	720	891	1872	900	1573
Enlarged by	224%		100%		63%		110%		75%	

L: left; R: right.

TABLE 2: Comparison of crown sizes of the mandibular teeth.

| Dimension (mm) | Mandibular arch | | | | | | | |
| | Lateral incisor | | Canine | | 1st premolar | | 2nd premolar | |
	L	R	L	R	L	R	L	R
Cervicoincisal	9	15	14	17	10	13	8	11
Mesiodistal	6	9	8	11	7	10	8	8
Labiolingual	4	7	6	9	6	7	7	8
Total surface volume (cu. mm)	216	945	672	1683	420	910	448	704
Enlarged by	337%		150%		116%		57.14%	

L: left; R: right.

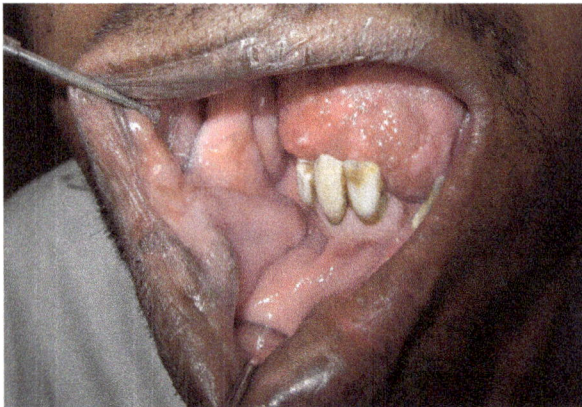

FIGURE 4: Intraoral photograph showing velvety buccal mucosa hanging in pendulous folds and granular gingival surface along with macrodontic permanent right lateral incisor and canine.

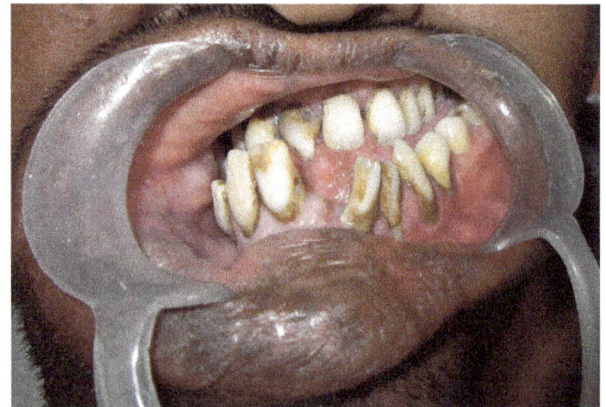

FIGURE 5: Intraoral photograph showing major variability between crown sizes of the teeth on the right and the left side with generalised crossbite relationship.

Computed tomographic (CT) scan of face revealed enlargement of the bony structures, including right half of maxilla, mandible, condyle, zygoma, bony walls of external auditory canal, and pterygoid bone (Figures 8 and 9). There was bony overgrowth of the glenoid fossa with irregularity of the articular surface. The right condyle was found to be irregular and flattened; however, the temporomandibular joint space was maintained. The right external auditory canal appeared stenosed due to bony overgrowth. The right frontal and parietal bones were thinned out with irregularity of inner table. The right foramen ovale, spinosum, rotundum, mental and infraorbital foramen, vidian canal, and greater and lesser palatine canals were widened as compared to those of the left side (Figure 10). An intracranial lipoma in the quadrigeminal cistern of the right side was also seen (Figure 11). Bony orbit on right side was deformed; however, globe, intra-, and extra-orbital structures were normal. Deformation and deviation of the nasal bone and chin were seen towards the left side due to enlargement of overlying soft tissues. Prominent vessels and few nodular serpiginous areas were seen within right parotid gland which was enlarged with heterogenous appearance (Figure 12). The right submental region, sub-mandibular region, parapharyngeal space, pterygopalatine fossa, soft palate, tongue, and floor of mouth were involved (Figure 12). All the muscles of mastication and the anterior belly of diagastric on the right side were enlarged with fatty

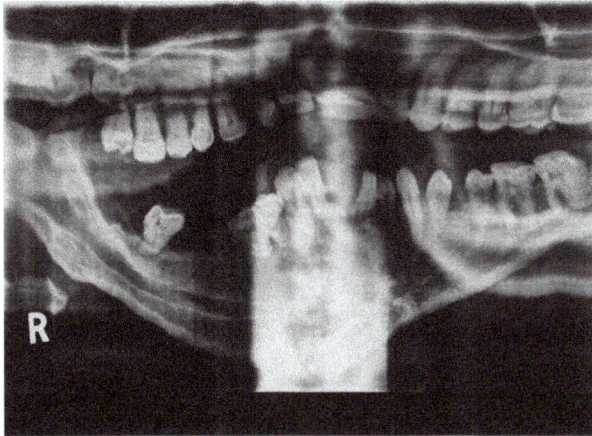

FIGURE 6: Panoramic radiograph showing widening of the right inferior alveolar canal.

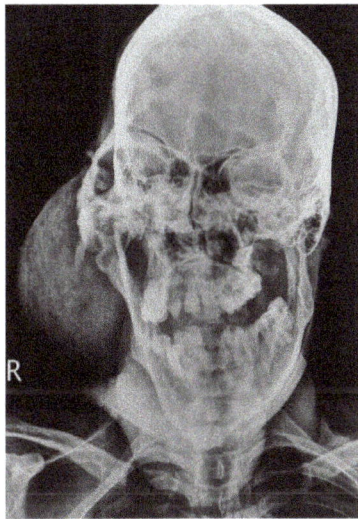

FIGURE 7: Posteroanterior view of the skull showing appreciable generalized bony and soft tissue enlargement of the right face.

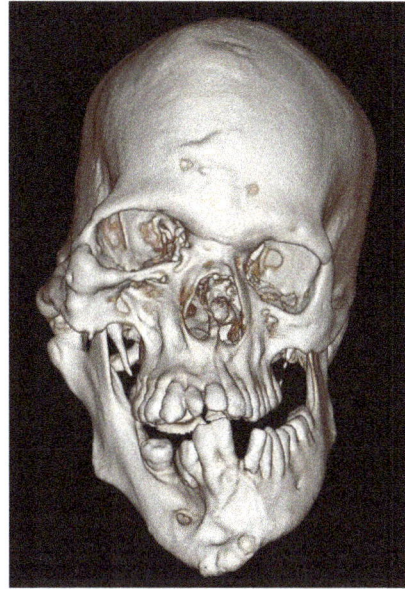

FIGURE 8: 3D volume rendered CT scan showing enlarged mandible, maxilla, and zygoma, with enlarged right mental foramen and teeth of the right side.

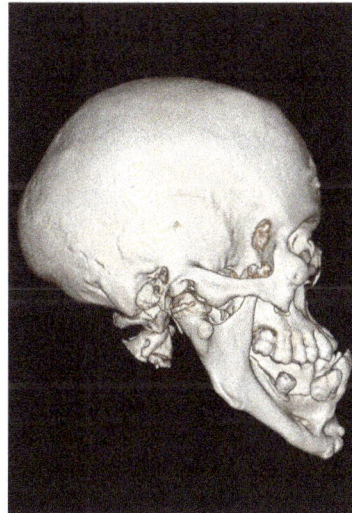

FIGURE 9: Lateral view of 3D volume rendered CT scan showing enlarged right condyle, coronoid process, mandibular body, and zygoma.

infiltration (Figure 13). Soft tissues of the right half of the face were hypertrophied, which demonstrated predominantly fat HU (Hounsfield unit) value (Figures 12 and 13). A 5.4 × 4.7 cm sized soft tissue swelling was seen in right high parietal region with fat HU value suggestive of lipoma (Figure 14).

Based on clinicoradiological findings, the diagnosis of THFH was established. Multiple reconstructive procedures were advised in view of correction of the massive facial deformity. The patient, however, refused to undertake the extensive surgeries, since the enlargement was asymptomatic.

3. Discussion

Subtle asymmetric variations of contralateral structures of the face and head are common occurrences and can be esthetically enhancing. However, marked unilateral overdevelopment of the hard and soft tissues of the head and face is

a rare congenital malformation variously described as facial hemihypertrophy, partial or unilateral gigantism, and hemifacial hyperplasia [5].

Hemifacial hyperplasia (HFH) was first reported by Friedreich in 1863 [6]. The prevalence rate of HFH is 1 : 86000 live births [7]. It affects men more commonly than women with the right side of the face more commonly affected than left side as observed in the present case [3]. Whites are more commonly affected than blacks [8]. HFH may be associated

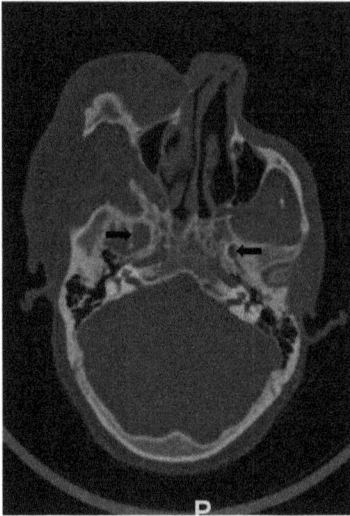

FIGURE 10: Axial CT scan with bone reconstructions showing widened foramen ovale (right side-arrow, left side-arrowhead).

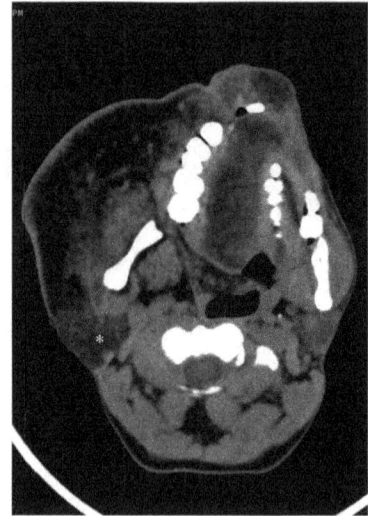

FIGURE 12: Axial CT scan showing lipomatous enlargement of the soft tissue on right side of face including buccal region, lips, tongue, soft palate, and right parotid gland (asterix).

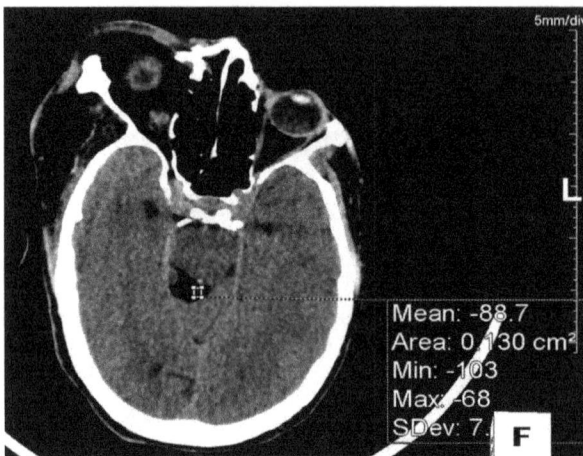

FIGURE 11: Axial CT scan showing a lipoma in the right quadrigeminal cistern.

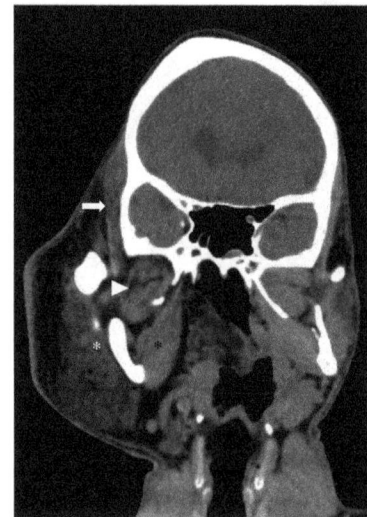

FIGURE 13: Coronal CT scan revealing hyperplasia of the right mandibular condyle, medial pterygoid (black asterisk), lateral pterygoid (arrowhead), masseter (white asterisk), and temporalis muscle (white arrow).

with other conditions, such as acromegaly and pituitary gigantism, or with hypertrophy of other parts of the body [8].

The etiology is unknown, but the condition has been ascribed to vascular & lymphatic malformations, endocrine disorders, neurocutaneous lesions, and central nervous system lesions leading to altered neurotropic action, abnormal intrauterine environment, somatic mutations, mechanical influences, and congenital syphilis [8]. Gesell suggested that the condition may result from a deviation of the normal process of twinning [9]. Noe and Berman have reviewed that fusion of two eggs following fertilization leads to unequal regulative ability in two halves, and mitochondrial damage to an overripe egg leads to overregeneration [10]. Pollock and colleagues have proposed a new embryologic hypothesis of asymmetrical development of the neural fold and hyperplasia of the neural crest cells as the basis for this disorder [4]. According to Yoshimoto et al., the basic fibroblast growth

factor (FGF) and its receptor may be selectively involved in the facial asymmetry, stimulating an osteoblast DNA synthesis of the affected side in a more pronounced manner than that of the unaffected side [11].

HFH is associated with a wide variety of abnormalities such as thickened skin and hair on the involved side, excessive secretion of sebaceous and sweat glands, and vascular and pigmentary defects of the affected side [12]. Different texture and colour variance of ipsilateral scalp hair have also been reported [4]. In addition skeletal abnormalities such as macrodactyly, polydactyly, syndactyly, ectrodactyly, scoliosis, tilting of pelvis, and clubfoot have also been described [13].

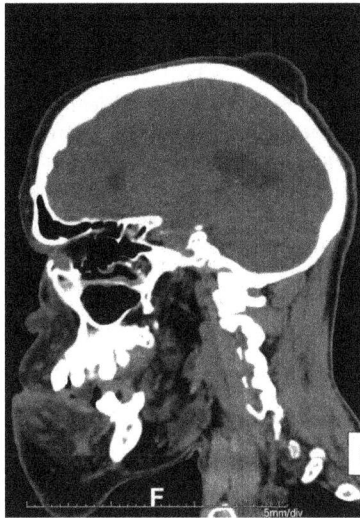

FIGURE 14: Sagital CT scan showing soft tissue swelling in right high parietal region.

Central nervous system involvement in the form of cerebral enlargement, epilepsy, strabismus, and mental retardation in 15–20% of patients has been reported in the literature [14]. Ipsilateral pinna and pupil may be enlarged, but an increase in size of the inner ear or globe of the eye has not been reported [4]. Occurrence of small exostoses of the posterior auditory canal has also been reported [12]. Adrenal cortical carcinoma, nephroblastoma (Wilm's tumour), and hepatoblastoma can be occasionally associated with this disorder [15]. Genitourinary system disorders, such as hypospadias, cryptorchidism, and medullary sponge kidney, were also noted occasionally [13].

Soft tissue like lips, uvula, and tonsils may be involved, and frequently the tongue exhibits enlarged lingual papillae with unilateral enlargement and displacement towards the normal side [4]. The buccal mucosa may also be involved exhibiting velvety surface and hangs in soft pendulous folds as reported by Miles [16]. Our patient presented with prominent enlargement of the tongue, lingual papillae, soft palate, and buccal mucosa. The mass of the ipsilateral parotid gland and that of the muscles of mastication were increased in our patient as reported by many authors [4, 13]. Widening of the palate and enlargement of the alveolar bone of the affected side were noted in the present case as described in the literature [4]. According to Rowe, the size and shape of the tooth crown and root size, as well as rate of development, are usually abnormal if the teeth are affected [3]. Random increase in tooth size frequently affecting cuspids, followed by premolars, molars, and incisors has been reported [17, 18]. Usually enlargement does not exceed 50% of normal side. The size of the teeth crown was considerably enlarged on the affected side than on the nonasffected side in our patient.

Hemifacial hyperplasia may occur as a part of crossed hemifacial hyperplasia in which facial asymmetry along with a coexistent enlargement of the opposite lower extremity is present [5]. Hemifacial lipomatosis may represent a possible subtype of partial hemifacial hyperplasia in which lipomatosis is a prominent feature [19]. Hemifacial myohyperplasia is also newly proposed and described as a separate entity in which there is predominantly hyperplasia of the facial musculature. In cases with hemifacial myohyperplasia, there is an enlargement of the muscle mass of the facial muscles with ipsilateral hypoplasia of the facial skeleton [20]. Our patient demonstrated both hyperplasia of the muscles of mastication and presence of lipomas along with involvement of bones and teeth. The enlargement of all tissues on the right side of the face and the absence of limb enlargement lead to the diagnosis of THFH.

While evaluating a patient with HFH, acquired causes of cranial asymmetry such as benign fibro-osseous lesion like fibrous dysplasia, Paget's disease, and dyschondroplasia (Ollier's disease), and malignant conditions like osteosarcoma and chondrosarcoma should be considered. Congenital hyperplasia shows overgrowth of bone and soft tissue with foraminal enlargement, while the other conditions do not show this feature [4]. There was enlargement of right foramen ovale, spinosum, rotundum, mental and infraorbital foramen, vidian, canal and greater and lesser palatine canals in our patient which distinguishes HFH from other entities. In addition, all these conditions have distinct features that differ from those of HFH radiographically and clinically. Occasionally, hemifacial atrophy (Parry-Romberg syndrome) can mimic hemifacial hyperplasia on the normal side; however, these patients present with atrophy later in life between 5–15 years of age. Sometimes HFH may resemble cystic hygroma, especially if the lymphatic anomaly is located inferior to the jaws and in the neck region. But HFH is a solid noncystic disease, whereas cystic hygroma is fluid filled and yields an aspirate which is high in fat content.

Other malformation syndromes and abnormalities such as neurofibromatosis, Proteus syndrome, Beckwith-Wiedemann syndrome, Schimmelpenning (epidermal nevus) syndrome, hyperpituitarism, Maffucci syndrome, Ollier's syndrome, Langer-Giedion syndrome, Klippel-Trenaunay-Weber syndrome, McCune-Albright syndrome, Russell Silver syndrome, triploid/diploid mixoploidy, multiple exostosis syndrome, and segmental odontomaxillary dysplasia may superficially resemble HFH. However, the unilateral distribution of dental anomalies and the concurrent unilateral tongue enlargement are the prominent features which make HFH an unique entity [3].

Our patient had the classical clinical features of THFH such as unilateral overgrowth of the orofacial soft tissues, tongue, teeth, and bones causing an obvious asymmetry of the right side of the face. CT scan of the present case demonstrated prominent facial asymmetry which was caused by the unilateral enlargement of both soft tissue structures and the underlying skeleton of the right side of the face, along with dental involvement, making this case unique in its presentation.

An extensive search of the English literature revealed no formal reports of malignant degeneration in HFH [8]. Hemifacial hyperplasia is generally associated with good prognosis. Treatment is not indicated for HFH unless cosmetic considerations are involved.

Conflict of Interests

The authors declare that they have no conflict of interests.

References

[1] J. F. Meckel, "Ueber die seitliche Asymmetric im tierischen Korper," in *Anatomische Physiologische Beobachtungen und Untersuchungen*, R. Halle, Ed., p. 147, 1822.

[2] H. L. Kottmeier and H. L. Wagner, "Über Hemihypertrophia und Hemiatrophia corporis totalis nebst spontane Extremitätengangräne bei Säuglingen im Anschluss zu einem ungewöhnlichen," *Fall Acta Paediatrica*, vol. 20, no. 4, pp. 530–543, 1938.

[3] N. H. Rowe, "Hemifacial hypertrophy—review of the literature and addition of four cases," *Oral Surgery, Oral Medicine, Oral Pathology*, vol. 15, no. 5, pp. 572–587, 1962.

[4] R. A. Pollock, M. Haskell Newman, A. R. Burdi, and D. P. Condit, "Congenital hemifacial hyperplasia: an embryologic hypothesis and case report," *Cleft Palate Journal*, vol. 22, no. 3, pp. 173–184, 1985.

[5] R. Nayak and M. S. Baliga, "Crossed hemifacial hyperplasia: a diagnostic dilemma," *Journal of Indian Society of Pedodontics & Preventive Dentistry*, vol. 25, no. 1, pp. 39–42, 2007.

[6] N. Friedrich, "Ueber congenitale halbseitige Kopfhypertrophie," *Archiv für Pathologische Anatomie und Physiologie und für Klinische Medicin*, vol. 28, no. 5-6, pp. 474–481, 1863.

[7] R. E. Marx and D. Stern, *Oral and Maxillofacial Pathology: A Rationale for Diagnosis and Treatment*, Quintessence, Chicago, Ill, usa, 1st edition, 2003.

[8] M. N. Islam, I. Bhattacharyya, J. Ojha, K. Bober, D. M. Cohen, and J. G. Green, "Comparison between true and partial hemifacial hypertrophy," *Oral Surgery, Oral Medicine, Oral Pathology, Oral Radiology and Endodontology*, vol. 104, no. 4, pp. 501–509, 2007.

[9] A. Gesell, "Hemihypertrophy and twinning," *The American Journal of the Medical Sciences*, vol. 173, no. 4, pp. 542–555, 1927.

[10] O. Noe and H. H. Berman, "The etiology of congenital hemihypertrophy and one case report," *Archives of Pediatrics*, vol. 79, pp. 278–288, 1962.

[11] H. Yoshimoto, H. Yano, K. Kobayashi et al., "Increased proliferative activity of osteoblasts in congenital hemifacial hypertrophy," *Plastic and Reconstructive Surgery*, vol. 102, no. 5, pp. 1605–1610, 1998.

[12] R. A. Azevedo, V. F. Souza, V. A. Sarmento, and J. N. Santos, "Hemifacial hyperplasia: a case report," *Quintessence International*, vol. 36, no. 6, pp. 483–486, 2005.

[13] J. N. Khanna and N. N. Andrade, "Hemifacial hypertrophy. Report of two cases," *International Journal of Oral & Maxillofacial Surgery*, vol. 18, no. 5, pp. 294–297, 1989.

[14] R. T. Miranda, L. M. Barros, L. A. N. D. Santos, P. R. F. Bonan, and H. Martelli Jr., "Clinical and imaging features in a patient with hemifacial hyperplasia," *Journal of oral science*, vol. 52, no. 3, pp. 509–512, 2010.

[15] C. E. Rudolph and R. W. Norvold, "Congenital partial hemihypertrophy involving marked malocclusion," *Journal of Dental Research*, vol. 23, no. 2, pp. 133–139, 1944.

[16] A. E. W. Miles, "A case of unilateral gigantism of the face and teeth," *British Dental Journal*, vol. 77, no. 7, pp. 197–199, 1944.

[17] P. H. Burke, "True hemihypertrophy of the face," *British Dental Journal*, vol. 91, no. 8, pp. 213–215, 1951.

[18] F. J. Hanley, C. E. Floyd, and D. Parker, "Congenital partial hemihypertrophy of the face. Report of three cases," *Journal of Oral Surgery*, vol. 26, no. 2, pp. 136–141, 1968.

[19] P. Bou-Haidar, P. Taub, and P. Som, "Hemifacial lipomatosis, a possible subtype of partial hemifacial hyperplasia: CT and MR imaging findings," *American Journal of Neuroradiology*, vol. 31, no. 5, pp. 891–893, 2010.

[20] D. F. Pereira-Perdomo, J. Vélez-Forero, and R. Prada-Madrid, "Hemifacial myohyperplasia sequence," *American Journal of Medical Genetics A*, vol. 152, no. 7, pp. 1770–1773, 2010.

14

Management of Crown Root Fracture by Interdisciplinary Approach

K. Radhakrishnan Nair,[1] **Anoop N. Das,**[1]
Manoj C. Kuriakose,[1] **and Nandakumar Krishnankutty**[2]

[1] *Department of Conservative Dentistry and Endodontics, Azeezia College of Dental Sciences and Research, Kollam 691537, India*
[2] *Department of Periodontics, Azeezia College of Dental Sciences and Research, Kollam 691537, India*

Correspondence should be addressed to K. Radhakrishnan Nair; radhnair@yahoo.com

Academic Editors: G. K. Kulkarni, P. Lopez Jornet, L. J. Oesterle, and E. F. Wright

Fracture of tooth after trauma is distressing to a person because of the discomfort and pain due to pulpal injury. Crown root fractures of anterior teeth cause concomitant periodontal injury and there will be concern about appearance, and aesthetics. Management of pulpal and periodontal tissue relieves pain and restoration of tooth form regains patients confidence. Restoration of fractured tooth will be accepted readily if it is minimally invasive, less expensive, and aesthetically acceptable. Reattachment is an option for restoration of anterior teeth compared to other artificial replacements because of its appearance as natural. This method is favourable when the fractured fragment is intact and available. Utilization of pulp space for retention of fragment is achieved by the insertion of a dentine bonding post. This case report describes a case of tooth reattachment after trauma in which the pulp space is utilized to bond a fiber-reinforced post for retention after periodontal tissue management.

1. Introduction

Tooth fracture can occur at any age due to trauma. Sports accidents and fights are more common among teenagers and automobile accidents are seen in all age groups. Impact of trauma on tooth varies from mild enamel chipping to complex crown root fractures. Aesthetic and functional implications of tooth fracture depend upon its severity and age of the patient. About 5% of all dental traumas are found to be associated with crown root fractures [1]. Severe pain arising from crown root fractures can be either due to pulpal exposure or due to concomitant periodontal injury or both.

Clinical considerations for the management of crown root fractures include extent and pattern of fracture, restorability of remaining tooth, availability of fractured fragment, and damage to the attachment apparatus [2, 3]. Extension of fracture subgingivally raises concern about biological width violation. Periodontal flap surgery combined with osteoplasty procedures is indicated for deep subgingival fractures to satisfy the requirement of biological width [4].

A conservative method for management of the crown root fracture when the intact fragment is available is the reattachment technique. It is a method which has been tried long before [5]. This method is gaining wide acceptance because of its several advantages over artificial replacements like composite resin or full coverage restorations. It can offer long lasting aesthetics and is reasonably a simple procedure [6, 7].

It is cost effective and can be completed in less chair side time. When endodontic therapy is indicated, the pulp space available after obturation can be used for retention of the fragment by using posts bonded to root canal. This case report describes an interdisciplinary approach to the management of two complicated crown root fractures of maxillary central incisors after an automobile accident.

2. Case Report

A forty-year-old male patient was referred to the Department of Conservative Dentistry and Endodontics with the complaint of broken front teeth. He had a history of road traffic accident with sustained hand and facial injuries and had fracture of two maxillary central incisors. He went to a nearby hospital immediately because of pain for medical aid and took some medications. He had no relevant medical history and reported to the department next day due to elevation of pain in the area.

Extra oral examination revealed lacerations with swelling of upper lips. Intraorally lacerations were present on buccal mucosa. Gingiva appeared to be erythematous in the upper front region and there was bleeding on probing. Both the upper central incisors were fractured with pulpal exposure. The horizontal fracture line was on the middle of the labial surface extending obliquely to the subgingival area on the palatal side (Figure 1). The incisal fragments were mobile and during talking, pain increased due to mobility. An IOPA radiograph showed the crown of 11 and 21 with fracture line extending subgingivally and the root and periapical area was found to be normal. This was diagnosed as a case of complicated crown root fracture with irreversible pulpitis.

The incisal fragments were removed after local anesthesia as a single piece and kept in normal saline immediately. The various options to restore the teeth were explained to the patient. After listening, the patient expressed the willingness to reattach the broken part. Single visit endodontics was done and root canal was obturated with gutta-percha using AH Plus as the sealer. Gingivectomy was done for 11 and 21 to bring the fracture line supragingival (Figure 2). The patient reported to the clinic after one day for the reattachment procedure. Root canal preparation for the post was done sequentially using the Tenax Fiber Trans drill (Coltene Whaledent). Corresponding fiber reinforced composite post was selected (Tenax Fiber Trans-Coltene Whaledent) to check the fit and occlusal clearance. The occlusal end of the post was shortened with a diamond disc to the desired length. The prepared root canal was conditioned using self-etching non rinse conditioner (ParaBond-Coltene Whaledent). Fixing of the post in the root canal was done using dual cure luting material (ParaCore-Coltene Whaledent). To facilitate polymerization, curing LED light (Woodpecker) was applied through the tip of the post into the root canal for 20 seconds. About 2 mm of the post was visible beyond the incisal margin after fixing (Figure 3).

A small recess was prepared in the pulp chamber of fractured segment of 11 and 21 and was tried against the remaining crown portion with the post for approximation. The opposite surface of the fractured crown was then etched with 37% phosphoric acid and the fragment was luted in the correct position using dual cure resin (ParaCore-Coltene Whaledent) with slight pressure. Excess of the material was removed using a sharp instrument from the edges and was light cured for 20 seconds for faster polymerization. A bevel was prepared on the margins of the approximating surfaces of 11 and 21 on the labial side and the margins were sealed with nanocomposite (Brilliant NG-Coltene Whaledent). Polishing of the surface was done with polishing disks which ensured an aesthetic blending of the margins (Figure 4).

Patient was recalled after six months and one year. On examination, 11 and 21 were found to be asymptomatic

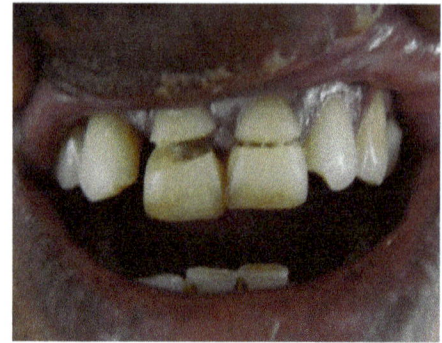

FIGURE 1: Preoperative view.

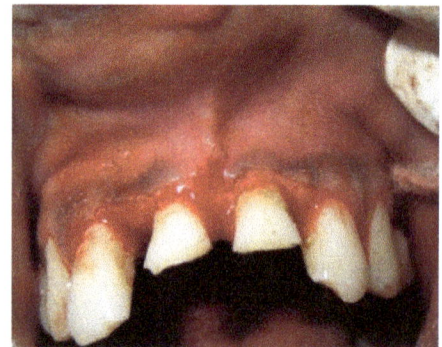

FIGURE 2: Gingivectomy of 11 and 21.

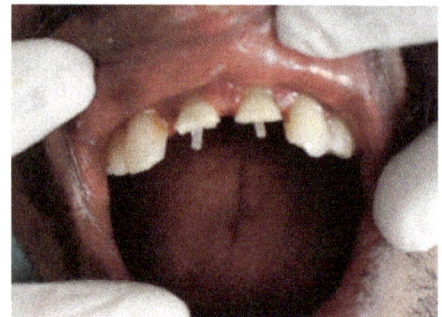

FIGURE 3: After fiber post fixation.

with satisfactory aesthetics. Periodontal status was good with 1 mm pocket. Gingival tissues had a normal texture with a normal contouring (Figure 5). Intraoral periapical radiograph showed intact tooth structure with intact lamina dura (Figure 6).

3. Discussion

Fracture of anterior teeth after trauma adversely affects the emotional well-being of a person in addition to the discomfort and pain. Complexity and extension of fracture along with the associated injury to the tooth influence the restorative design. Reattachment of the tooth is an option when the broken fragment is intact and available. It has several

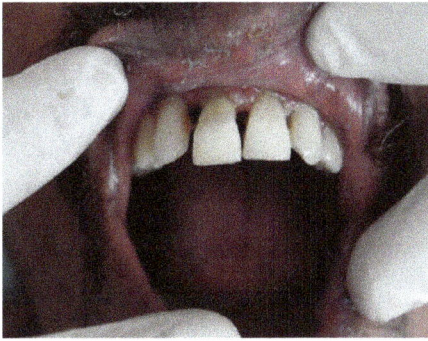

FIGURE 4: Immediate postoperative view.

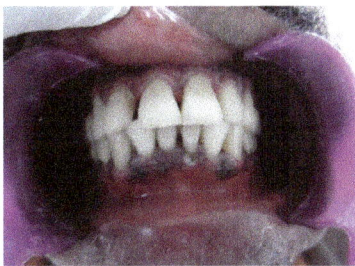

FIGURE 5: Postoperative view after one year.

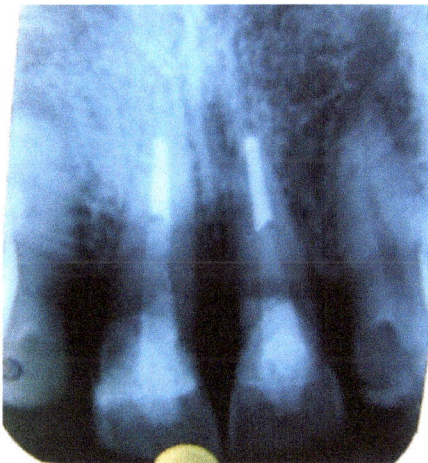

FIGURE 6: Postoperative radiograph after one year.

advantages over conventional methods of restoration. It retains the translucency of natural tooth and its abrasive resistance is better than composites.

It is less time consuming and is cost effective. Several studies have shown that the impact strength of reattached tooth is not significantly different from that of intact natural tooth [8, 9].

Reattachment procedure is often multidisciplinary dictated by the extension of tooth fracture and injury to the attachment apparatus. This case was a subgingival fracture and gingivectomy was done to bring the fracture line supragingival. Pulp space after root canal treatment was utilized to attach a post for auxiliary retention. Metallic and nonmetallic posts are available with different properties. Fiber posts which have the modulus of elasticity similar to that of root dentin are used here to bond with the root and are preferred to metal posts because of less stress concentration on the root and there is low incidence of root fracture [10]. There is less tooth preparation with a fiber post compared to cast post; thus, the tooth is conserved more. Failures of post and core occur by debonding of the core and due to root fracture [11].

Available clinical evaluation for longevity of reattachment shows medium-term prospects for this technique [12, 13]. A seven-year follow-up of crown reattachment showed mild discoloration of crown without any evidence of fracture [14]. Long-term followup is required to assess the longitivity of reattachment technique. Improvement in adhesive technology may provide a long-lasting bonding of the fragments to improve the prospects of this technique in future.

References

[1] J. D. Andreason, F. M. Andreason, and L. Andersson, *Textbook and Colour Atlas of Traumatic Injuries to Teeth*, Blackwell, Oxford, UK, 4th edition, 2007.

[2] S. Olsburgh, T. Jacoby, and I. Krejci, "Crown fractures in the permanent dentition: pulpal and restorative considerations," *Dental Traumatology*, vol. 18, no. 3, pp. 103–115, 2002.

[3] A. Reis, C. Francci, A. D. Loguercio, M. R. Carrilho, and L. E. R. Filho, "Re-attachment of anterior fractured teeth: fracture strength using different techniques," *Operative Dentistry*, vol. 26, no. 3, pp. 287–294, 2001.

[4] L. N. Baratieri, S. Monteiro, C. A. Cardoso, and M. A. C. Andrada, "Coronal fracture with invasion of the biologic width: a case report," *Quintessence International*, vol. 24, no. 2, pp. 85–91, 1993.

[5] A. Chosack and E. Eidelman, "Rehabilitating of a fractured incisor using the patient's natural crown: a case report," *Journal of Dentistry for Children*, vol. 71, pp. 19–21, 1994.

[6] A. Reis, A. D. Loguercio, A. Kraul, and E. Matson, "Reattachment of fractured teeth: a review of literature regarding techniques and materials," *Operative Dentistry*, vol. 29, no. 2, pp. 226–233, 2004.

[7] E. A. V. Maia, L. N. Baratieri, M. A. C. de Andrada, S. Monteiro Jr., and E. M. de Araújo Jr., "Tooth fragment reattachment: fundamentals of the technique and two case reports," *Quintessence International*, vol. 34, no. 2, pp. 99–107, 2003.

[8] B. Farik, E. C. Munksgaard, and J. O. Andreasen, "Impact strength of teeth restored by fragment-bonding," *Dental Traumatology*, vol. 16, no. 4, pp. 151–153, 2000.

[9] B. Farik and E. C. Munksgaard, "Fracture strength of intact and fragment-bonded teeth at various velocities of the applied force," *European Journal of Oral Sciences*, vol. 107, no. 1, pp. 70–73, 1999.

[10] B. Akkayan and T. Gülmez, "Resistance to fracture of endodontically treated teeth restored with different post systems," *Journal of Prosthetic Dentistry*, vol. 87, no. 4, pp. 431–437, 2002.

[11] E. Asmussen, A. Peutzfeldt, and T. Heitmann, "Stiffness, elastic limit, and strength of newer types of endodontic posts," *Journal of Dentistry*, vol. 27, no. 4, pp. 275–278, 1999.

[12] I. A. Öz, M. C. Haytaç, and M. S. Toroğlu, "Multidisciplinary approach to the rehabilitation of a crown-root fracture with

original fragment for immediate esthetics: a case report with 4-year follow-up," *Dental Traumatology*, vol. 22, no. 1, pp. 48–52, 2006.

[13] C. L. Capp, M. I. Rodo, R. Tawaki, G. M. Castanho, M. A. Carmago, and A. A. deClara, "Reattachment of rehydrated dental fragment using two techniques," *Dental Traumatology*, vol. 25, pp. 95–99, 2009.

[14] J. C. M. de Castro, W. R. Poi, D. Pedrini, A. R. F. Tiveron, D. A. Brandini, and M. A. M. de Castro, "Multidisciplinary approach for the treatment of a complicated crown-root fracture in a young patient: a case report," *Quintessence International*, vol. 42, no. 9, pp. 729–734, 2011.

15

Apicotomy as Treatment for Failure of Orthodontic Traction

Leandro Berni Osório,[1,2] **Vilmar Antonio Ferrazzo,**[3]
Geraldo Serpa,[4] **and Kívia Linhares Ferrazzo**[5]

[1] *Stomatology Department, Pediatric Dentistry, School of Dentistry, Federal University of Santa Maria,*
97015-370 Santa Maria, RS, Brazil

[2] *Department of Orthodontics, Pontifícia Universidade Católica do Rio Grande do Sul, 90619-900 Porto Alegre, RS, Brazil*

[3] *Stomatology Department, Orthodontics, School of Dentistry, Federal University of Santa Maria, 97015-370 Santa Maria, RS, Brazil*

[4] *Stomatology Department, Radiology, School of Dentistry, Federal University of Santa Maria, 97015-370 Santa Maria, RS, Brazil*

[5] *Oral Medicine and Oral Pathology, School of Dentistry, Franciscan University Center, 97015-370 Santa Maria, RS, Brazil*

Correspondence should be addressed to Leandro Berni Osório; leandro.osorio@ufsm.br

Academic Editors: J. H. Campbell, C. Evans, A. Y. Gamal, and A. Milosevic

Objective. The purpose of this study was to present a case report that demonstrated primary failure in a tooth traction that was subsequently treated with apicotomy technique. *Case Report.* A 10-year-old girl had an impacted upper right canine with increased pericoronal space, which was apparent on a radiographic image. The right maxillary sinus showed an opacity suggesting sinusitis. The presumptive diagnosis was dentigerous cyst associated with maxillary sinus infection. The plan for treatment included treatment of the sinus infection and cystic lesion and orthodontic traction of the canine after surgical exposure and bonding of an orthodontic appliance. The surgical procedure, canine position, root dilaceration, and probably apical ankylosis acted in the primary failure of the orthodontic traction. Surgical apical cut of the displaced teeth was performed, and tooth position in the dental arch was possible, with a positive response to the pulp vitality test. *Conclusion.* Apicotomy is an effective technique to treat severe canine displacement and primary orthodontic traction failure of palatally displaced canines.

1. Introduction

Impacted teeth are common abnormalities of development and the prevalence ranges from 5% to 18% [1–3]. The maxillary permanent canine is the second most prevalent impacted tooth in the human dentition (8%–10%), after third molars [4, 5]. Girls are more often affected than boys [6], and palatally positioned canines are more frequent than buccally positioned ones, at a ratio of 3 : 1, respectively [7].

The displacement of an upper canine is determined by distinct etiopathogenesis. Lack of space in the dental arch, trauma, and loss of primary teeth as well as a genetic component are pointed out as etiological factors [8, 9]. The facial impaction of a maxillary permanent canine is usually more frequent in crowded dental arches, while palatal impaction usually shows no association with any particular malocclusion [7]. This fact contributes to the late recognition of the wrong position of these teeth and can be a determining

factor in the failure of orthodontic movement of palatal-impacted canines. Sometimes, bring these teeth into the correct position represents a challenge [10].

Surgical access to a displaced tooth is the key factor in treatment success, and the intervention should be carefully planned. There are three main types of surgery that are possible for managing impacted teeth: extraction, exposure for spontaneous eruption, and exposure for orthodontic traction with bonding devices [6, 11, 12]. For orthodontic traction, the surgical techniques can still be divided in apically positioned flap, for buccally positioned canines, closed eruption technique, for canines in the middle of the alveolar bone, and tunnelization for palatal-impacted teeth [5, 13].

Becker et al. [14] classified the reasons for the failure of orthodontic traction at dependent factors of the patient, of the orthodontist, and of the surgeon. Patient-dependent factors are age, anatomical local factors, such as root anomalies, angle of tooth eruption, and associated complications, such

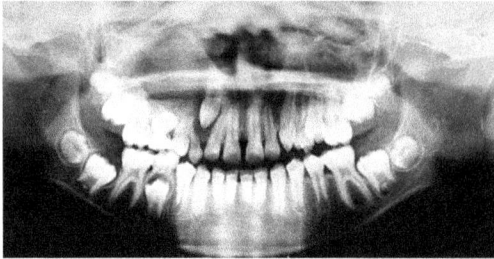

FIGURE 1: Initial panoramic radiography: retention of the upper right second premolar and upper right canine with increased pericoronal space, vertical impaction, and root dilaceration; root resorption of primary teeth; opacity of the right maxillary sinus.

as lack of compliance. Orthodontist-dependent factors can be identified as misdiagnosis of tooth position, improper directional force, and the use of inefficient appliances. Surgeon-dependent factors include the misdiagnosis of tooth position, exposing the wrong side, damage on the impacted tooth, injury to an adjacent tooth, and surgery without orthodontic planning.

In those cases in which the tooth has local factors contributing to lack of orthodontic movement, a new surgical intervention can be necessary. Ankylosis is often the main local cause for failure of the movement of the impacted tooth [14]. Mobilization of the ankylosed tooth with forceps is a technique used to help orthodontic movement, but, in some cases, the root anatomy is unfavorable, avoiding the tooth movement.

The apicotomy is a technique described in 1987 that aims to liberate the part of the tooth with root dilacerations or ankylosis, thus allowing the traction and eruption. The technique consists of surgical fracture of the apical portion of the root and may be indicated after failure of conservative techniques to promote the correct position of the canine [15, 16].

The purpose of this study was to present a case report that showed primary failure in the tooth traction and was treated using the apicotomy technique.

2. Case Report

This case report was submitted and approved by the Research Ethical Committee of the Franciscan University Center, under number CEP/UNIFRA 346.2010.2. A 10-year-old girl was referred to the Integrated Clinic of the Franciscan University Center, Santa Maria, Brazil, with the complaint of recurrent rhinorrhea that has not responded after two months of antibiotic therapy. Extra oral physical examination revealed a slight facial asymmetry with swelling over the right maxillary sinus and nasal obstruction. The intraoral examination showed the presence of a deciduous canine and a maxillary right first molar.

The absence of primary teeth roots was identified in image exams (panoramic radiograph and computed tomography). Moreover, impactions of the upper right second premolar and of the upper right canine, associated with

increased pericoronal space, were observed. The right maxillary sinus showed opacity (Figures 1 and 2(a)). The presumptive diagnosis was dentigerous cyst associated with maxillary sinus infection. Planning for this case has included the treatment of the sinus infection and of the cystic lesion, orthodontic traction of the canine after surgical exposure, and bonding of an orthodontic appliance to allow the traction of the canine.

The surgeon performed a Caldwell-Luc incision [17] under general anesthesia to access the right maxillary sinus. The cavity was washed with saline solution, and a fragment of the cystic capsule was obtained for histopathological examination. The cystic lesion caused a large amount of bone loss, and so, a conservative treatment was performed by surgical decompression, and a Penrose drain was inserted in the canine region. The primary teeth (canine and first molar) were extracted. The histopathological analysis revealed a stratified squamous epithelium of a few layers, confirming the dentigerous cyst hypothesis.

Amoxicillin with clavulanate potassium was used for 2 weeks. The drain was monitored for 3 months until there was no more secretion. At the time, no signs of sinus infection in imaging exams were observed (Figure 2(b)). After removing the drain, an attachment was bonded in the canine for orthodontic traction. Extractions of four first premolars were planned, but initially only the right maxillary premolar has been removed.

Two years of orthodontic treatment were not able to change the impacted canine position. This behavior was determined because of the apical dilaceration in the canine's root (Figure 3). For this reason, a new surgical intervention was necessary, and the apicotomy of the dilacerated canine root was carried out [15, 16]. The technique consists of promoting an apical fracture of the impacted root's tooth. In this way, the periodontal area was reduced and mechanical retention was avoided by separating the dilacerated portion of the root and the tooth. The orthodontist could move the canine to a better position after the surgery and the upper canine retained was repositioned after five months of orthodontic movement (Figure 4). The pulp sensitivity test with cold responded positively and the tooth remained vital even in five years of followup. The canine root length was reduced as a consequence of the apicotomy.

3. Discussion

The canines occupy a strategic position in the upper arch developing an important role in the masticatory function. The lateral excursion with the canine-protected occlusion has been advocated as the best relationship for the mandibular excursion guide. This is due to the concave shape of the palatine surface of the canine, which is a good guide for the lateral movements, and due to the size of the canine root surface, which is able to resist the masticatory forces and provide a greater number of periodontal mechanoreceptors [18, 19]. Furthermore, it is easier to establish the deocclusion with orthodontic movement in a single tooth than with movement of a group of teeth. For these reasons, the canine

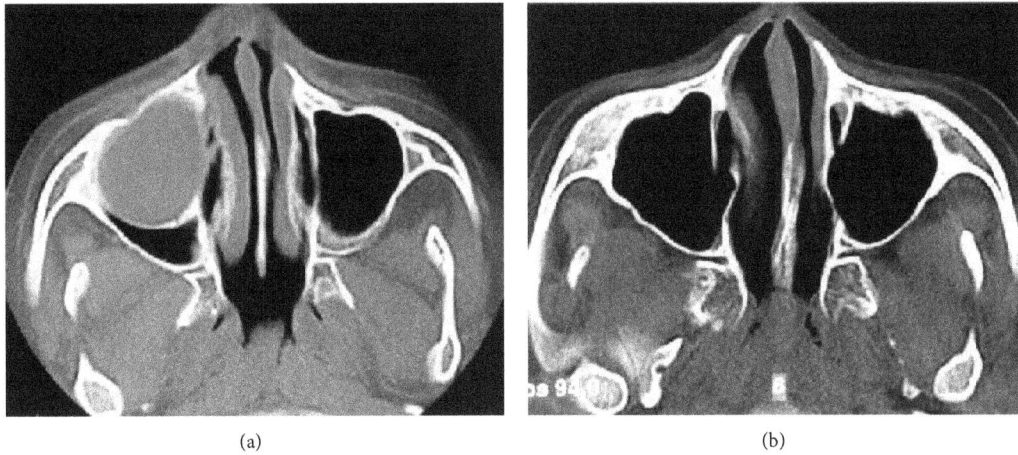

FIGURE 2: CT axial images showing opacity of the right maxillary sinus in the diagnostic phase (a); maxillary sinus cleared after 3 months of treatment (b).

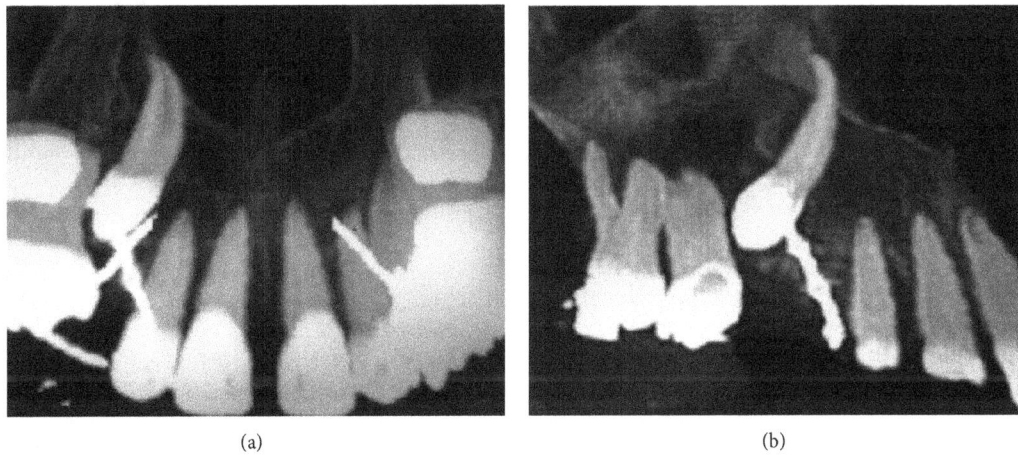

FIGURE 3: Right maxillary canine with large dilaceration root and orthodontic appliance for orthodontic traction.

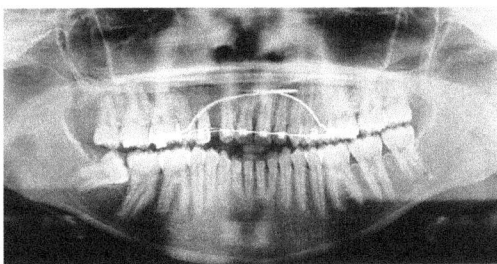

FIGURE 4: Final panoramic radiography: upper right canine positioned in the dental arch showing reduced root length.

is considered the most important tooth to be positioned in orthodontic treatment, which aims to promote a proper contour of the face and a final aesthetic smile [6].

Becker et al. recommend extraction of palatal canines severely impacted in height, when they are vertically positioned above the apices of the incisors [20]. The canine displacement in the present report was very severe, and the infection associated with the dentigerous cyst, as well as the apical dilaceration, was complicating factor. Despite that, the maintenance of the tooth was performed because the reduced bone volume in the affected canine could compromise the facial aesthetic at the end of the treatment. The eruption process promotes alveolar bone growth and, in this case, it helped the healing of the anterior maxilla.

The appropriate direction of eruption for a palatally impacted canine is essential for correcting the impaction and bringing the tooth to its correct position. It is important to remember that the presence of the periodontal ligament is necessary to allow tooth movement. This way, the main movement direction of the displaced tooth must be following its long axis, regardless of whether it will occur far from the correct position. The simple lateral traction of the tooth toward the edentulous alveolar ridge finds immediate resistance due to the compression of the canine crown against the adjacent palatine bone [10]. The consequence can be bone necrosis by compression and very slow movement, which can lead to a resorption process in the crown, and, thus, canine enamel damage can occur [21, 22]. These facts should be observed in order to minimize the orthodontic movement failure, as proposed by Becker et al. [14]. They concluded that the inaccuracy in diagnosis of location and orientation of impacted teeth and the failure to recognize anchorage demands were the major reasons for failure in the treatment of palatally displaced canines. However, in the same research, ankylosis was pointed out as a significant etiological factor that interfered in the success rate, corresponding to 32.4% of impacted canine failures. The ankylosis of the displaced teeth can be a consequence of the action of the low-speed drill during the surgery, chemical injury, and cervical periodontal ligament trauma by the magnitude and direction of orthodontic force [21]. Extensive surgery can be an additional factor compromising the cervical root area and promoting root resorption. The gaps formed by resorption are difficult to identify radiographically, and if the region is not repaired by cementoblasts, the bone can be deposited at the site, causing a lack of response to extrusive traction [20, 23].

Undoubtedly, the apicotomy allows traction of teeth with anatomical complications, but it is not always a simple procedure. The major difficulty in performing the apicotomy was sectioning the apical portion of the root without compromising the pulp tissue or with minimal injury to this tissue, as advocated by the technique [15, 16]. In the present case, the tooth was in a vertical position, located in the center of the alveolar crest, with the crown inclined for palatine. Moreover, the tooth was in a high position and the root was located more deeply, making it difficult to access the apical portion of the root. Despite the difficulty, it was possible to perform surgery successfully, which can be demonstrated by the position of the tooth in the dental arch and the positive response to the pulp vitality test. Importantly, the length of the canine root can be shortened, especially when the root dilaceration is extensive. This must be taken into account by the orthodontist, since the canine supports the load of the occlusion movement, as previously discussed.

4. Conclusion

Apicotomy is an effective technique for treating severe canine displacement and primary orthodontic traction failure of palatally displaced canines.

References

[1] A. Fardi, A. Kondylidou-Sidira, Z. Bachour, N. Parisis, and A. Tsirlis, "Incidence of impacted and supernumerary teeth— a radiographic study in a North Greek population," *Medicina Oral, Patologia Oral y Cirugia Bucal*, vol. 16, no. 1, Article ID 16791, pp. e56–e61, 2011.

[2] R. Hou, L. Kong, J. Ao et al., "Investigation of impacted permanent teeth except the third molar in chinese patients through an X-ray study," *Journal of Oral and Maxillofacial Surgery*, vol. 68, no. 4, pp. 762–767, 2010.

[3] M. D. Campoy, A. Gonzalez-Allo, J. Moreira, J. Ustrell, and T. Pinho, "Dental anomalies in a Portuguese population," *International Orthodontics*, vol. 11, no. 2, pp. 210–220, 2013.

[4] P. S. Grover and L. Lorton, "The incidence of unerupted permanent teeth and related clinical cases," *Oral Surgery, Oral Medicine, Oral Pathology*, vol. 59, no. 4, pp. 420–425, 1985.

[5] A. R. Chapokas, K. Almas, and G.-P. Schincaglia, "The impacted maxillary canine: a proposed classification for surgical exposure," *Oral Surgery, Oral Medicine, Oral Pathology, Oral Radiology and Endodontology*, vol. 113, no. 2, pp. 222–228, 2011.

[6] W. D. Johnston, "Treatment o f palatally impacted canine teeth," *American Journal of Orthodontics*, vol. 56, no. 6, pp. 589–596, 1969.

[7] E. Mercuri, M. Cassetta, C. Cavallini, D. Vicari, R. Leonardi, and E. Barbato, "Dental anomalies and clinical features in patients with maxillary canine impaction," *The Angle Orthodontist*, vol. 83, no. 1, pp. 22–28, 2013.

[8] A. Becker, "Etiology of maxillary canine impactions," *American Journal of Orthodontics*, vol. 86, no. 5, pp. 437–438, 1984.

[9] D. D. Chung, M. Weisberg, and M. Pagala, "Incidence and effects of genetic factors on canine impaction in an isolated Jewish population," *American Journal of Orthodontics and Dentofacial Orthopedics*, vol. 139, no. 4, pp. e331–e335, 2011.

[10] V. G. Kokich, "Preorthodontic uncovering and autonomous eruption of palatally impacted maxillary canines," *Seminars in Orthodontics*, vol. 16, no. 3, pp. 205–211, 2010.

[11] G. F. Andreasen, "A review of the approaches to treatment of impacted maxillary cuspids," *Oral Surgery, Oral Medicine, Oral Pathology*, vol. 31, no. 4, pp. 479–484, 1971.

[12] D. Clark, "The management of impacted canines: free physiologic eruption," *The Journal of the American Dental Association*, vol. 82, no. 4, pp. 836–840, 1971.

[13] V. G. Kokich and D. P. Mathews, "Surgical and orthodontic management of impacted teeth," *Dental Clinics of North America*, vol. 37, no. 2, pp. 181–204, 1993.

[14] A. Becker, G. Chaushu, and S. Chaushu, "Analysis of failure in the treatment of impacted maxillary canines," *American Journal of Orthodontics and Dentofacial Orthopedics*, vol. 137, no. 6, pp. 743–754, 2010.

[15] E. Puricelli, "Apicotomy: a root apical fracture for surgical treatment of impacted upper canines," *Head and Face Medicine*, vol. 3, no. 33, 2007.

[16] E. Puricelli, "Treatment of retained canines by apicotomy," *RGO*, vol. 35, no. 4, pp. 326–330, 1987.

[17] E. Kim and J. Duncavage, "Caldwell-Luc procedure," *Operative Techniques in Otolaryngology—Head and Neck Surgery*, vol. 21, no. 3, pp. 163–165, 2010.

[18] M. Q. Wang and N. Mehta, "A possible biomechanical role of occlusal cusp-fossa contact relationships," *Journal of Oral Rehabilitation*, vol. 40, no. 1, pp. 69–79, 2013.

[19] J. R. Clark and R. D. Evans, "Functional occlusion: I. A review," *Journal of Orthodontics*, vol. 28, no. 1, pp. 76–81, 2001.

[20] A. Becker and S. Chaushu, "Palatally impacted canines: the case for closed surgical exposure and immediate orthodontic traction," *American Journal of Orthodontics and Dentofacial Orthopedics*, vol. 143, no. 4, pp. 451–459, 2013.

[21] S. I. Koutzoglou and A. Kostaki, "Effect of surgical exposure technique, age, and grade of impaction on ankylosis of an impacted canine, and the effect of rapid palatal expansion on eruption: a prospective clinical study," *American Journal of Orthodontics and Dentofacial Orthopedics*, vol. 143, no. 3, pp. 342–352, 2013.

[22] D. P. Mathews and V. G. Kokich, "Palatally impacted canines: the case for preorthodontic uncovering and autonomous eruption," *American Journal of Orthodontics and Dentofacial Orthopedics*, vol. 143, no. 4, pp. 450–458, 2013.

[23] A. Becker, I. Abramovitz, and S. Chaushu, "Failure of treatment of impacted canines associated with invasive cervical root resorption," *The Angle Orthodontist*, vol. 83, no. 5, pp. 870–876, 2013.

16

A Multidisciplinary Approach in the Treatment of Tempromandibular Joint Pain Associated with Qat Chewing

Mansoor Shariff,[1] Mohammed M. Al-Moaleem,[1] and Nasser M. Al-Ahmari[2]

[1] *Prosthodontic Department, College of Dentistry, King Khalid University, P.O. Box 3263, Abha 61471, Saudi Arabia*
[2] *College of Dentistry, King Khalid University, P.O. Box 3263, Abha 61471, Saudi Arabia*

Correspondence should be addressed to Mansoor Shariff; mansoor_shariff@hotmail.com

Academic Editors: A. Kasaj, C. Ledesma-Montes, A. Markopoulos, and A. Milosevic

Pain of the tempro-mandibular joint (TMJ) has a direct bearing to missing teeth and excessive physical activity. Consumption of qat requires chewing on the leaves to extract their juice for long hours. A 65-year-old male Yemeni patient, a Qat chewer, reported to the university dental hospital at King Khalid University complaining of pain in left temporomandibular joint with missing mandibular anterior teeth. A multidisciplinary approach for the overall treatment of the patient was decided. Initial treatment was the relief of patient's pain with the help of a night guard. This was followed by a fabrication of anterior FPD. The case was under maintenance and follow-up protocol for a period of 8 months with no complaint of pain discomfort.

1. Introduction

Qat-chewing habit in Yemen is widely spread and practiced by a majority of the populace [1]. Qat is the leaves of the shrub *Catha edulis* which are chewed like tobacco or used to make tea; it has the effect of a euphoric stimulant. Fresh qat leaves are usually chewed during social and cultural gatherings and held in the lower buccal pouch unilaterally in a bolus for long hours [2, 3]. Chewing Qat has been practiced for central stimulant effects; the pleasurable central stimulant properties of Qat are commonly believed to improve work capacity, during travelling, by students preparing for exams and counteract fatigue [4]. TMJ pain is the most common compliant seen among TMJ dysfunction patients especially Qat chewers. The pain is commonly originated from TMJ and masticatory muscle dysfunction. An occlusal appliance/a splint is a removable device, usually made of hard acrylic, that fits over the occlusal and incisal surfaces of teeth in one arch, creating precise occlusal contact with the teeth of the opposing arch [5]. It may be used for occlusal stabilization, for treatment of TMJ disorder, or to prevent wear of the dentition [6]. Qat was reported to cause dental attrition, staining of teeth, TMJ disorders (pain and clicking), cervical caries, and increased periodontal problems [4–7]. If signs and symptoms of occlusal abnormalities are present, therapy should be initiated prior to any permanent prosthetic treatment. Replacement of the missing teeth by FPD should be in harmony with the existing occlusal relationship [8]. This paper describes a sequence of treatment for a qat-chewing patient with pain in left side TMJ and missing lower anterior teeth.

2. Case Report

A 65-year-old male Yemeni patient presented to College of Dentistry, King Khalid University, dental clinics. The patient complained of chronic pain, dull in nature around his left ear and the left side of his face. The pain starts late in the night and early mornings. Reviewing his personal history, he habitually has been chewing Qat for over 30 years. The extraoral examination elicited pain in left masseter and TMJ. There was evidence of a hypertrophic left Masseter muscle (Figure 1). The intraoral examination showed server generalized attrition of all present teeth and a history of bruxism. Class I molar relationship and occlusal group function were observed. Teeth numbers 26, 41, 42, and 43 were missing (Figure 2). The radiographic interpretation revealed mild bone loss; flat anatomy of glenoid fossa and condyle on

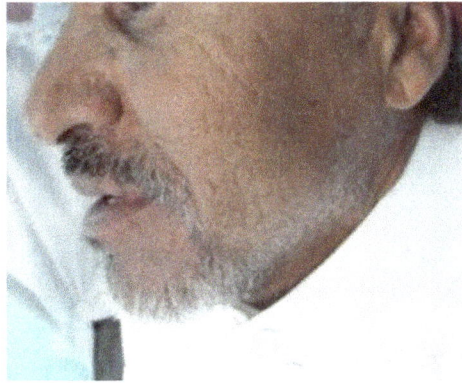

FIGURE 1: Left lateral view of the patient with hypertrophic masseter muscle.

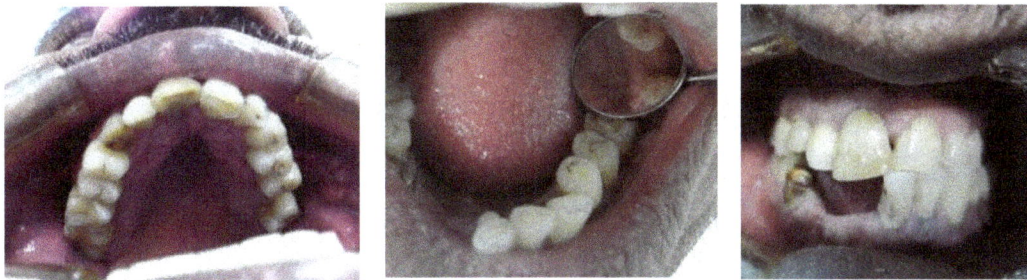

FIGURE 2: Intraoral view.

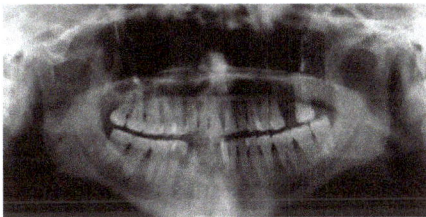

FIGURE 3: Preoperative OPG.

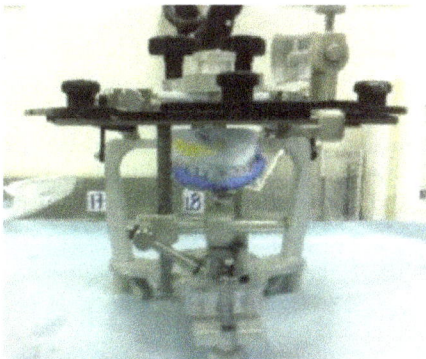

FIGURE 4: Face bow mounted on articulator.

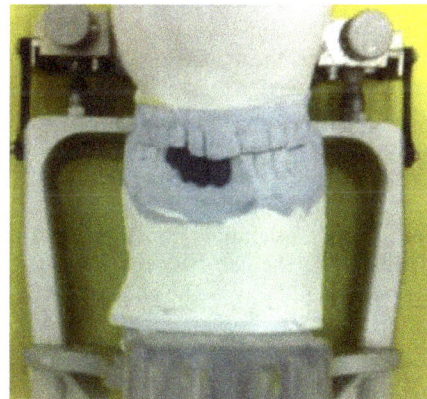

FIGURE 5: Diagnostic wax-up on mandibular arch.

The treatment was initiated with periodontal therapy and oral hygiene instruction. Maxillary and mandibular impressions were made for diagnostic casts, which were mounted on semiadjustable Whip-Mix articulator (Waterpik Technologies, Fort Collins, Co, USA) after face bow transfer (Figure 4). The diagnostic wax-up was done in harmony with centric occlusion, protrusive and extrusive movements (Figure 5). Relaxation soft splint was constructed and given to the patient starting from 0.9 mm increasing to 2 mm (Figure 6). The premature contacts were identified and selective grinding was done intraorally with articulating paper 8 microns in thickness.

the left side was obvious. The position of the right condyle is slightly anteriorly bracing the articular eminence with normal anatomy of glenoid fossa (Figure 3).

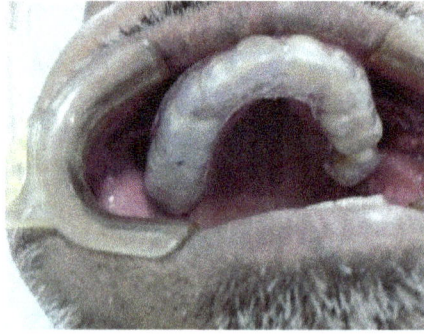

FIGURE 6: Soft splint on the maxillary teeth.

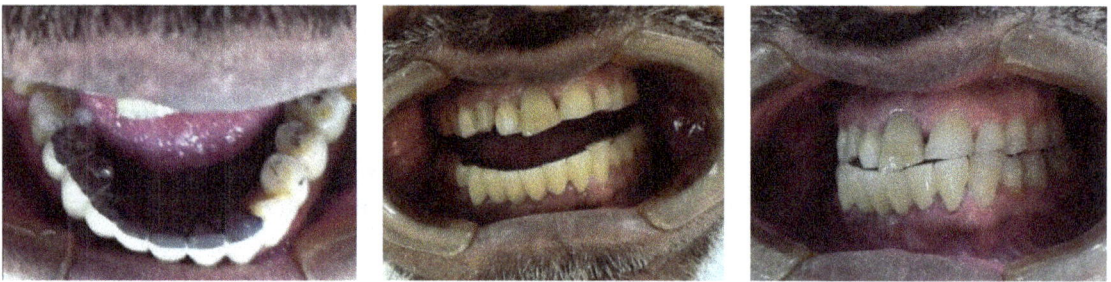

FIGURE 7: Definitive prosthesis after metal try-in and cemented FPD with metal occlusal surface.

After a one-month followup, there was considerable im–provement in pain with only slight stiffness in the left TMJ in the early morning. After the second month, there was no pain and discomfort. Root canal treatment of tooth number 44 was done, followed by post and core buildup. A definitive fixed prosthesis was planned for replacing missing teeth number 43, 42, and 41. Provisional bridge was given to the patient in group function. After one month from the placement of the provisional bridge, definitive prosthesis was tried and cemented (Figure 7). The case was recalled after 3 and 6 months for maintenance phase. The patient was free of pain and discomfort.

3. Discussion

The harmony and sequence of the treatment are essential to be considered in this case. The preliminary assessment and relief of presenting symptoms, removal of etiological factors, RCT, prosthodontic treatment, and maintenance with follow-up program were needed for satisfactory outcome.

Before commencing any appliance therapy for a TMD, the clinician should be confident that the patient will benefit from the therapeutic approach. However, much controversy exists over the exact mechanism by which occlusal appliances reduce symptoms. Most conclusions are that they decrease muscle activity (particularly parafunctional activity) [5]. The prosthetic treatment of seriously damaged, endodontically treated teeth often requires an endodontic post as an additional retention element for core buildup prior to crown restoration [9]. Tooth number 44 was root-canal-treated;

then fiber resin post was selected for reinforcing of the coronal as well as the radicular portion of the badly broken tooth. Mandibular canine lies outside the interabutment axis and forms the strongest point of force, so complex fixed partial denture with an additional abutment tooth in the arch was considered for replacement of the mandibular right anterior teeth. Tooth number 26 was extracted 13 years ago. Missing tooth should not be routinely replaced, especially in the presence of long-standing edentulous space with no drifting, elongation of adjacent or opposing teeth (stable occlusion). Porcelain abrades the opposing natural teeth because of their hardness; this causes a significant problem if the porcelain surface is roughened by occlusal adjustments [10]. Hence, metallic occlusal surface provides stable occlusal contacts without causing loss of the opposing tooth structure.

The clinical significance of this treatment is the relief of the pain by removing the cause with the replacement of missing teeth by a prosthesis in harmony with the existing occlusion.

4. Conclusion

A planned logical sequence was followed in the treatment of this case. Identifying the patient's chief complaint with symp-tomatic relief (occlusal therapy) followed by stabilization and correction of the occlusion with definitive fixed prosthesis and follow-up care was executed. The severe attrition and group function were considered during the construction and fabrication of fixed partial denture.

Acknowledgment

This case was supported by a Grant from the Collaborative Center of Creative Maxillofacial Research and Treatment Modalities (Max Center), College of Dentistry, King Khalid University, Abha, Saudi Arabia.

References

[1] A. K. Al-Sharabi, "Conditions of oral mucosa due to takhzeen al-qat," *Yemeni Journal for Medical Sciences*, vol. 5, pp. 1–6, 2011.

[2] F. N. Hattab and N. Al-Abdulla, "Effect of Khat chewing on general and oral health," *Journal of Oral Medicine*, pp. 33–35, 2011.

[3] A. G. Imran and A. H. Murad, "The effect of qat chewing on periodontal tissues and buccal mucosa membrane," *Damascus University Medical Science Journal*, no. 1, pp. 493–504, 2009.

[4] N. A. G. M. Hassan, A. A. Gunaid, and I. M. Murray-Lyon, "Khat (*Catha edulis*): health aspects of khat chewing," *Eastern Mediterranean Health Journal*, vol. 13, no. 3, pp. 15–24, 2007.

[5] R. G. Deshpande and S. Mahatre, "TMJ disorders and occlusal splint therapy—a review," *International Journal of Dental Clinics*, vol. 2, pp. 22–29, 2010.

[6] Glossary of Prosthodontics Terms # 8.

[7] K. Almas, K. Al Wazzan, I. Al Hussain, K. Y. Al-Ahdal, and N. B. Khan, "Temporomandibular joint status, occlusal attrition, cervical erosion and facial pain among substance abusers," *Odonto-Stomatologie Tropicale*, vol. 30, no. 117, pp. 27–33, 2007.

[8] S. Rosenstiel, M. Land, and J. Fujimoto, *Contemporary Fixed Prosthodontic*, p. 174–6, The Mosby, St. Louis, Mo, USA, 4th edition, 2006.

[9] M. Jain and V. Vinayak, "Post-endodontic rehabilitation using glass fiber nonmetallic posts: a review," *Indian Journal of Stomatology*, vol. 2, no. 2, pp. 117–119, 2011.

[10] H. Shillingburg, S. Hobb, L. Whitsett, R. Jacobi, and S. Brackett, *Fundamentals of Fixed Prosthodontics*, Quintessence Publishing, Hong Kong, China, 3rd edition, 1997.

17

Oromaxillary Prosthetic Rehabilitation of a Maxillectomy Patient Using a Magnet Retained Two-Piece Hollow Bulb Definitive Obturator; A Clinical Report

Jafar Abdulla Mohamed Usman,[1] Anuroopa Ayappan,[2] Dhanraj Ganapathy,[3] and Nilofer Nisha Nasir[4]

[1] Subsitutive Dental Sciences, College of Dentistry, King Khaled University, P.O. Box 3263, Abha 61471, Saudi Arabia
[2] Department of Prosthodontics, Sree Mookambika Institute of Dental Sciences, Kulashekaram, India
[3] Derartment of Prosthodontics, Saveetha Dental College, Chennai, India
[4] Department of Conservative Dentistry and Endodontics, Rajah Mutthiah Dental College, Annamalai University, Chidambaram, Tamilnadu, India

Correspondence should be addressed to Jafar Abdulla Mohamed Usman; drjafara@gmail.com

Academic Editors: Y.-K. Chen and Y. Nakagawa

Resection of a malignant lesion involving the maxilla produces severe oromaxillary defect that can seriously jeopardize the normal phonetics of the patient. These defects are effectively managed by well-designed and fabricated obturator. This paper discusses the oromaxillary prosthetic rehabilitation of a maxillectomy patient using a magnet retained two-piece hollow bulb definitive obturator.

1. Introduction

Palatal defects impart significant physical and psychological damage to the ailing patient. The various etiological factors constituting these defects can be segregated into two broad categories, namely, the congenital and the acquired defects. The acquired defects could be due to trauma, infection, and iatrogenic as a result of surgical resection of malignant as well as nonmalignant lesions. The oromaxillary defect causes transportation of oral and nasal microflora, regurgitation of oral fluids, alteration in voice due to asynchrony in resonance, and difficulty in speech as well as swallowing. Hence effective treatment modalities to treat these defects become mandatory as a clinical protocol.

2. Case Report

A male patient aged fifty years was referred to the hospital with the history of swelling in left maxillary posterior region and mobility of teeth from second premolar to third molar.

The patient was examined both clinically and radiographically. The lesion was sent for biopsy and histodiagnosed as squamous cell carcinoma involving the left maxillary antrum. The patient underwent a total maxillectomy of the left maxilla along with block dissection of lymph nodes in the neck. After surgery, the patient was rehabilitated with an interim obturator for a month and surgical site was allowed to heal. The patient reported after a month to the department of prosthodontics with complaints of change in voice, regurgitation of fluids to nose, and burning sensation in the mouth and nose.

On clinical examination, a defect due to maxillectomy was present from the midline to the soft palate on the left side. The tissue showed good signs of healing and the defect was classified as Aramany class two defect which measured 2 cm mediolaterally and 3.5 cm superoinferiorly (Figure 1) [1]. The remaining teeth exhibited significant periodontal breakdown and mild supraeruption. The treatment plan was ruled out and a definitive prosthesis was decided to be given to the patient. The defect was packed with gauze so as

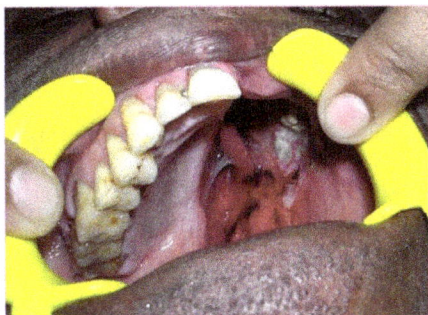

FIGURE 1: Maxillectomy defect.

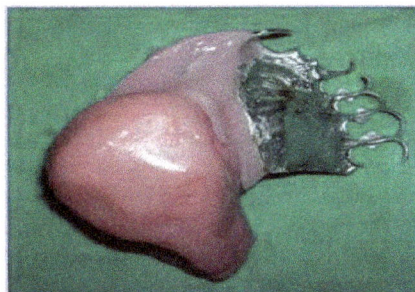

FIGURE 3: Completed prosthesis.

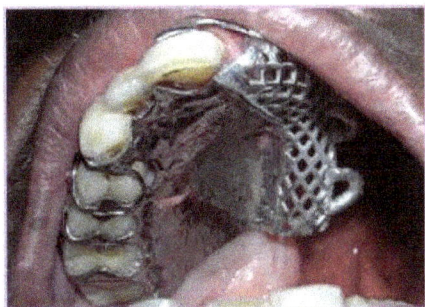

FIGURE 2: Framework try-in.

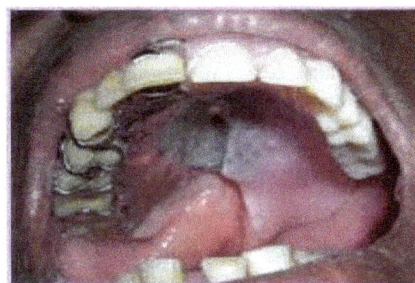

FIGURE 4: Insertion of the prosthesis.

to prevent the ingress of the impression material into the nasal cavity. Primary impression was made with irreversible hydrocolloid (Zelgan 2000) and casts were obtained. The casts were surveyed with Jelenko dental surveyor and the undercuts were established and direct retainers in the form of embrasure clasps were planned in teeth numbers 15, 16, 17, and 18 [2]. Complete coverage palatal maxillary major connector with chrome cobalt alloy and mesh type denture base minor connector were selected (Figure 2).

Careful surveying revealed the defect and the palatal plate major connector had varied paths of insertion. Hence a two-piece hollow bulb obturator was planned for treating the patient. Special trays were constructed with suitable tissue stops from the primary cast. The secondary impressions were secured by twin stage impression procedure where the impression of the defect was made with putty consistency polyvinyl siloxane (Aquasil) and was picked up by a full arch impression with medium consistency polyvinyl siloxane and poured with type IV stone (ultra rock) and a secondary cast was obtained. The lateral undercuts in the defective area were blocked out and a hollow bulb obturator was processed using a lost salt technique. The hollow bulb obturator was tried in patient's mouth for retention and comfort. Then the cast partial denture framework with the prosthetic teeth was tried in the patient's mouth and evaluated for extension, retention, stability, occlusion, and phonetics (Figure 3). Cobalt samarium magnets of 4 mm dimension were placed over the tissue side of cast partial denture framework and the corresponding pair was fixed on the obturator using autopolymerising acrylic resin (DPI, India). The retention

was excellent with magnetic keepers. The obturator was subsequently relined with permanent soft liner (Perma Soft) to completely obturate the lateral defects. This was tried in the patient (Figure 4). The patient was reviewed periodically for 12 months. The patient experienced great comfort, enhanced mastication, and phonetics with the prosthesis.

3. Discussion

Acquired maxillary defects due to various etiologic factors pose a great challenge to the clinician. The patient suffers a severe deficit in the masticatory and phonetics function. Salvaging teeth during the surgical procedure reduces the number of occlusal units in the oral cavity and significantly hampers masticatory efficiency [3]. It also substantially compromises pronunciation of words which occurs in the form of nasal twang and increased cubicle space resulting in poor articulation with linguodental and linguopalatal consonants [4]. One of the serious dysfunction caused by acquired palatomaxillary defect is the intertransportation of micro organisms between the oral and nasal cavity. The nasal cavity is lined by pseudo stratified ciliated columnar epithelium and goblet cells present there aggressively attract oral flora [5]. In addition, regurgitation and transportation of food and fluids from the oral cavity to nasal cavity via the defect cause severe discomfort to the patient.

The obturator prosthesis is designed to seal the defect, functions efficiently as it prevents the infiltration of food, fluids, and flora from the oral to nasal chambers and vice versa. It tremendously improves the quality of voice as it completely seals the lateral palatal defect as well as the maxillary defect. One of the problems associated with oromaxillary obturators is insertion of the prosthesis due to compromised anatomic morphology in different planes [6]. Hence it is mandatory to design an obturator in two sections wherein the obturator is inserted initially followed by oropalatal metal framework [7]. The two sections are retained together in function as one unit by retentive devices subsequently.

There are several retentive devices available to secure the two sections in position [8]. Among the various retentive devices magnetic attachments are more user friendly and cost effective when compared to internal attachments which required extreme precision and good neuromuscular coordination from the patient to insert and use the prosthesis. When compared to conventional iron boron magnets, cobalt samarium magnets undergo less corrosion and hence they were selected for this case. The disadvantage of magnetic attachment is the possible loss of magnetism during function during extended period of time. But they can be magnetized with reasonable ease and can be induced to function immediately [9].

Another problem with maxillofacial obturator is the increased weight of the prosthesis due to the bulk of the resin occupied in the defect area and hence the weight was reduced by fabrication of hollow bulb obturator using lost salt technique [10]. The palatal obturator in the defect which is subsequently relined with a soft liner greatly enhances the comfort of the patient as it is flexible and protects the integrity of the adjoining moving tissues. A proper maintenance regimen with chlorhexidine mouth wash and a comprehensive education on the manipulation of the prosthesis increases the success and survival rate of oromaxillary obturator.

4. Conclusion

This paper discussed the prosthetic management of acquired Oromaxillary defect with a two-piece cast partial hollow bulb definitive obturator with magnetic attachment and tissue liners.

References

[1] G. R. Parr, G. E. Tharp, and A. O. Rahn, "Prosthodontic principles in the framework design of maxillary obturator prostheses," *The Journal of Prosthetic Dentistry*, vol. 93, no. 5, pp. 405–411, 2005.

[2] A. G. Wagner and E. G. Forgue, "A study of four methods of recording the path of insertion of removable partial dentures," *The Journal of Prosthetic Dentistry*, vol. 35, no. 3, pp. 267–272, 1976.

[3] M. Matsuyama, Y. Tsukiyama, M. Tomioka, and K. Koyano, "Subjective assessment of chewing function of obturatorprosthesis wearer," *International Journal of Prosthodontics*, vol. 20, no. 1, pp. 46–50, 2007.

[4] T. J. Salinas, L. R. Guerra, and W. A. Rogers, "Aesthetic considerations for maxillary obturators retained by implants," *Practical Periodontics and Aesthetic Dentistry*, vol. 9, no. 3, pp. 265–276, 1997.

[5] L. H. Abdullah and C. W. Davis, "Regulation of airway goblet cell mucin secretion by tyrosine phosphorylation signaling pathways," *The American Journal of Physiology*, vol. 293, no. 3, pp. L591–L599, 2007.

[6] B. Rilo, J. L. Dasilva, I. Ferros, M. J. Mora, and U. Santana, "A hollow-bulb interim obturator for maxillary resection. A case report," *Journal of Oral Rehabilitation*, vol. 32, no. 3, pp. 234–236, 2005.

[7] W. S. Oh and E. D. Roumanas, "Optimization of maxillary obturator thickness using a double-processing technique," *Journal of Prosthodontics*, vol. 17, no. 1, pp. 60–63, 2008.

[8] M. Fukuda, T. Takahashi, H. Nagai, and M. Iino, "Implant-supported edentulous maxillary obturators with milled bar attachments after maxillectomy," *Journal of Oral and Maxillofacial Surgery*, vol. 62, no. 7, pp. 799–805, 2004.

[9] T. Takahashi, M. Fukuda, K. Funaki, and K. Tanaka, "Magnet-retained facial prosthesis combined with an implant-supported edentulous maxillary obturator: a case report," *International Journal of Oral and Maxillofacial Implants*, vol. 21, no. 5, pp. 805–807, 2006.

[10] F. M. Blair and N. R. Hunter, "The hollow box maxillary obturator," *The British Dental Journal*, vol. 184, no. 10, pp. 484–487, 1998.

18

Hypodontia and Delayed Dentition as the Primary Manifestation of Cleidocranial Dysplasia Presenting with a Diagnostic Dilemma

Radhika Chopra,[1] **Mohita Marwaha,**[1] **Payal Chaudhuri,**[1]
Kalpana Bansal,[1] **and Saurabh Chopra**[2]

[1] *Department of Pedodontics and Preventive Dentistry, SGT Dental College & Research Institute, Budhera 123505,*
  Gurgaon, Haryana, India
[2] *Department of Pediatrics, Subharti Medical College, Meerut 250005, India*

Correspondence should be addressed to Radhika Chopra, drradhikachopra@gmail.com

Academic Editors: S. Anil and P. R. Warren

Cleidocranial dysplasia is a rare autosomal disorder which manifests as partial or complete absence of clavicles, multiple supernumerary teeth, and delayed closure of fontanelle. Classical cases of cleidocranial dysplasia are easily diagnosed very early in the life. However, cases with partial manifestation of the syndrome and noncontributory family history are difficult to diagnose. Here, we report a case of 8.5-year-old girl child who presented with delayed tooth development (without any supernumerary teeth), anterior open fontanelle, and normal clavicles, thus resulting in a diagnostic dilemma.

1. Introduction

Cleidocranial dysplasia (CCD) is a dominant, inherited autosomal bone disorder with a wide range of expressivity, primarily affecting bones undergoing intramembranous ossification and characterized by clavicular aplasia or hypoplasia, retarded cranial ossification, supernumerary teeth, short stature, and a variety of other skeletal abnormalities [1].

The classical features of this syndrome are partial or complete absence of the clavicles, multiple supernumerary teeth [2], and delayed closure of the sagittal fontanelle [3]. Other features include a bell-shaped thorax, enlargement of frontal and occipital bones, hypoplasia of the pelvis and distal phalanges, short stature, hypertelorism [4], and impacted permanent teeth. Less common findings of CCD patients include shortened or absent nasal bones, reduced or absent paranasal sinuses, thickening of some segments of the calvaria, underdevelopment of maxilla, and delayed union of mandibular symphysis [5].

Here, we report a case of 8.5-year-old female child who did not manifest the classical features of CCD, thus resulting in diagnostic dilemma.

2. Case Report

A 8.5-year-old girl was referred to the department of pedodontics and preventive dentistry with the chief complaint of delayed eruption of permanent teeth. She was born prematurely at 8 months to healthy parents, and her birth weight was 2.9 kg. The family history was unremarkable.

General examination of the patient revealed a weight of 22 kgs, height of 109 cms, and head circumference of 53 cm. On extraoral examination, the patient presented with frontal bosselation, hypertelorism, epicanthal fold with respect to left eye, and depressed nasal bridge (Figure 1). Open fontanelle could be palpated in the anterior region of the head. Intraoral examination revealed the presence of a set of deciduous dentition with missing primary mandibular right and left lateral incisors and none of the permanent teeth had erupted as yet (Figure 2).

An orthopantomogram revealed absence of permanent tooth buds of permanent mandibular right and left lateral incisors and permanent mandibular right central incisor (Figure 3) and there was a generalized delay in the development of permanent tooth buds. Delayed root formation

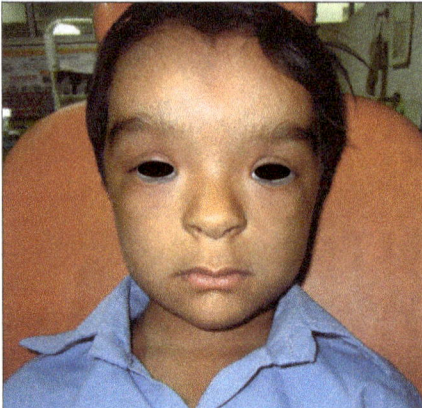

FIGURE 1: Facial photograph.

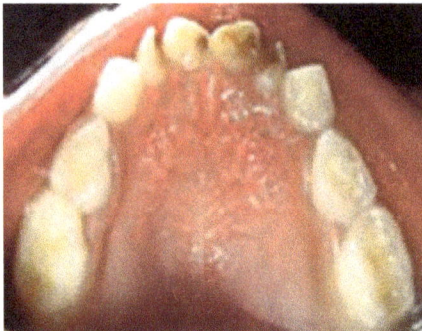

(a)

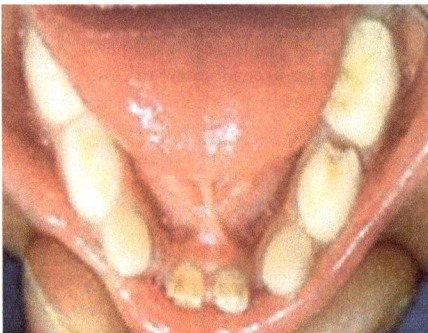

(b)

FIGURE 2: Intraoral photograph.

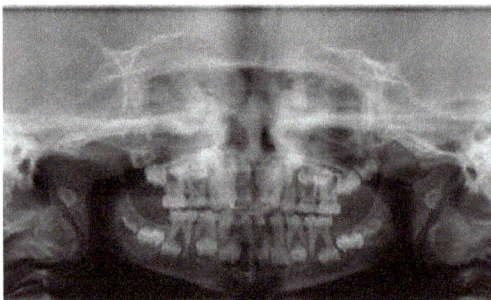

FIGURE 3: OPG.

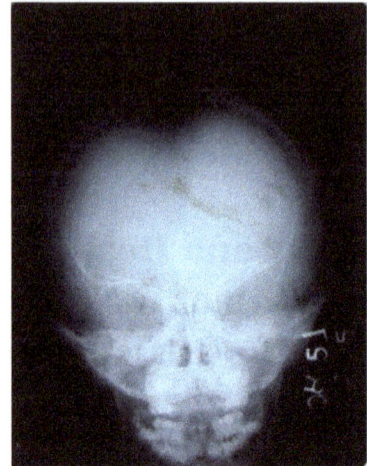

FIGURE 4: PA view skull.

of permanent first molars was noted. No supernumerary teeth were seen in the radiograph. PA skull revealed delayed closure of fontanelle (Figure 4). CT scan of skull was done revealing focal defect in frontal bone measuring upto 3.8 cm (Figure 5).

The posteroanterior view of chest radiograph showed normally developed clavicles. Hand wrist radiograph showed short distal phalanges and the bone age was found to be on the lower limit for her age (Figure 6). Thyroid function test was also normal.

So the prominent findings in our case were delayed development of permanent dentition, frontal bossing, and anterior open fontanelle. These findings did not correlate with any other syndrome except for CCD.

Thereafter, all the family members were screened for any manifestation of CCD. Only the younger sister showed hypermobility of the shoulders. Complete physical and radiologic assessment revealed abnormal clavicles with a small right clavicle and two pieces of left clavicle (Figure 7). There was no other dental or skeletal abnormality detected.

Based on this finding, a diagnosis of cleidocranial dysplasia was made. The decayed anterior teeth of the patient were restored and the patient is being kept under regular followup to evaluate the eruption of permanent teeth. The orthodontic and prosthodontic intervention will be planned as required.

3. Discussion

CCD was first described by Pierre Marie and Paul Sainton in 1898 [6]. CCD is also known as Marie-Sainton disease, mutational dysostosis, and cleidocranial dysostosis. This condition is usually caused by a mutation of the Core binding factor alpha 1 (Cbfa1) gene, located at chromosome 6p21, which is essential for osteoblasts and odontoblasts differentiation as well as for bone and tooth formation [7].

CCD is a relatively uncommon disorder with a prevalence of 0.5 per 100,000 live births [8]. Clinically, the diagnosis is often made at birth but may not occur until later, when persistence of the widely open anterior fontanelles and sutures or short stature incites parental concern. Individuals

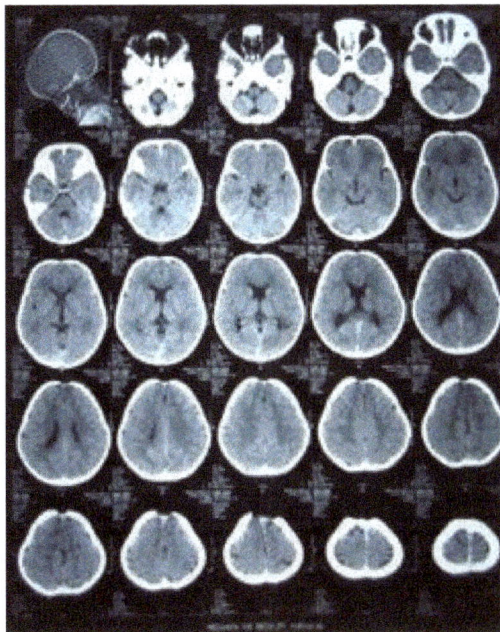

Figure 5: CT scan skull.

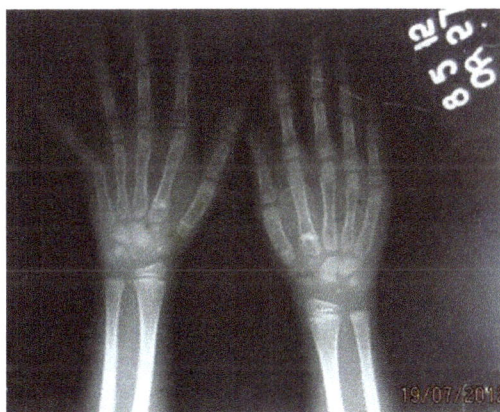

Figure 6: Hand wrist radiograph.

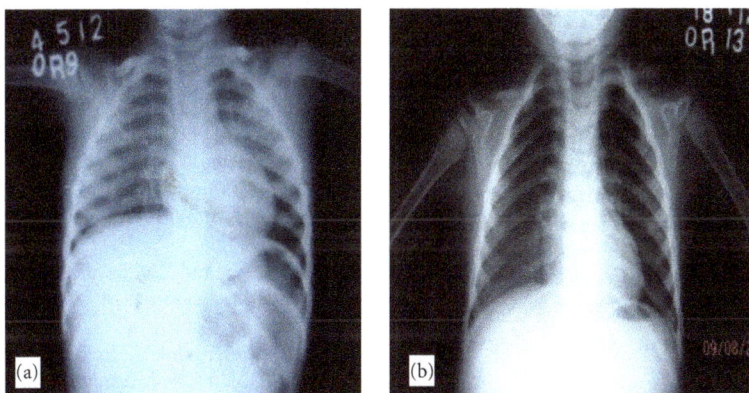

Figure 7: Chest radiograph: (a) patient and (b) sister.

with this disorder present with some or all of very characteristic features. Skeletal abnormalities commonly found include clavicular aplasia/hypoplasia, bell-shaped thorax, enlarged calvaria with frontal bossing and open fontanelles, Wormian bones, brachydactyly with hypoplastic distal phalanges, hypoplasia of the pelvis with widened symphysis pubis, severe dental anomalies, and short stature. Our patient showed no pathology in the clavicular and pelvic bones but there was a presence of open fontanelle, frontal bossing, and hypoplastic distal phalanges. Clavicles are underdeveloped to varying degrees in these patients and are completely absent in approximately 10 percent [1, 9, 10]. Patients with normal clavicles have also been described in previous studies [11].

Dental changes occur frequently and are very characteristic of CCD. The large number of supernumerary teeth that form a more or less complete third dentition (up to 30 extra teeth in some cases) is one of the most striking findings in CCD. Contrary to this, delayed eruption without supernumerary teeth was present in our case which made it difficult to reach a definite diagnosis, as such findings are also frequently observed in other conditions such as osteopetrosis or pycnodysostosis. CCD is also associated with a delay of root development in permanent dentition and a lessened but not entirely absent eruptive potential [12]. These features were in accordance with the findings in our case.

In CCD, many of the deciduous teeth are retained throughout life and lie among the permanent teeth. The permanent teeth generally lose their eruption stimulus and stay embedded, while the deciduous teeth are retained. Suggested factors for overretained deciduous teeth are lack of eruption potential and lack of cellular cementum on roots of permanent teeth, delayed mineralization of teeth, physical barrier-abnormal density of bone overlying the succedaneous teeth, and failure of bony crypt to resorb [13]. In our patient there was delayed eruption of permanent teeth and tooth buds of 32, 41, 42 were missing.

CCD involves mutation in the transcription factor, Runx2/Cbfa1, located on chromosome 6p21 [7]. There is a notably phenotypic variation of CCD even within one and the same family. In approximately 40% of CCD patients, a genetic transition cannot be identified, and the condition develops spontaneously [5, 14]. In our report, both the sisters were affected with CCD with variable manifestations. The patient showed hypodontia and delayed permanent dentition, open fontanelle with normal clavicles while the sister had only defective clavicles without any other manifestations of CCD.

Osseous development is severely delayed in the newborn period and manifested by the delayed ossification of skull and the pubis, absence of nasal bones, and the incomplete fusion of the vertebral arches [4, 15]. The abnormal modeling of bone is manifested in the calvaria, by delayed ossification, causing secondary ossification centres to form and the bones of the skull to be thin and with abnormal margins. This causes the sutures to be widely spaced and late closing [4, 15]. Our patient showed a large defect in the frontal bone measuring upto 3.8 cms.

The planning of treatment for patient with CCD is complicated by a number of factors and largely depends on both chronological and dental ages of the patient. The timing of diagnosis is not only important for choosing an appropriate treatment plan but also for obtaining successful treatment results. A team approach to management of dental abnormalities on a long-term basis is necessary. The overall goal is to provide an aesthetic facial appearance and functional occlusion by late adolescence or early adulthood.

References

[1] B. S. González López, C. Ortiz Solalinde, T. Kubodera Ito, E. Lara Carrillo, and E. Ortiz Solalinde, "Cleidocranial dysplasia: report of a family," *Journal of Oral Science*, vol. 46, no. 4, pp. 259–266, 2004.

[2] P. D. Quinn, J. Lewis, and L. M. Levin, "Surgical management of a patient with cleidocranial dysplasia: a case report," *Special Care in Dentistry*, vol. 12, no. 3, pp. 131–133, 1992.

[3] L. A. Brueton, A. Reeve, R. Ellis, P. Husband, E. M. Thompson, and H. M. Kingston, "Apparent cleidocranial dysplasia associated with abnormalities of 8q22 in three individuals," *American Journal of Medical Genetics*, vol. 43, no. 3, pp. 612–618, 1992.

[4] B. L. Jensen and S. Kreiborg, "Craniofacial abnormalities in 52 school-age and adult patients with cleidocranial dysplasia," *Journal of Craniofacial Genetics and Developmental Biology*, vol. 13, no. 2, pp. 98–108, 1993.

[5] J. L. Tanaka, E. Ono, E. M. Filho, J. C. Castilho, L. C. Moraes, and M. E. Moraes, "Cleidocranial dysplasia: importance of radiographic images in diagnosis of the condition," *Journal of Oral Science*, vol. 48, no. 3, pp. 161–166, 2006.

[6] E. Kalliala and P. J. Taskinen, "Cleidocranial dysostosis. Report of six typical cases and one atypical case," *Oral Surgery, Oral Medicine, Oral Pathology*, vol. 15, no. 7, pp. 808–822, 1962.

[7] T. Yoshida, H. Kanegane, M. Osato et al., "Functional analysis of RUNX2 mutations in Japanese patients with cleidocranial dysplasia demonstrates novel genotype-phenotype correlations," *American Journal of Human Genetics*, vol. 71, no. 4, pp. 724–738, 2002.

[8] T. R. Yochum and L. J. Rowe, *Essentials of Skeletal Radiology*, Williams and Wilkins, Baltimore, Md, USA, 2nd edition, 1996.

[9] V. Gombra and S. Jayachandran, "Cleidocranial dysplasia: report of four cases and review," *Journal of Indian Academy of Oral Medicine and Radiology*, vol. 20, pp. 23–27, 2008.

[10] S. K. Verma, P. Jain, and N. C. Sharma, "Scheuthauer-Marie-Sainton syndrome—a rare entity imaging findings," *Indian Journal of Radiology and Imaging*, vol. 14, no. 2, pp. 175–176, 2004.

[11] W. R. Cole and S. Levine, "Cleidocranial dysostosis," *The British Journal of Radiology*, vol. 24, no. 286, pp. 549–555, 1951.

[12] B. L. Jensen and S. Kreiborg, "Development of the dentition in cleidocranial dysplasia," *Journal of Oral Pathology and Medicine*, vol. 19, no. 2, pp. 89–93, 1990.

[13] D. N. Mehta, R. V. Vachhani, and M. B. Patel, "Cleidocranial dysplasia: a report of two cases," *Journal of Indian Society of Pedodontics and Preventive Dentistry*, vol. 29, no. 3, pp. 251–254, 2011.

[14] R. K. Garg and P. Agrawal, "Clinical spectrum of cleidocranial dysplasia: a case report," *Cases Journal*, vol. 1, no. 1, p. 377, 2008.

[15] B. L. Jensen and S. Kreiborg, "Development of the skull in infants with cleidocranial dysplasia," *Journal of Craniofacial Genetics and Developmental Biology*, vol. 13, no. 2, pp. 89–97, 1993.

19

Orthodontic Elastic Embedded in Gingiva for 7 Years

Shruti Tandon,[1] **Abdul Ahad,**[1] **Arundeep Kaur,**[1]
Farrukh Faraz,[1] **and Zainab Chaudhary**[2]

[1] *Department of Periodontics and Oral Implantology, Maulana Azad Institute of Dental Sciences,*
  Bahadur Shah Zafar Marg, New Delhi 110002, India
[2] *Department of Oral and Maxillofacial Surgery, Maulana Azad Institute of Dental Sciences,*
  Bahadur Shah Zafar Marg, New Delhi 110002, India

Correspondence should be addressed to Shruti Tandon; drst@in.com

Academic Editors: Y.-K. Chen and R. Crespi

Dental materials especially orthodontic elastics often get embedded in gingival tissues due to iatrogenic factors. If retained for a long time, inflammatory response starts as asymptomatic crestal bone loss and may progress to severe periodontal abscess. Unsupported orthodontic elastics used for diastema closure may result in exfoliation of teeth, while elastic separators may get embedded in interdental gingiva if banding is performed without removing it. These cases of negligence are detrimental for survival of affected teeth. This paper highlights a case of orthodontic elastic embedded in interproximal gingiva of a 23-year-old healthy female for 7 years after completion of fixed orthodontic treatment. Surprisingly, there was no clinical sign of inflammation around elastic band and it was removed easily without any local anaesthesia. However, mild crestal bone loss was observed on periapical radiograph. The gingiva healed completely after sub gingival debridement.

1. Introduction

The presence of foreign bodies in gingiva, leading to inflammatory response, is unusual but not a rare condition. Most of the cases in the literature have been reported to be iatrogenic, commonly associated with use of elastic bands and separators for orthodontic treatment [1–3]. Other dental materials like amalgam, composite, cements, and prophylaxis paste have also been found to be embedded in gingiva [4]. The resulting inflammatory response varies from asymptomatic mild crestal bone loss to severe periodontal destruction causing abscess formation [5, 6].

Most of the cases in literature have been reported to be most common in mandibular posterior region (34%), followed by maxillary posterior (29%) and maxillary anterior regions (26%). Probably this incidence correlates with more dental treatments received in these regions [7].

Unsupported orthodontic elastics creeping into gingival sulcus have been reported frequently in the literature [8–10]. Some authors have also reported the presence of elastic separators in interproximal area that are used for relieving contact before band placement [5, 6, 11–13]. This report describes a case of intact orthodontic elastic found embedded in interproximal gingiva between mandibular first and second molars, 7 years after completion of orthodontic treatment.

2. Case Presentation

A 23-year-old female reported for routine oral prophylaxis. She complained of occasional bleeding from gums on brushing. There was no history of pain; however she reported to have noticed a yellow growth on gingiva between right mandibular posterior teeth, for last 1 month. The medical history was not significant. The patient had completed fixed orthodontic treatment for crowded anterior teeth when she was 16 years old. On examination, oral hygiene was found to be fair except mild deposits of calculus. As reported by the patient, a yellow coloured material was found protruding through interdental papilla between right mandibular first and second molars (Figure 1). When held with forceps, an intact elastic band came out easily, without bleeding or any discomfort to the patient (Figure 2). An indentation of the elastic band was found on the buccal aspect of interdental

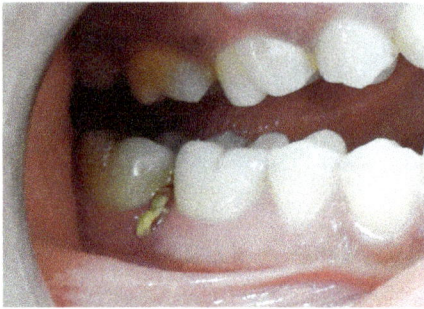

FIGURE 1: Elastic band protruding through interdental gingiva between right mandibular first and second molars.

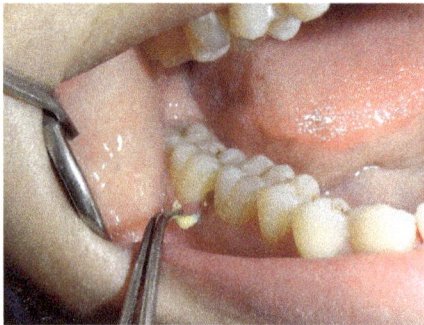

FIGURE 2: Elastic band was easily removed using forceps.

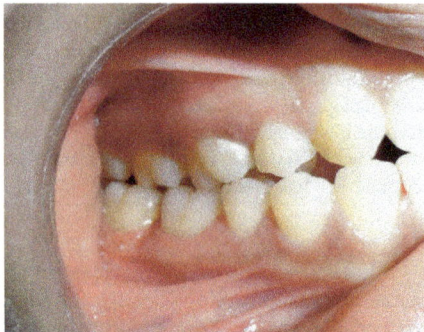

FIGURE 3: Indentation of elastic band on interdental papilla after its removal.

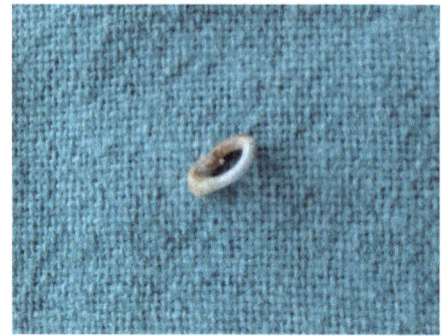

FIGURE 4: Intact elastic band. Half of the band was covered with heavy plaque while the other half was relatively cleaner.

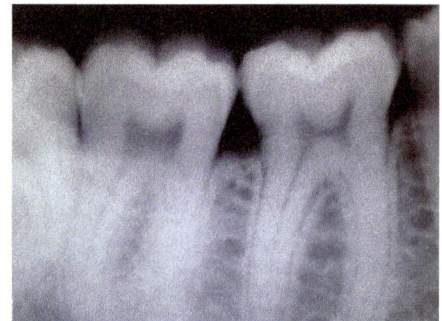

FIGURE 5: Periapical radiograph showing mild crestal bone loss between first and second molars.

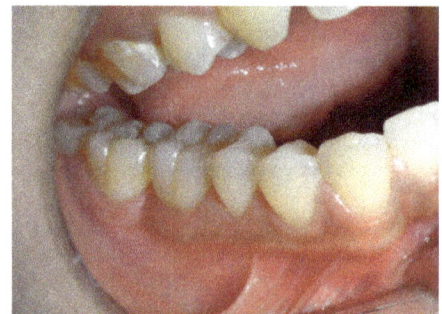

FIGURE 6: Completely healed gingiva after 1 month.

papilla (Figure 3). Heavy plaque was present on the part of the elastic band that was protruding out while the other part was relatively cleaner (Figure 4). To rule out any other foreign bodies, an IOPA radiograph was taken that revealed only mild crestal bone loss (Figure 5). The area was debrided using Gracey curettes nos. 11-12 and nos. 13-14 (Hu-Friedy, Chicago, IL, USA) and irrigated with normal saline. Patient was advised to do warm saline rinses 3 times daily for 1 week. Patient was recalled after 1 week, and she reported no incidence of pain or any discomfort in the area. After 1 month, there was complete healing of gingiva (Figure 6).

3. Discussion

Elastic bands are commonly used in orthodontics for space closure, derotation, correction of cross bite, and as separator before band placement. Ideally, elastics other than separators should be stabilized by bonded attachments or brackets and evaluated at regular intervals. It is recommended that under no circumstances any unsupported elastic be looped around teeth for diastema closure [8]. However, this is still in practice by clinicians and due to negligence or failure to follow up, this often results in creeping of elastic band apically into gingival sulcus, along the root surface [9]. In the case reported here, it was unusual that the patient was oblivious of the elastic embedded in the gingiva for the last 7 years, although a part of it was protruding out of the interdental papilla. The gingiva had grown around the elastic in a tunnel-like manner, such that pulling it out with forceps did not require local anaesthesia, nor caused any bleeding. The part of the elastic band that was protruding out of the gingiva was covered with plaque, imparting a yellowish colour and rough surface to otherwise blue and smooth elastic. Although the patient had noticed a yellowish "growth" on her gums, but since it was symptom-free, she did not report to a dentist.

The presence of foreign bodies in the gingiva may result in inflammatory response in surrounding tissues and subsequent loss of attachment apparatus, as reported in various case reports [5, 6, 8–10, 13]. This inflammation is independent of the degree of plaque colonization [14]. The condition may initially remain asymptomatic but usually presents clinically as pain, oedema, mobility, and/or pus discharge from the sulcus [6, 9, 13]. Becker and Neronov [5] reported abscess formation due to an elastic separator embedded in interdental space that healed completely after removal of elastic and periodontal curettage, leaving only mild alveolar bone loss. They emphasized the importance of appropriate imaging for diagnosis of such cases, which otherwise may remain unnoticed and continue periodontal destruction [5]. For effective and predictable management of such cases, early diagnosis of the condition is essential. In case the separator is missing at the time of banding, the patient should be asked about it. If the patient is unaware, then the area should be explored clinically and radiographically before banding. It is recommended that radiopaque and brightly coloured material be used for making orthodontic elastics, separators, and ligature bands to easily identify them on radiographs. Since clinical features are nonspecific and radiographs often fail to reveal the elastic bands, although metallic foreign bodies can easily be traced, a detailed history of previous dental treatments is of utmost importance. Depending on severity of the case, various treatment options may be tried. The area needs to be debrided of all the foreign bodies, granulation tissues, and calculus. The affected teeth may sometimes require splinting before surgical intervention. It may be required to raise a full thickness flap as in the case of Nettem et al. [6]. They reported a case of elastic band embedded between mandibular first and second molars that resulted in a deep pocket and abscess formation in otherwise healthy dentition of a 20-year-old female. They performed incision and drainage followed by raising a flap for retrieval of elastic. The area healed completely 1 week after surgery [6]. In severe cases, interdisciplinary approach may be required as reported by Al-Qutub [9]. He described the surgical management of a maxillary central incisor with grade III mobility, resulting from severe bone loss due to creeping of elastic placed for closure of midline diastema in a 9-year-old female child. After splinting, a full thickness flap was reflected to retrieve the elastic, followed by complete debridement, bone grafting, and placement of a resorbable membrane. Patient later required orthodontic intrusion after the tooth was found to be stable 6 months postoperatively. In most of the reported cases, antibiotic and analgesics were also prescribed to control the infection and pain. Specialized individual oral home care and regular monitoring of these areas are also important to prevent further breakdown of the periodontal attachment.

Fortunately, in this case, no significant periodontal destruction had occurred. Apparently, fair maintenance of oral hygiene in the affected area kept inflammation only subclinical. Still, the negligence in this case cannot be ignored, as it might have resulted in more severe conditions, jeopardizing the survival of teeth as reported in previous literature.

4. Conclusion

Elastic bands are commonly used for various purposes in orthodontics. It is advisable to do a thorough examination particularly in the interproximal areas for any residual material left at the completion of orthodontic treatment. Any area with periodontal destruction and history of orthodontic treatment should be inspected for the presence of foreign bodies. If diagnosed early, bone loss can be arrested and may even be regenerated if anatomy of defect is favourable.

Conflict of Interests

The authors report no conflict of interests related to this case report.

References

[1] N. I. Zager and M. L. Barnett, "Severe bone loss in a child initiated by multiple orthodontic rubber bands: case report," *Journal of Periodontology*, vol. 45, no. 9, pp. 701–704, 1974.

[2] Y. Zilberman, A. Shteyer, and B. Azaz, "Iatrogenic exfoliation of teeth by the incorrect use of orthodontic elastic bands," *The Journal of the American Dental Association*, vol. 93, no. 1, pp. 89–93, 1976.

[3] W. F. Waggoner and K. D. Ray, "Bone loss in the permanent dentition as a result of improper orthodontic elastic band use: a case report," *Quintessence international*, vol. 20, no. 9, pp. 653–656, 1989.

[4] M. A. Lochhead and K. Gravitis, "Foreign body gingivitis: a literature review," *Canadian Journal of Dental Hygiene*, vol. 40, no. 6, pp. 318–324, 2006.

[5] T. Becker and A. Neronov, "Orthodontic elastic separator-induced periodontal abscess: a case report," *Case Reports in Dentistry*, vol. 2012, Article ID 463903, 3 pages, 2012.

[6] S. Nettem, S. K. Nettemu, K. K. Kumar, G. V. Reddy, and P. S. Kumar, "Spontaneous reversibility of an iatrogenic orthodontic elastic band-induced localized periodontitis following surgical intervention—case report," *The Malaysian Journal of Medical Sciences*, vol. 19, no. 4, pp. 77–80, 2012.

[7] H. S. Koppang, A. Roushan, A. Srafilzadeh, S. Ø. Stølen, and R. Koppang, "Foreign body gingival lesions: Distribution, morphology, identification by X-ray energy dispersive analysis and possible origin of foreign material," *Journal of Oral Pathology and Medicine*, vol. 36, no. 3, pp. 161–172, 2007.

[8] K. F. Lim, "Latex elastic-induced periodontal damage: a case report on the subsequent orthodontic management," *Quintessence International*, vol. 27, no. 10, pp. 685–690, 1996.

[9] M. N. Al-Qutub, "Orthodontic elastic band-induced periodontitis—a case report," *Saudi Dental Journal*, vol. 24, no. 1, pp. 49–53, 2012.

[10] Y. Lin, Y. Huang, S. Chang, and H. Hong, "Sequelae of iatrogenic periodontal destruction associated with elastics and permanent incisors: literature review and report of 3 cases," *Pediatric Dentistry*, vol. 33, no. 7, pp. 516–521, 2011.

[11] G. St George and M. A. Donachie, "Case report: orthodontic separators as periodontal ligatures in periodontal bone loss,"

The European Journal of Prosthodontics and Restorative Dentistry, vol. 10, no. 3, pp. 97–99, 2002.

[12] Z. Harrington and U. Darbar, "Localised periodontitis associated with an ectopic orthodontic separator," *Primary Dental Care*, vol. 14, no. 1, pp. 5–6, 2007.

[13] A. E. Vishwanath, B. K. Sharmada, S. S. Pai, and N. Nelvigi, "Severe bone loss induced by orthodontic elastic separator: A Rare Case Report," *Journal of Indian Orthodontic Society*, vol. 47, no. 2, pp. 97–99, 2013.

[14] P. Diedrich, I. Rudzki-Janson, H. Wehrbein, and U. Fritz, "Effects of orthodontic bands on marginal periodontal tissues: a histologic study on two human specimens," *Journal of Orofacial Orthopedics*, vol. 62, no. 2, pp. 146–156, 2001.

20

Gorlin-Goltz Syndrome

Padma Pandeshwar,[1] **K. Jayanthi,**[2] **and D. Mahesh**[3]

[1] *Sri Venkateshwara Dental College and Hospital, Kariyappanahalli, Anekal Road, Bannerughatta, Bangalore 560083, India*
[2] *Oral Medicine, Diagnosis and Radiology, Bangalore Institute of Dental Sciences, Lakkasandra, Wilson Garden, Bangalore, India*
[3] *Dayananda Sagar College of Dental Sciences, Shivage Malleshwara Hills, Kumarswamy Layout, Bangalore, India*

Correspondence should be addressed to Padma Pandeshwar, padmapandeshwar9@gmail.com

Academic Editors: J. J. Segura-Egea and M. J. Wahl

The Gorlin-Goltz syndrome (GGS) (the nevoid basal cell carcinoma syndrome—NBCCS) is a rare autosomal dominant syndrome caused due to mutations in the *PTCH* (patched) gene found on chromosome arm 9q. The syndrome, characterized by increased predisposition to develop basal cell carcinoma and associated multiorgan anomalies, has a high level of penetrance and variable expressiveness. GGS is a multidisciplinary problem, early diagnosis of which allows introduction of secondary prophylaxis and following an appropriate treatment to delay the progress of the syndrome. The following report emphasizes the need for awareness of the diagnostic criteria of this syndrome in cases with no typical skin lesions.

1. Introduction

GGS, also known as nevoid basal cell carcinoma syndrome (NBCCS), is an infrequent multisystemic disease with an autosomal dominant trait, with a complete penetrance and variable expressivity, though sporadic cases have been described [1, 2]. GGS shows a predisposition to neoplasms and other developmental abnormalities. The estimated prevalence varies from 1/57,000 to 1/256,000 among various studies, with a male-to-female ratio of 1 : 1 [2].

The first report of the syndrome was made in 1894 by Jarisch and White in a patient with multiple basal cell carcinomas, scoliosis, and learning disability. Binkley and Johnson in 1951, and Howell and Caro in 1959 suggested a relationship between basal cell epitheliomas and developmental malformations. It was delineated only in 1960 by Robert James Gorlin and William Goltz [3, 4] who established the classical triad (multiple basocellular epitheliomas, keratocysts in the jaws and bifid ribs) that characterizes the diagnosis of this syndrome. This triad was later modified by Rayner et al., who established that the diagnostic criteria would require cysts to appear in combination with calcification of the falx cerebri or palmar and plantar pits [5–7].

In addition to the classical triad described by Gorlin and Goltz, calcification of the falx cerebri, palmar and plantar epidermal pits, spine and rib anomalies, relative macrocephaly, facial milia, frontal bossing, ocular malformation, medulloblastomas, cleft lip and/or palate, and developmental malformations have also been established as features of the syndrome [5–7].

The pathogenesis of GGS is attributed to be the consequence of abnormalities in the *PTCH* gene. The loss of human patched gene (PTCH1 gene), a tumor suppressor gene, forms the molecular basis of the syndrome [8]. This gene is significant for embryonic structuring and cellular cycle, thus its mutation leads to the development of the disease including neoplasms. The syndrome exhibits abnormalities similar to those seen in people exposed for long periods to UV radiation. Several different mutations of the PTCH1 gene have also been identified in patients with GGS [2, 3].

It is important to establish an earlier diagnosis to prevent fatal consequences, due to multiple skin cancers and other tumors associated with the syndrome [8]. Furthermore, our case emphasizes the role of the dentist in recognizing

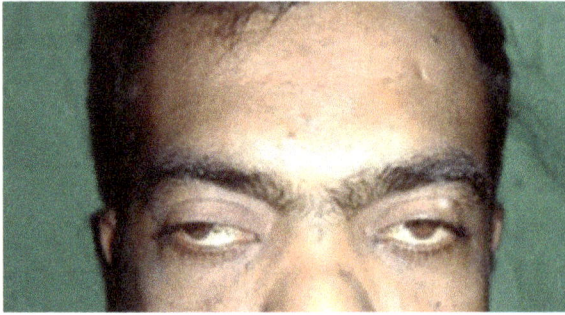

FIGURE 1: Broad nasal bridge.

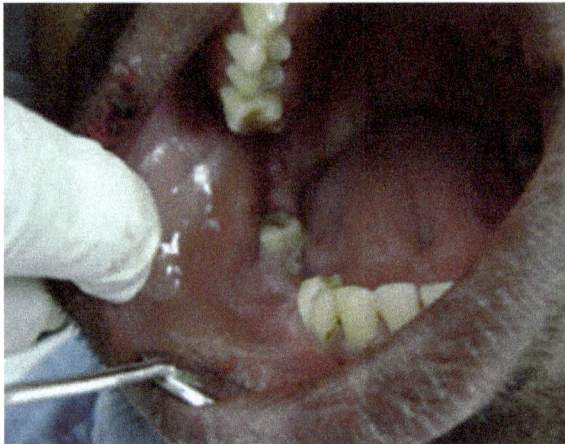

FIGURE 2: Intraoral swelling in relation to 46, 45.

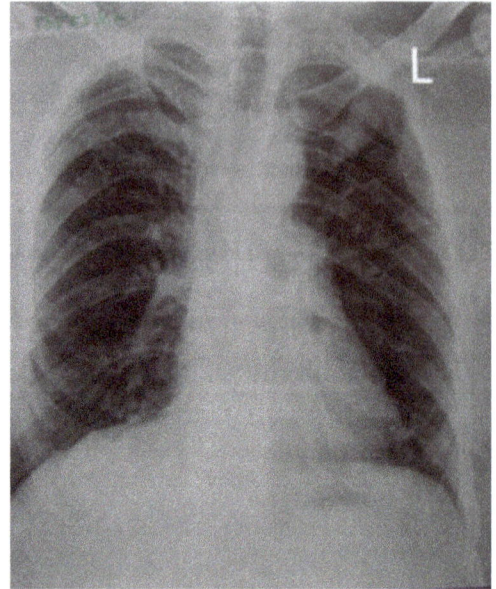

FIGURE 3: Bifid rib right 4th and 8th rib anteriorly.

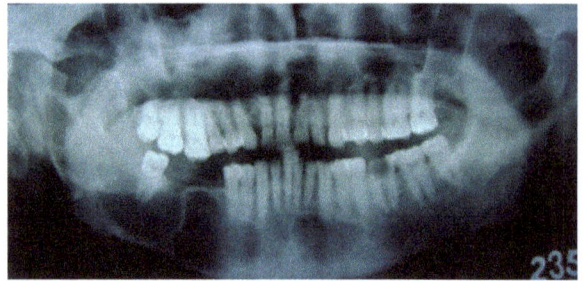

FIGURE 4: Panoramic radiograph showing cystic lesions in the mandible.

these features in order to arrive at an early diagnosis and a multidisciplinary approach in treating the condition.

2. Case Report

A 38-year-old male patient reported to the OPD of our department with a chief compliant of swelling in the right lower back tooth region since 3 months and gave a history of extraction with respect to 46 and 47 (carious teeth) 7 months ago. This was followed by persistent pus discharge from the region of extraction. Three months back he was referred to a hospital but was refused treatment owing to medical risk (Asthmatic). In the meanwhile the swelling had not increased in size and had no associated pain or discomfort. There was h/o regular discharge of creamy viscous fluid from the gingival sulcus of adjacent teeth.

Patient was a known case of asthma for which he was undergoing treatment. Patient was asked for CVS, hematologic, neurological abnormalities, and for allergies with no relevant history. Personal history was insignificant, but family history revealed his 9-year-old daughter had similar bilateral mandibular swelling, but no further investigations had been done. Extraoral examination revealed an increased fronto-occipital circumference of the head (57 cm), frontal bossing, hypertelorism, and strabismus with the right eye (Figure 1). Intraoral examination of the right posterior

mandibular region in relation to 44, 45, and 46 showed a diffuse solitary swelling measuring 2 × 4 cm in size which was soft and fluctuant in consistency (Figure 2).

On OPG 3 cystic lesions were seen in the mandible with the apical regions of 33, 34, 35, 44, 45, and 48. Both the condylar and coronoid processes on the right side were deformed in comparison to those of the left side (Figure 4). The maxillary alveolar bone in relation to the apical regions of 14, 15, and 16 showed a diffuse area of mixed radiolucent and radiopaque lesion with ground glass appearance. Chest radiograph showed bifid right 4th and 8th rib anteriorly (normal variant) (Figure 3). CT scan of the brain showed lamellar calcification along the falx and tentorium (Figure 5). A mottled appearance in the skull vault was seen in the parietal region bilaterally. CT scan of the face revealed an enlargement of the right mandible with two osteolytic lesions (Figure 6) and ground glass appearance of the marrow with calcific densities within. Aspiration was performed with the mandibular lesion and showed a cheesy fluid which was sent for histopathological evaluation.

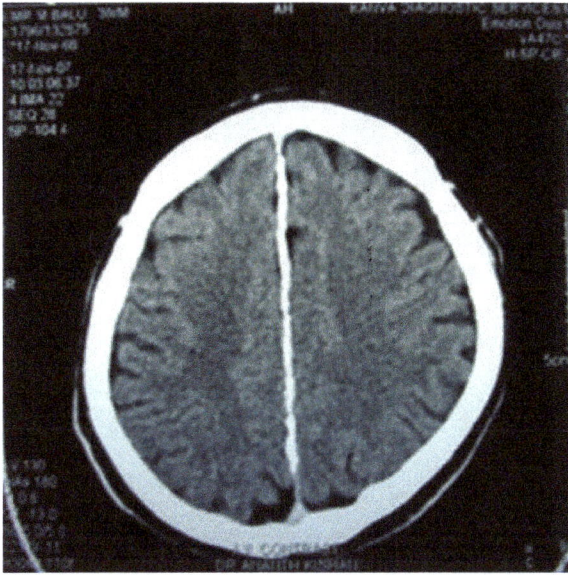

FIGURE 5: Axial CT of brain showing calcification of falx cerebri.

Based on the patient's history, clinical findings, and radiological findings a provision diagnosis of Gorlin-Goltz syndrome was given. Differential diagnosis of Bazex Syndrome and Torre's syndrome was given. The patient later underwent enucleation of the cystic lesions of both the maxilla and the mandible, with primary closure. The specimens were sent for histopathological evaluation which confirmed the diagnosis of multiple odontogenic cysts.

The final diagnosis of Gorlin-Goltz syndrome with fibrous dysplasia of the skull bones was reached.

3. Discussion

In the case of GGS it is important to make an early diagnosis as these patients show increased propensity to multiple malignant neoplasms and are also sensitive to ionizing radiation including UV radiation [3]. Patients' undergoing regular and detailed checkups can reduce the severity of complications, such as malignant skin, brain tumors, and maxillofacial deformities due to odontogenic keratocysts.

Diagnosis is based upon established major and minor clinical and radiological criteria and is ideally confirmed by DNA analysis [8]. The diagnostic criteria for nevoid basal cell carcinoma, established by Evans et al. and modified by Kimonis et al. in 1997, state that when two major or one major and two minor criteria should be present for diagnosis, as described below [3–9].

(I) Major Criteria

(i) More than two basal cell carcinomas or one basal cell carcinoma at younger than 30 years of age or more than 10 basal cell nevi.

(ii) Any odontogenic keratocyst (proven on histology) or polyostotic bone cyst.

(iii) Three or more palmar or plantar pits (present in about 65% of patients).

(iv) Bifid, fused, or markedly splayed ribs.

(v) Ectopic calcification: lamellar or early at younger than 20 years of age.

(vi) Falx cerebri calcification.

(vii) Positive family history of nevoid basal cell carcinoma.

Some authors take plurilamellar appearance of the falx cerebri calcification as a pathognomonic symptom of Gorlin-Goltz syndrome.

(II) Minor Criteria

(i) Macrocephaly determined after adjustment with height.

(ii) Skeletal anomalies: hemivertebrae, scoliosis, syndactyly, polydactyly, and shortened 4th metacarpal.

(iii) Radiological abnormalities like bridging of sella turcica, vertebral anomalies, and modelling defect of hands and feet.

(iv) Medulloblastoma.

(v) Ovarian Fibroma.

(vi) Congenital malformations: cleft lip or palate, polydactylism or eye anomalies (cataract, coloboma, and microphthalmus).

In the above case, two major criteria (odontogenic keratocysts of the jaw and calcification of falx cerebri and tentorium) and one minor (skeletal anomalies (bifid rib)) were detected, suggesting that the patient had GGS.

Appropriate management depends on early recognition of the disease, a detailed family history, and a thorough evaluation of signs and symptoms. A multidisciplinary approach team consisting of various specialists is required for a successful treatment.

Treatment involves removal of tumors by surgical excision, laser ablation, photodynamic therapy, or topical chemotherapy, while radiotherapy is a contraindication. Chemoprevention involves use of vitamin A analogs. Recurrent odontogenic cysts (up to 60% of cases) require repeated surgical excisions. 5–10% of the patients may develop brain medulloblastoma, a potential cause of early death, thus requiring intervention by a neurologist. Though survival in Gorlin-Goltz patients is not affected significantly, morbidity from complications can be considerable. Nowadays gene mutation analysis, if feasible, can confirm diagnosis. Antenatal diagnosis is possible with ultrasound scans and DNA analysis. Thus, a genetic counsellor is of importance in the ongoing care of the patient [8, 10].

A new treatment strategy, based on the understanding of the Hh signaling pathway and the premise that tumors arise due to its overactivity, supposes that inhibition of this pathway with specific pharmacological treatment might suppress tumor growth [3, 11].

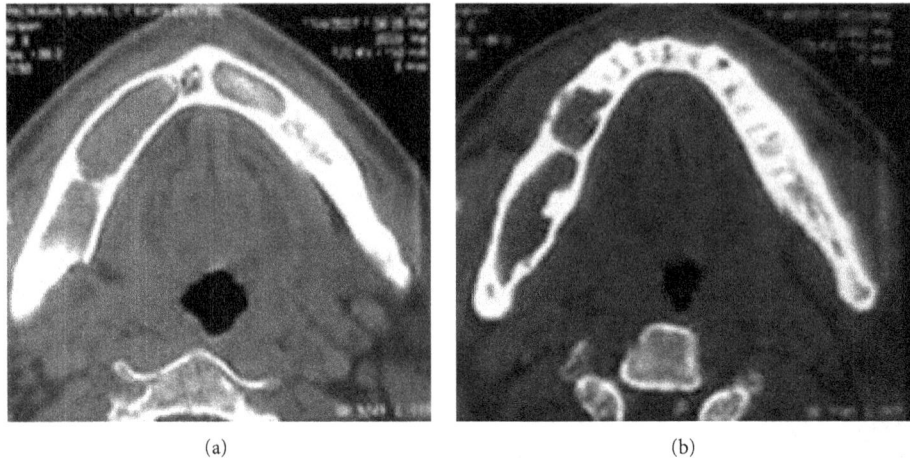

(a)   (b)

FIGURE 6: CT scan showing cystic lesions of body and condyle of the mandible.

4. Conclusion

The case illustrates the need for awareness of the syndrome among dentists in relation to younger age patients with no lesions of the skin. Proper evaluation and characterization of clinical features are essential for the correct diagnosis and management. Ongoing surveillance as well as treatment for sequelae of Gorlin-Goltz syndrome (GGS) requires regular followups (3-4 times a year or more) to detect new odontogenic cysts and basal cell carcinomas that occur continuously [8, 10, 11]. This, along with genetic counseling in family members of patients with GGS, as in the above case who has a daughter with related symptoms, in whom the diagnosis is possible but not confirmed, helps to detect necessary diagnostic criteria and thus improves their survival through well-directed treatment.

References

[1] A. R. Casaroto, D. C. N. Rocha Loures, E. Moreschi et al., "Early diagnosis of Gorlin-Goltz syndrome: case report," *Head and Face Medicine*, vol. 7, no. 1, article 2, 2011.

[2] I. Yordanova, D. Gospodinov, V. Kirov, V. Pavlova, and G. Radoslavova, "A familial case of gorlin-goltz syndrome," *Journal of IMAB*, vol. 13, no. 1, pp. 59–63, 2007.

[3] M. Ljubenovi, D. Ljubenovi, I. Bini, D. Jovanovi, and M. Stanojevi, "Gorlin-Goltz syndrome," *Acta Dermatoven APA*, vol. 16, no. 4, pp. 166–169, 2007.

[4] A. O. G. de Amezaga, O. G. Arregui, S. Z. Nuño, A. A. Sagredo, and J. M. A. Urizar, "Gorlin-Goltz syndrome: clinicopathologic aspects," *Medicina Oral, Patologia Oral y Cirugia Bucal*, vol. 13, no. 6, pp. E338–E343, 2008.

[5] L. Lo Muzio, "Nevoid basal cell carcinoma syndrome (Gorlin syndrome)," *Orphanet Journal of Rare Diseases*, vol. 3, no. 1, article 32, 2008.

[6] V. E. Kimonis, A. M. Goldstein, B. Pastakia et al., "Clinical manifestations in 105 persons with nevoid basal cell carcinoma syndrome," *American Journal of Medical Genetics*, vol. 69, pp. 299–308, 1997.

[7] N. Santana, B. K. Yashodha Devi, and D. Jatti, "Gorlin Goltz syndrome—a case report," *Journal of the Indian Dental Association*, vol. 5, no. 4, p. 521, 2011.

[8] C. Kalogeropoulou, P. Zampakis, S. Kazantzi, P. Kraniotis, and N. S. Mastronikolis, "Gorlin-Goltz syndrome: incidental finding on routine ct scan following car accident," *Cases Journal*, vol. 2, no. 11, article 9087, 2009.

[9] L. Chandra Shekar, R. Sathish, S. Beena, and S. Ganeshan, "Gorlin Goltz syndrome," *Journal of Dental Sciences and Research*, vol. 2, no. 2, pp. 1–5.

[10] P. Garg, F. Karjodkar, and S. K. Garg, "Gorlin-Goltz Syndrome—Case Report," http://www.jcdr.net/.

[11] B. Daniel, Nevoid Basal Cell Carcinoma Syndrome, Follow up [Internet], 2010, http://emedicine.medscape.com/article/1101196-follow-up.

21

Plasmablastic Lymphoma of Gingiva Mimicking a Reactive Lesion

Neeta Bagul, G. S. Mamatha, and Aditi Mahalle

Department of Oral Pathology and Microbiology, Dr. D. Y. Patil Dental College and Hospital, Pimpri, Pune 411018, India

Correspondence should be addressed to Neeta Bagul, neeta.bagul@gmail.com

Academic Editors: R. S. Brown, I. El-Hakim, and M. Manfredi

Oral plasmablastic lymphoma (PBL) is a rare malignancy, associated with HIV or other immunocompromised conditions. The lesion constituted a new subtype of diffuse large B-cell lymphoma and proposed a distinct entity based on its basic morphology, its clinical behaviour involving predominantly extramedullary sites (particularly oral cavity), and its limited antigenic phenotype data suggesting plasmacytic differentiation. Authors here report a case of apparently healthy individual aged 35 years, presenting one-month history of swelling associated with loosened teeth around upper anteriors. Following incisional biopsy, routine histopathologic and immunohistochemical studies, the diagnosis of plasmablastic lymphoma was given.

1. Introduction

Plasmablastic lymphoma is a unique AIDS-related lymphoma, which was first described in the jaws and oral cavity of HIV-infected persons [1, 2]. The disease accounts for 2.6% of all HIV-related non-Hodgkin lymphomas [3]. The lymphoma has also been reported in HIV-negative persons, particularly those who have immunosuppression. The lymphoma is listed in the World Health Organization 2001 classification as a variant of diffuse large B-cell lymphoma [4].

It usually develops in middle-aged adults [4], but can also occur in the pediatric age group [5]. The lymphoma involves predominantly the gingival and palatal mucosa, causing thickening and ulceration with a tendency to infiltrate adjacent bone [3]. The clinical appearance may mimic periodontal disease, Kaposi sarcoma, or melanoma [6]. Radiographic changes include widening of the periodontal ligament space and loss of the lamina dura [7].

Plasmablastic lymphoma of oral mucosa contains a monomorphic population of plasmablasts with no or minimal plasmacytic differentiation. The histological findings of a diffuse infiltrative growth pattern, brisk mitotic activity, and necrosis, along with the fact that they are rapidly growing destructive tumors, supports their designation as a high-grade malignant lymphoma.

Plasmablasts are lymphoid cells that morphologically resemble B-cell immunoblasts but have acquired a plasma cell immunophenotype (i.e., loss of B-cell markers and surface immunoglobulin with the acquisition of plasma cell surface markers). Thus, unlike immunoblasts, plasmablasts fail to express CD45 (leukocyte common antigen) as well as the B-cell marker CD20 and are only variably immunoreactive for CD79a—a broader-spectrum B-cell marker. They are also negative for pan-T-cell markers. Positive staining for plasma cell markers such as VS38c, CD38, MUM-1, and CD138 indicates a phenotype akin to plasma cells [8, 9]. Newer B-lineage markers (e.g., OCT.2 and BOB.1) may prove useful in determining a B-cell origin in plasmablastic lymphomas [10, 11].

Treatment includes radiotherapy, chemotherapy, surgery, or a combination of these modalities. The lymphoma is known to be rapidly progressive with a poor prognosis for persons with HIV/AIDS, with a median survival of 6 months. After the institution of highly active antiretroviral therapy, an increase in survival time has been noticed [12–14].

2. Case Report

A 35-year-old, apparently healthy individual reported to the Department of Oral Pathology complaining of a painless

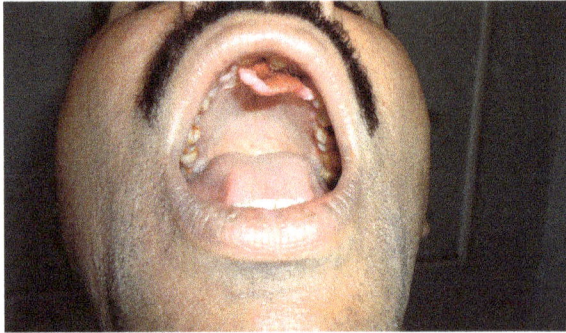

Figure 1: Exophytic gingival growth in the maxillary anterior palatal region.

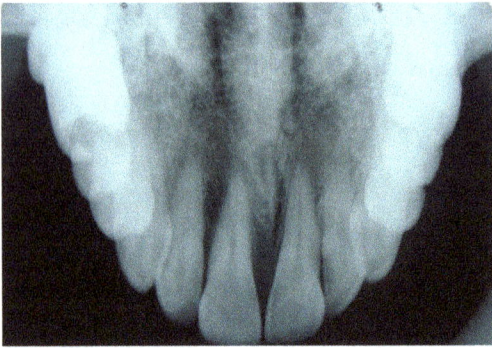

Figure 2: Interdental bone loss in relation to maxillary central and lateral incisors.

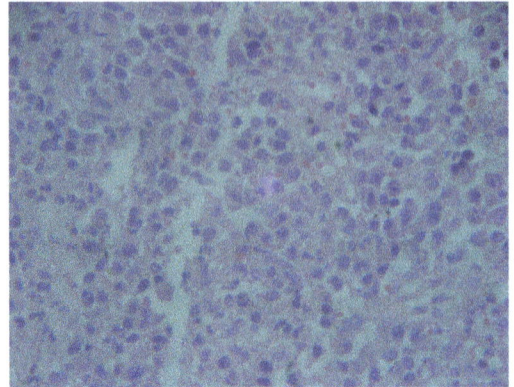

Figure 3: Diffuse large lymphoid cells with abundant eosinophilic cytoplasm, centrally or few eccentrically placed nuclei, and pleomorphic basophilic nucleoli ($\times 40$).

growth in the upper jaw since 1 month that gradually grew in size. No other symptoms were reported before the onset of the swelling. The patient did not notice loosening of the teeth associated with the growth. Extraorally no abnormalities were detected There was no history of trauma or spontaneous bleeding. The patient did not give a history of tobacco smoking, alcohol consumption, or drug use.

Intraoral hard tissue examination revealed an exophytic, lobulated mass, irregular in consistency, in the maxillary palatal aspect extending from the right maxillary lateral incisor to the left maxillary first premolar region. Ulcerated growth was noted with the palatal aspect of 11, 12, 21, and 22. The growth was soft in consistency, and bleeding on probing was evident (Figure 1).

Routine haematological examinations were carried out which revealed normal numbers of red blood cells and white blood cells. Platelet count was also within normal limits. The HIV status of the patient was negative.

The radiographic investigations included occlusal and intraoral periapical radiography of the anterior part of the upper jaw which revealed interdental bone loss with 11, 21 and 21, 22 (Figure 2).

An incisional biopsy of intraoral mass was performed. Histopathological examination of haematoxylin and eosin stained section showed covering of parakeratinized stratified squamous epithelium with ulceration at places. There was no evidence of dysplasia in the epithelium. Underlying connective tissue stroma revealed diffusely arranged large round tumor cells. Majority of the tumor cells showed open face nuclei with prominent nucleoli, while few others showed eccentric nuclei (Figure 3). The distribution of nucleoli was located either in the center or peripherally near the nuclear membrane. Admixed among these tumor cells, macrophages were also seen. On immunohistochemical analysis, tumor cells were positive for LCA, CD-138, and CD-56 (Figures 4(a), 4(b), and 4(c)) and negative for CD20, CD30, ALK1, Cyclin D1, and EMA.

3. Discussion

Non-Hodgkin's lymphoma finds its mention in oral manifestations of HIV/AIDS for the first time in Pindborg's classification [15], and plasmablastic lymphoma was first described by Delecluse et al. in 1997 [1]. Originally it was described to be a disease specifically involving the oral cavity of immunodeficient patients, but, number of cases have been reported in various extraoral sites including nasopharynx, stomach, small bowel, anus, lungs, skin, and so forth. Some of the cases are even reported in immunocompetent patients [16].

Oral NHL may appear as swelling, ulceration, exophytic masses, delayed healing of extraction sites, or trigeminal neuropathy. Recognition of this distinctive type of lymphoma confined to gingiva is important to avoid confusion with other gingival enlargements as PBL may mimic benign/reactive gingival enlargements like pyogenic granuloma and peripheral giant cell granuloma [17].

Thus, it is imperative to include PBL in the differential diagnosis of solitary gingival enlargement, as seen in our case.

The morphological hallmark of plasmablastic lymphoma is diffuse submucosal proliferation of monomorphic large-sized tumor cells with deep ulceration of the overlying mucosa. The tumor cells typically demonstrate high nuclear-cytoplasmic ratio, moderate amount of amphophilic, or basophilic cytoplasm with squared or rounded borders and centrally or eccentrically placed round nucleus with smooth nuclear outlines [18]. Plasmablasts are a type of lymphoid cells that have retained the morphology of an immunoblast

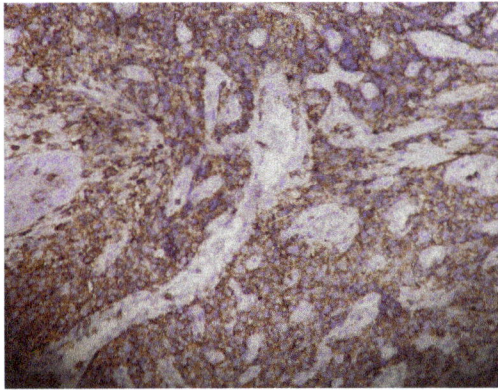

(a) Tumor cells expressing strong positivity for LCA (×40)

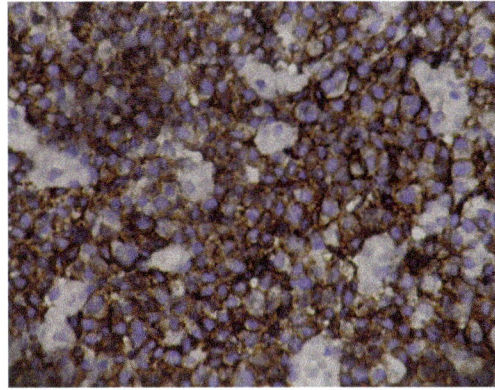

(b) Tumor cells expressing strong positivity for CD 138 (×40)

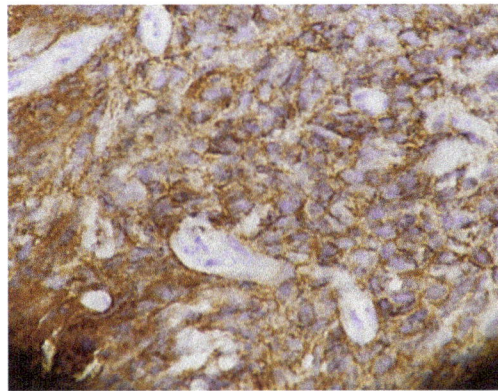

(c) Tumor cells expressing strong positivity for CD 56 (×40)

FIGURE 4

but have already acquired the immunophenotype of a plasma cell [1]. Plasmablastic lymphoma may show plasma cells, but these are always reactive in nature and never neoplastic. Morphologically, a neoplastic plasma cell population is characterized by an intimate admixture of mature plasma cells with varying proportion of bi/multinucleated pleomorphic and immature plasma cells at all stages of maturity forming a sort of morphological continuum [2].

Kane et al. proposed minimum morphological criteria to diagnose plasmablastic lymphoma which includes the following. Predominant population of plasmablasts which are large monomorphic cells with high nuclear: cytoplasm ratio, moderate amount of amphophilic cytoplasm, and round nucleus with prominent central nucleolus; high mitotic and/or apoptotic index; absence of neoplastic plasma cells in the background [18].

PBL patients have been treated heterogeneously, and well-defined guidelines are lacking. Chemotherapy, radiotherapy with or without surgical excision, has been reported with various degrees of success [19, 20].

The prognosis of PBL is reported to be poor with or without treatment, and death is predicted in 1–24 months with average survival time of 6 months, though it has been suggested that addition of highly active antiretroviral therapy (HAART), chemotherapy is capable of significantly improving the prognosis [20].

4. Summary

In conclusion, this paper has detailed the case of plasmablastic lymphoma clinically mimicking a reactive lesion of gingiva; PBL should be considered in differential diagnosis of gingival enlargements. Patients with gingival enlargements are seen very commonly in daily clinical practice, but to differentiate neoplastic lesions from nonneoplastic/reactive lesions is essential in treating planning. Biopsy of these gingival enlargements, histopathological examination, and immunohistochemical analysis will aid in accurate diagnosis and treatment. Patient was referred to the higher centre after the final diagnosis.

Acknowledgment

The authors would like to thank Medilinkers Research Consultancy for their guidance in the preparation of the paper.

References

[1] H. J. Delecluse, I. Anagnostopoulos, F. Dallenbach et al., "Plasmablastic lymphomas of the oral cavity: a new entity associated with the human immunodeficiency virus infection," *Blood*, vol. 89, no. 4, pp. 1413–1420, 1997.

[2] A. Carbone, A. Gloghini, V. Canzonieri, U. Tirelli, and G. Gaidano, "AIDS-related extranodal non-Hodgkin's lymphomas with plasma cell differentiation," *Blood*, vol. 90, no. 3, pp. 1337–1338, 1997.

[3] G. S. Folk, S. L. Abbondanzo, E. L. Childers, and R. D. Foss, "Plasmablastic lymphoma: a clinicopathologic correlation," *Annals of Diagnostic Pathology*, vol. 10, no. 1, pp. 8–12, 2006.

[4] E. S. Jaffe, N. L. Harris, H. Stein, and J. W. Vardiman, *World Health Organization WHO Classification of Tumours, Pathology and Genetics of Tumours of Haematopoietic and Lymphoid Tissue*, IARC Press, Lyon, France, 2001.

[5] R. Radhakrishnan, S. Suhas, R. V. Kumar, G. Krishnanand, R. Srinivasan, and N. N. Rao, "Plasmablastic lymphoma of the oral cavity in an HIV-positive child," *Oral Surgery, Oral Medicine, Oral Pathology, Oral Radiology and Endodontology*, vol. 100, no. 6, pp. 725–731, 2005.

[6] J. B. Epstein, R. J. Cabay, and M. Glick, "Oral malignancies in HIV disease: changes in disease presentation, increasing understanding of molecular pathogenesis, and current management," *Oral Surgery, Oral Medicine, Oral Pathology, Oral Radiology and Endodontology*, vol. 100, no. 5, pp. 571–578, 2005.

[7] I. Hewson, "Oral plasmablastic lymphoma: a case report," *Australian Dental Journal*, vol. 56, no. 3, pp. 328–330, 2011.

[8] S. A. Jaffar, G. Pihan, B. J. Dezube, and L. Pantanowitz, "Differentiating HIV-associated lymphomas that exhibit plasmacellular differentiation," *HIV and AIDS Review*, vol. 4, no. 3, pp. 43–49, 2005.

[9] A. Carbone, A. Gloghini, L. M. Larocca et al., "Expression profile of MUM1/IRF4, BCL-6, and CD138/syndecan-1 defines novel histogenetic subsets of human immunodeficiency virus-related lymphomas," *Blood*, vol. 97, no. 3, pp. 744–751, 2001.

[10] L. Colomo, F. Loong, S. Rives et al., "Diffuse large B-cell lymphomas with plasmablastic differentiation represent a heterogeneous group of disease entities," *American Journal of Surgical Pathology*, vol. 28, no. 6, pp. 736–747, 2004.

[11] R. Chetty, N. Hlatswayo, R. Muc, R. Sabaratnam, and K. Gatter, "Plasmablastic lymphoma in HIV+ patients: an expanding spectrum," *Histopathology*, vol. 42, no. 6, pp. 605–609, 2003.

[12] N. A. Hessol, S. Pipkin, S. Schwarcz, R. D. Cress, P. Bacchetti, and S. Scheer, "The impact of highly active antiretroviral therapy on non-AIDS-defining cancers among adults with AIDS," *American Journal of Epidemiology*, vol. 165, no. 10, pp. 1143–1153, 2007.

[13] S. D. Nasta, G. M. Carrum, I. Shahab, N. A. Hanania, and M. M. Udden, "Regression of a plasmablastic lymphoma in a patient with HIV on highly active antiretroviral therapy," *Leukemia and Lymphoma*, vol. 43, no. 2, pp. 423–426, 2002.

[14] R. Lester, C. H. Li, P. Phillips et al., "Improved outcome of human immunodeficiency virus-associated plasmablastic lymphoma of the oral cavity in the era of highly active antiretroviral therapy: a report of two cases," *Leukemia and Lymphoma*, vol. 45, no. 9, pp. 1881–1885, 2004.

[15] J. J. Pindborg, "Classification of oral lesions associated with HIV infection," *Oral Surgery Oral Medicine and Oral Pathology*, vol. 67, no. 3, pp. 292–295, 1989.

[16] C. Cattaneo, F. Facchetti, A. Re et al., "Oral cavity lymphomas in immunocompetent and human immunodeficiency virus infected patients," *Leukemia and Lymphoma*, vol. 46, no. 1, pp. 77–81, 2005.

[17] R. S. Desai, S. S. Vanaki, R. S. Puranik, G. Giraddi, and R. V. Pujari, "Plasmablastic lymphoma presenting as a gingival growth in a previously undiagnosed HIV-positive patient: a case report," *Journal of Oral and Maxillofacial Surgery*, vol. 65, no. 7, pp. 1358–1361, 2007.

[18] S. Kane, A. Khurana, G. Parulkar et al., "Minimum diagnostic criteria for plasmablastic lymphoma of oral/sinonasal region encountered in a tertiary cancer hospital of a developing country," *Journal of Oral Pathology and Medicine*, vol. 38, no. 1, pp. 138–144, 2009.

[19] P. Rafaniello Raviele, G. Pruneri, and E. Maiorano, "Plasmablastic lymphoma: a review," *Oral Diseases*, vol. 15, no. 1, pp. 38–45, 2009.

[20] S. C. Sarode, G. A. Zarkar, R. S. Desai, V. S. Sabane, and M. A. Kulkarni, "Plasmablastic lymphoma of the oral cavity in an HIV-positive patient: a case report and review of literature," *International Journal of Oral and Maxillofacial Surgery*, vol. 38, no. 9, pp. 993–999, 2009.

22

Recurrent Giant Pilomatrixoma of the Face

Mohammed Nadershah,[1] Ahmad Alshadwi,[2] and Andrew Salama[3]

[1] *Department of Oral and Maxillofacial Surgery, Boston Medical Center, Boston University, 850 Harrison Avenue, Boston, MA 02118, USA*
[2] *Oral and Maxillofacial Surgery Department, Boston Medical Center, Boston University, 100 East Newton street, Boston, MA 02118, USA*
[3] *Boston Medical Center, Boston University, 850 Harrison Avenue, Boston, MA 02118, USA*

Correspondence should be addressed to Mohammed Nadershah, mnadershah@gmail.com

Academic Editors: M. Manfredi, G. Sammartino, and E. F. Wright

Pilomatrixoma, also known as pilomatricoma, is a benign tumor that originates from the matrix of the hair root. It usually presents as a single, slow-growing subcutaneous or intradermal firm nodule with a general size of less than 3 centimeters (cm) in diameter. However, giant pilomatrixomas (more than 5 cm) have been reported infrequently. It is more common in females and usually presents during the first two decades of life (60%) as an asymptomatic, mobile, hard, elastic mass. Most of the cases are benign and affect the face. The authors report a rare case of a giant pilomatricoma of the cheek and discuss the surgical management of these lesions, histopathological findings, and review of the literature.

1. Introduction

Pilomatrixoma, also known as pilomatricoma or calcifying epithelioma of Malherbe, was first described in 1880 by Malherbe and Chenantais [1]. In 1961, Forbis and Helwig proposed the term pilomatrixoma to emphasize the lesion origin, the matrix of the hair root [2]. pilomatrixoma is a benign skin neoplasm that usually presents as a single, slow-growing subcutaneous or intradermal firm nodule with a general size of less than 3 centimeters (cm) in diameter. However, giant pilomatrixomas (more than 5 cm) have been reported infrequently. It is more common in females and usually presents during the first two decades of life (60%) as an asymptomatic, mobile, hard, elastic mass. Most of the cases are benign and affect the face [3, 4]. We report a rare case of a giant pilomatricoma of the cheek and discuss the surgical management of these lesions, histopathological findings, and review of the literature.

2. Case Report

A 28-year-old male was referred to the department of oral and maxillofacial surgery for evaluation and management of a left facial mass. He had no other medical problems and no known food or drug allergies. At the age of 15 years, he noticed a mass on his left cheek eminence, which was excised and was told that it was a sebaceous cyst. Three years later, he had a local recurrence of the facial mass that was surgically excised again showing the same pathology. A third recurrence in the same area occurred 4 years later and was excised with the overlying skin. However, at this time the pathology specimen proved to be pilomatrixoma. The mass recurred again few years later and has been growing slowly over the past 3 years prior to presentation.

Clinical examination of the face showed a firm, non-tender mass infiltrating the overlying skin of the left buccal subunit measuring about 5 × 3 cm. The overlaying skin had bluish discoloration (Figure 1). There was no limitation of the mandibular range of motion. Cranial nerve exam was grossly intact. The neck was supple with no palpable masses or cervical lymphadenopathy. Intraoral exam was unremarkable.

Another incisional biopsy was done under local anesthesia, which confirmed the diagnosis and ruled out malignant transformation. A contrast enhanced magnetic resonance

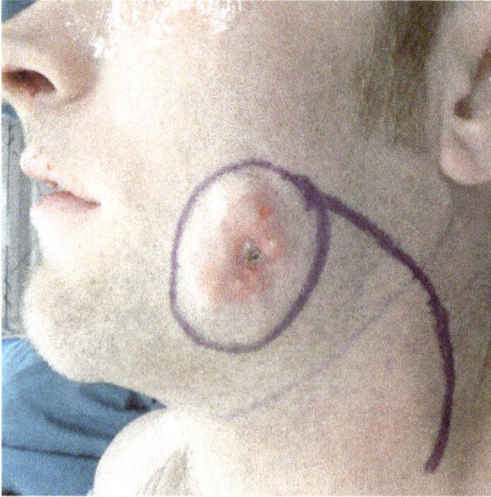

FIGURE 1: Clinical view of the lesion with calcified portion protruding from the central part of the lesion.

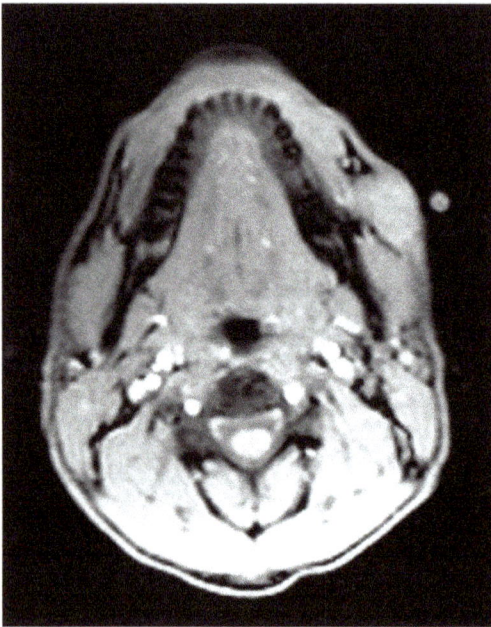

FIGURE 2: Axial view of a T2 magnetic resonance image at the level of the mandible showing a heterogeneous mass on the left side of the face with no evidence of deep invasion.

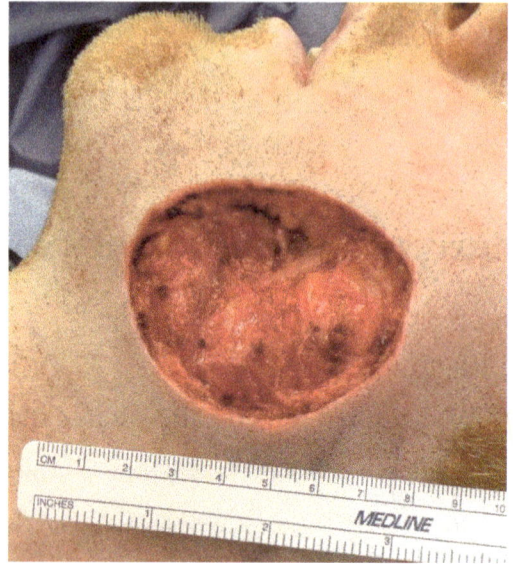

FIGURE 3: Intraoperative picture of the surgical defect measuring about 5×6 cm.

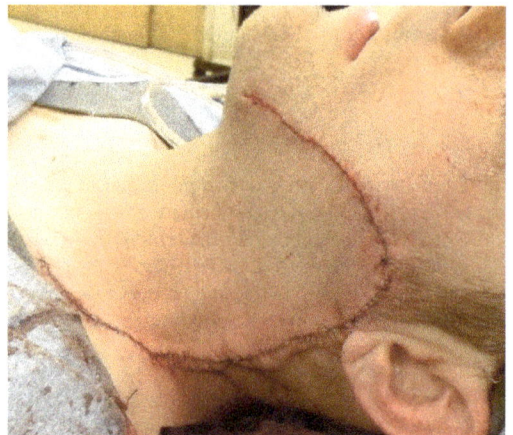

FIGURE 4: The surgical defect was reconstructed with cervicofacial advancement flap.

imaging (MRI) study showed a heterogeneously enhancing mass in the subcutaneous tissues overlying the left platysma muscle at the level of the mandible (Figure 2). The adjacent musculature and bone marrow maintained their normal signal intensity. The mass was surgically excised including the overlying skin with a safety margin of 1 cm. About 6×5 cm skin was marked over the pilomatrixoma and was included in the specimen. The incision was carried through the skin, subcutaneous tissues, and the superficial musculoaponeurotic system (SMAS). The buccal and marginal mandibular branches of the left facial nerve were

identified and preserved. The resulting cheek defect measured about 6×5 cm (Figure 3) and was reconstructed using a cervicofacial flap (Figure 4). Postoperatively, the patient recovered well without any appreciable facial nerve deficits or wound complications. He had no evidence of disease recurrence in his one-year follow up.

3. Histopathologic Findings

Pilomatrixomas appear as well-demarcated, lobulated lesions situated in the dermis or subcutaneous tissue. The tumor is composed of ghost cells, basaloid cells, and giant cell, in addition to keratin debris and intracellular and stromal calcifications (Figure 5) [5]. Uncommon histological features include pigmentation, transepidermal elimination, and

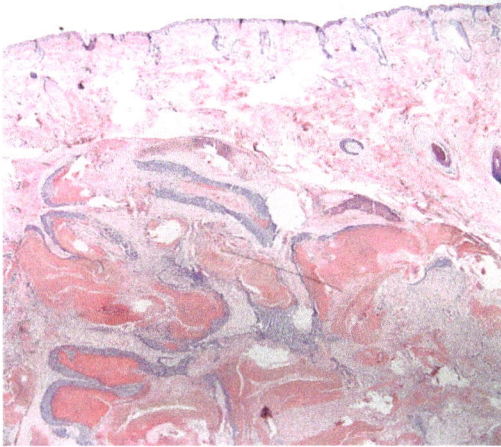

FIGURE 5: Low magnification H&E stained histopathological slide showing islands of epithelial cells with areas of calcification.

aggressiveness with infiltrative growth pattern [6]. Malignant transformation is rare [7, 8].

4. Discussion

Pilomatrixoma is an unusual neoplasm of hair germ matrix origin. Head and neck pilomatrixoma represent 50% of the reported cases with the cervical, frontal, temporal, eyelids, and preauricular regions being the most frequent locations [3]. A female predominance has been reported with a male : female ratio of 2 : 3, and the vast majority of patients in the literature are Caucasian [3]. There has been association between multiple lesions with Gardner syndrome, myotonic dystrophy, and Turner's syndrome [9, 10].

Pilomatrixoma usually presents as an asymptomatic nodular single mass. The skin overlying the lesion is usually normal or may have reddish or bluish discoloration. These lesions are usually well circumscribed, spherical, or ovoid, and sometimes encapsulated. The behavior of pilomatrix carcinoma resembles that of basal cell carcinoma, but with the potential for metastasis. According to Bremnes et al., only 55 cases of pilomatrix carcinoma have been reported in the literature [8]. Rare cases of malignant pilomatrixoma with distant metastasis have been reported [11].

The diagnosis is usually established based on an incisional biopsy. However, fine needle aspiration cytology (FNAC) has been described as a preoperative diagnostic tool, but the results can be misleading and, at times, can lead to the erroneous diagnosis of a malignant neoplasm [12]. These tumors do not regress spontaneously and they require surgical excision. The surgeon should focus on preservation of the facial nerve branches that underlie the tumor without compromising adequate excision of the tumor. Few authors advised for a wide safety margin of 2 cm but this may be excessive given the rarity of malignant transformation of these tumors [13, 14]. Although this case report demonstrates multiple recurrences, pilomatrixoma has generally low recurrence rate (0–3%) [13–16]. This may

be explained by inadequate conservative excision of previous lesions due to its sensitive location. Reconstruction is best achieved using local flaps because its good color match and simplicity.

In summary, pilomatrixoma is a benign skin neoplasm that usually presents as a single, slow-growing subcutaneous or intradermal nodule. It is usually less than 3 cm and commonly affects the face. Giant pilomatrixoma (>5 cm), as in the presented case, is unusual. Malignant transformation has been reported but it is very rare. The diagnosis is established based on an incisional biopsy with questionable value of FNAC. The treatment of choice is surgical excision with a clear margin with every effort to preserve the branches of the facial nerve. Recurrence with adequate treatment is low.

Conflict of Interests

The authors declare that they have no conflict of interests.

References

[1] A. Malherbe and J. Chenantais, "Note sur l'épithélioma calcifiédes glandes sébacées," *Progressi in Medicina*, vol. 8, pp. 826–837, 1880.

[2] R. Forbis and E. B. Helwig, "Pilomatrixoma (calcifying epithelioma)," *Archives of Dermatology*, vol. 83, pp. 606–618, 1961.

[3] F. W. Moehlenbeck, "Pilomatrixoma (calcifying epithelioma). A statistical study," *Archives of Dermatology*, vol. 108, no. 4, pp. 532–534, 1973.

[4] B. Rink, "Pilomatrixoma in the oro-facial region," *International Journal of Oral and Maxillofacial Surgery*, vol. 20, no. 4, pp. 196–198, 1991.

[5] R. P. Agarwal, S. D. Handler, M. R. Matthews, and D. Carpentieri, "Pilomatrixoma of the head and neck in children," *Otolaryngology—Head and Neck Surgery*, vol. 125, no. 5, pp. 510–515, 2001.

[6] D. V. Nield, M. N. Saad, and M. H. Ali, "Aggressive pilomatrixoma in a child: a case report," *British Journal of Plastic Surgery*, vol. 39, no. 1, pp. 139–141, 1986.

[7] N. G. Mikhaeel and M. F. Spittle, "Malignant pilomatrixoma with multiple local recurrences and distant metastases: a case report and review of the literature," *Clinical Oncology*, vol. 13, no. 5, pp. 386–389, 2001.

[8] R. M. Bremnes, J. M. Kvamme, H. Stalsberg, and E. A. Jacobsen, "Pilomatrix carcinoma with multiple metastases: report of a case and review of the literature," *European Journal of Cancer*, vol. 35, no. 3, pp. 433–437, 1999.

[9] P. S. Harper, "Calcifying epithelioma of Malherbe. Association with myotonic muscular dystrophy," *Archives of Dermatology*, vol. 106, no. 1, pp. 41–44, 1972.

[10] H. Noguchi, K. Kayashima, S. Nishiyama, and T. Ono, "Two cases of pilomatrixoma in Turner's syndrome," *Dermatology*, vol. 199, no. 4, pp. 338–340, 1999.

[11] H. P. Niedermeyer, K. Peris, and H. Höfler, "Pilomatrix carcinoma with multiple visceral metastases: report of a case," *Cancer*, vol. 77, no. 7, pp. 1311–1314, 1996.

[12] L. B. Lemos and R. W. Brauchle, "Pilomatrixoma: a diagnostic pitfall in fine-needle aspiration biopsies. A review from a small county hospital," *Annals of Diagnostic Pathology*, vol. 8, no. 3, pp. 130–136, 2004.

[13] C. T. Sasaki, A. Yue, and R. Enriques, "Giant calcifying epithe-lioma," *Archives of Otolaryngology*, vol. 102, no. 12, pp. 753–755, 1976.

[14] P. Solanki, I. Ramzy, N. Durr, and D. Henkes, "Pilomatrixoma. Cytologic features with differential diagnostic considerations," *Archives of Pathology and Laboratory Medicine*, vol. 111, no. 3, pp. 294–297, 1987.

[15] C. G. Julian and P. W. Bowers, "A clinical review of 209 pilo-matricomas," *Journal of the American Academy of Dermatology*, vol. 39, no. 2, pp. 191–195, 1998.

[16] M. Y. Lan, M. C. Lan, C. Y. Ho, W. Y. Li, and C. Z. Lin, "Pilomatricoma of the head and neck: a retrospective review of 179 cases," *Archives of Otolaryngology—Head and Neck Surgery*, vol. 129, no. 12, pp. 1327–1330, 2003.

23

The Correlation between Chronic Periodontitis and Oral Cancer

Maximilian Krüger,[1] **Torsten Hansen,**[2] **Adrian Kasaj,**[3] **and Maximilian Moergel**[1]

[1] *Department of Oral and Maxillofacial Surgery-Plastic Surgery, Johannes Gutenberg University of Mainz,*
 Medical Center, Augustusplatz 2, 55131 Mainz, Germany
[2] *Institute of Pathology, University of Mainz, Medical Surgery, Langenbeckstraße 1, 55131 Mainz, Germany*
[3] *Department of Operative Dentistry and Periodontology, Johannes Gutenberg-University, Augustusplatz 2, 55131 Mainz, Germany*

Correspondence should be addressed to Maximilian Krüger; maximilian.krueger@unimedizin-mainz.de

Academic Editors: D. W. Boston, A. C. B. Delbem, and A. Milosevic

Infections are increasingly considered as potential trigger for carcinogenesis apart from risk factors like alcohol and tobacco. The discussion about human papilloma virus (HPV) in oral squamous cell carcinoma (OSCC) points at a general role of infection for the development of oral carcinomas. Furthermore, first studies describe a correlation between chronic periodontitis and OSCC, thus, characterizing chronic inflammation as being a possible trigger for OSCC. In front of this background, we present four well-documented clinical cases. All patients showed a significant anatomical relation between OSCC and clinical signs of chronic periodontitis. The interindividual differences of the clinical findings lead to different theoretical concepts: two with coincidental appearance of OSCC and chronic periodontitis and two with possible de novo development of OSCC triggered by chronic inflammation. We conclude that the activation of different inflammatory cascades by chronic periodontitis negatively affects mucosa and bone. Furthermore, the inflammatory response has the potential to activate carcinogenesis. Apart from a mere coincidental occurrence, two out of four patients give first clinical hints for a model wherein chronic periodontitis represents a potential risk factor for the development of OSCC.

1. Introduction

Squamous cell carcinoma is the most frequent malignancy in the oral cavity and with nearly 400.000 new diagnosed patients worldwide each year; it represents the sixth frequent malignant tumor. Despite multimodality approaches for the treatment comprising surgery and adjuvant chemo- and radiation therapy, the disease still has a low overall survival rate of about 50% [1, 2]. The development of new therapeutic strategies with improved treatment options or possible prevention of oral squamous cell carcinoma (OSCC) requests a substantial understanding of its etiology. The last years have revealed more detailed information about different risk factors for the development of OSCC. Important risk factors of the general accepted multistep carcinogenesis model are genetic predisposition [3], presence of premalignant lesions [4], and environmental or behavioural carcinogenic triggers, for example, the ingestion of tobacco and alcohol [5]. Recently, the influence of infection and

inflammation for cancer development has been discussed. Associations between human papilloma virus (HPV) infection and oropharyngeal carcinomas have been documented [6]. These patients are typically Caucasians, nonsmokers, nondrinkers, and one decade younger on average than people suffering from HPV negative carcinomas. Intriguingly, patients with HPV-positive oropharyngeal carcinomas had a significant better prognosis than the HPV negative collective [7, 8]. This finding might point at subtypes of infection-induced carcinomas with different clinical behaviours, thus, stressing the need of further characterization. Comparably, the predominant infection within the oral cavity is chronic periodontitis, and its role for the development of oral cancer was likewise recently discussed [9, 10]. Herein, periodontitis occurs as chronic inflammatory process characterized by specific bacteria and the loss of attached gingiva and alveolar bone, with consecutive development of periodontal pockets and loss of teeth [11]. A recently published work by Tezal et al. found the loss of bone as clinical sign for chronic periodontitis being an independent risk factor for the development of carcinoma within the oral cavity [12]. In front of this background, the case series at hand comprises four patients treated at our clinical Department for OSCC. Within these, the synopsis of clinical appearance, radiologic findings, and cross-sectional resection specimen offer an association of the carcinoma to the periodontal space with signs of chronic inflammation. The different clinical aspects are discussed comprising the available literature on this topic.

2. Case Presentations

Case 1. A 59-year-old woman presented herself with an exophytic mass of 2 cm adherent to the mandible and localized distally of tooth 36. The tooth revealed signs of chronic periodontitis with bleeding on probing, attachment loss and a 5 mm deep pocket, and significant mobility on clinical examination. Polymerase chain reaction (Micro-ident, Hain Lifescience GmbH D-72147 Nehren) (PCR) revealed an infection with *Porphyromonas gingivalis* and *Tannerella forsythia* (*red complex*). The expansion of the tumor reached from the sulcus glossoalveolaris with its center along the alveolar crest to the adjacent buccal mucosa (Figure 1). The patient reported herself to be a never smoker and never ingested alcohol. Oral hygiene habits were sufficient. No other precursor lesions like leukoplakia, erythroplakia, or signs of oral lichen planus were found on examination. The visit of our department was induced by progressive pain and increasing swelling. The preoperatively taken orthopantomography (OPTG) revealed a considerable generalized horizontal type of bone loss within the upper and the lower jaw, as also a distinct inter- and periradicular osteolytic lesion at the region of 36 (Figure 2). A both-sided selective neck dissection [13] and partial resection of the mandible followed. The clinical appearance (Figure 1) showed an exophytic mass with contact to the distal root of 36. Intriguingly, the OPTG showed no arrosion of the distal mandible but apparently an inhomogeneous radiolucency between the roots of the molar. The cross-section specimen (Figure 3) furthermore highlights the interradicular spreading of the tumor without an infiltration of cancellous bone or the distal alveolar crest. HPV status by p16 immunostaining was negative.

Taking all clinical findings together, the present case supports the hypothesis of a possible de novo development of malignancy from the interradicular periodontium.

Case 2. A 48-year-old man presented himself with a histological verified squamous cell carcinoma of the left mandible adjacent to the partially retained tooth 37 surrounded by a bony defect of 3 mm. Analysis of the bacteria (Micro-ident, Hain Lifescience GmbH D-72147 Nehren) inside the pocket showed an infection with *Peptostreptococcus micros* and *Fusobacterium nucleatum* (*orange complex*) as well as *Eikenella corrodens* and *Capnocytophaga* sp. (*green complex*). The patient reported recurring inflammation in the left lower quadrant for a period of six weeks. Prior to the planned osteotomy of the wisdom tooth, the dentist had taken a scalpel biopsy, giving evidence for OSCC. Clinical examination revealed an ulcerous lesion with dominant signs

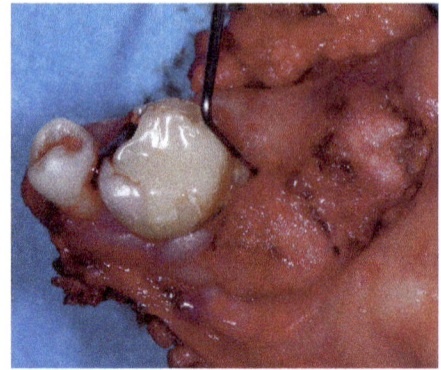

FIGURE 1: Case 1—resection specimen of the mandible. The probe reveals the loss of clinical attachment within the periodontal space, and the tumor seems to emerge from the periodontal compartment.

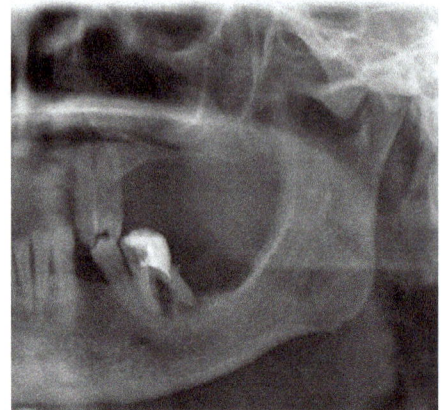

FIGURE 2: Case 1—the preoperative OPTG exhibits severe horizontal and vertical bone loss of the jaws. In addition, peri- and interradicular osteolytic lesions around tooth 36 are present. A soft radiopacity as projection of the tumor mass can be identified along the intact alveolar crest distal of 36. Radiolucency, suspect for bone invasion is solely present at the interradicular and distal aspect of the roots.

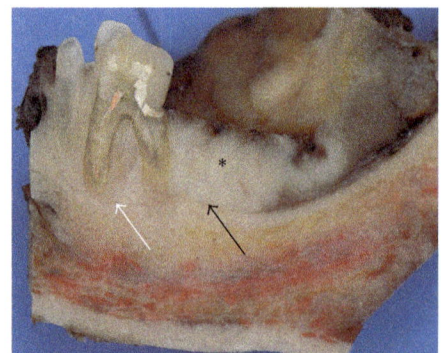

FIGURE 3: Case 1—cross section specimen. The black arrow highlights the close relation of the distal root to the tumor mass (∗) with preserved cortical bone distal to the tooth. The white arrow points at a tumor formation along the mesial root filling out the interradicular space.

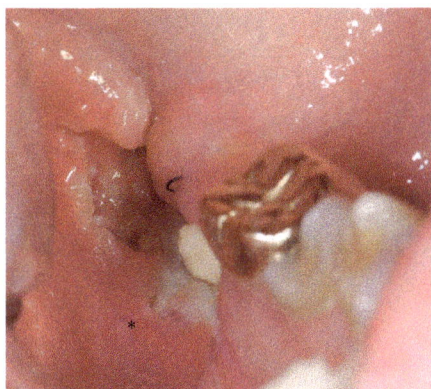

FIGURE 4: Case 2—the clinical aspect consists of a fibrin-coated ulcer in region of the wisdom tooth at the left lower mandible. The adjacent mucosa shows perifocal signs of inflammation (∗).

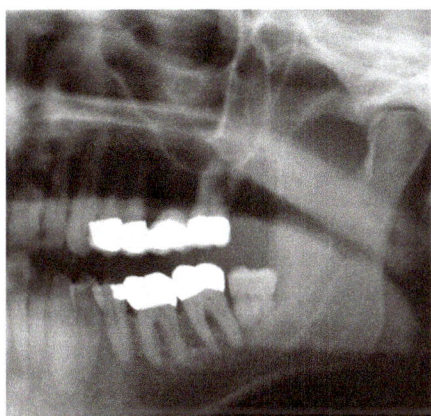

FIGURE 5: Case 2—Preoperative OPTG—A large formation of enhanced translucency is found in projection of the radices 36 and 37 as also at the pericoronal aspect of the partially retained wisdom tooth.

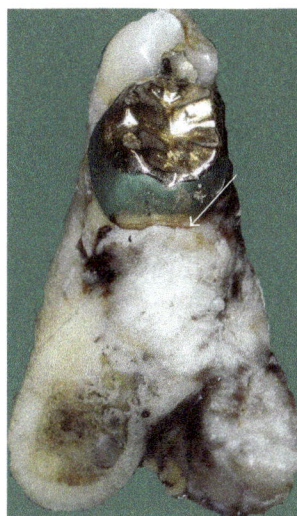

FIGURE 6: Case 2—cross section specimen with a sectional view from distal after removal of the bony aspect that contained the wisdom tooth. The tumor is in broad contact to the periodontium (arrow) with infiltration of the adjacent cancellous bone and the floor of the mouth.

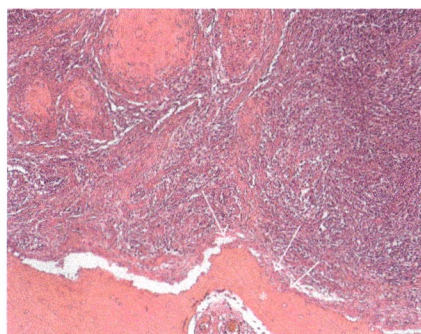

FIGURE 7: Case 2—histological view of the cross section specimen after Haematoxglin-Eosin staining. The arrows mark the arrosion of the bone (∗) by the tumor cells.

of perifocal inflammation. The ulcer was delineated by a rigid wall of mucosa attached to the alveolar crest related to 37 and 38 (Figure 4). The patient declared to be a nonsmoker but admitted occasional alcohol consumption. Oral hygiene was assessed to be average, and no other precursor lesions were present. The preoperatively taken OPTG (Figure 5) revealed considerable periradicular bone loss in regions 37 and 36 analogous to typical radiologic findings in patients with moderate to advanced chronic periodontitis. The patient underwent radical intended resection of the tumor. Figure 6 shows the resection specimen from a distal view. The tumor is mainly localized in the interdental space of 37 and 36 with distinct relation to the periodontal space of the crown 36. The beginning infiltration of the mouth floor becomes apparent. Figure 7 shows the microscopic view with arrosion of the bone by the tumor cells. HPV status by p16 immunostaining was negative.

Case 3. A 50-year-old man was referred to our clinic by a maxillofacial surgeon with diagnosis of a squamous cell carcinoma of the right mandible. The clinical examination revealed a tumor of 4 cm in diameter, localized at the alveolar crest distal of 46 with extensions to the adjacent floor of the mouth. Around the ulcer, fields of homogeneous leukoplakia were detectable (Figure 8). The patient suffered from generalized advanced chronic periodontitis, exhibiting pocket depths up to 7 mm with bleeding on probing. Analysis of bacteria (Micro-ident, Hain Lifescience GmbH D-72147 Nehren) revealed infection with *Porphyromonas gingivalis*, *Tannerella forsythia*, *Treponema denticola* (*red complex*), *Peptostreptococcus micros*, *Fusobacterium nucleatum* (*orange complex*), and *Campylobacter rectus* (*orange-associated complex*). Oral hygiene was extremely poor with high amounts of soft and hard debris on the furthermore carious teeth. The patient reported to be a heavy smoker (60 pack years) and drinker (>3 L beer a day). The OPTG (Figure 9) exhibited severe general bone loss with a basin-like translucency comprising

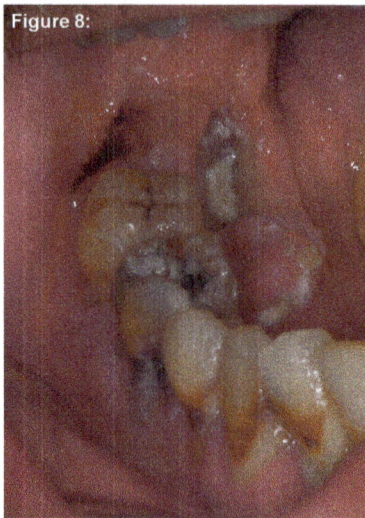

FIGURE 8: Case 3—clinical situation. A partially ulcerous tumour formation covered the lingual aspect of the alveolar crest adjacent to the two distal molars (46 and 47). Nearly all teeth of this quadrant show clearly the sequelae of nearly nonexistent oral hygiene habits. Striae of leukoplakia are found on the wall of the ulcer, the tongue, and also along the vestibular papillae.

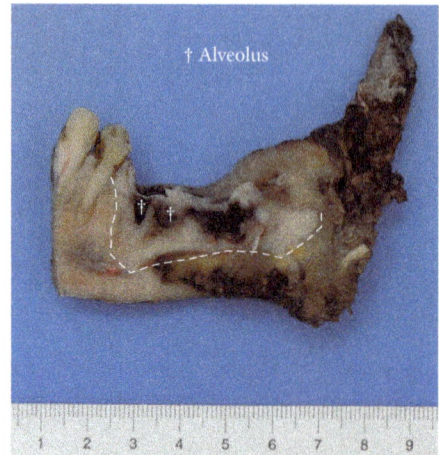

FIGURE 10: Case 3—the sagittal split preparation of the resection specimen from a lingual view clearly shows the association of the tumor (borders marked with lines) to the dental alveoli (†) of the distal molars. The teeth 36 and 37 are lost due to the preparation process.

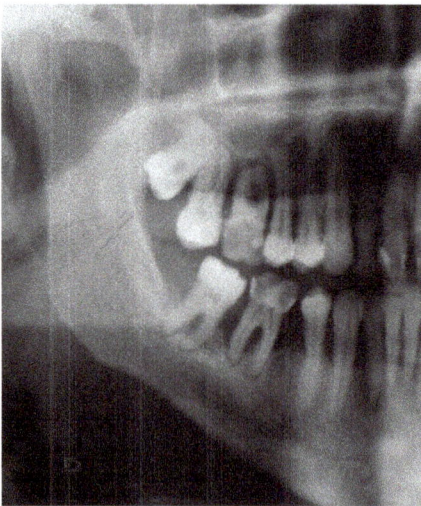

FIGURE 9: Case 3—preoperative OPTG. Beside multiple carious lesions the present X-ray examination reveals signs of chronic periodontal disease with a general loss of horizontal bone level, liberation of both dental roots, and bifurcations. The local maximum of destruction is found in the region of the last two molars. The retromolar triangle, however, appears to be intact.

the last distal molars of the right mandible. A radical intended operation followed. Figure 10 shows a transverse section of the resected mandible from a lingual view. Herein, the tumor surrounds the empty alveoli of the artificially removed right molars with considerable infiltration of the alveolar bone. HPV status by p16 immunostaining was negative.

Case 4. A 53-year-old man was admitted to our clinic with the histological verified diagnosis of a squamous cell carcinoma of the anterior floor of the mouth. The patient noticed an indolent growing mass five weeks before admission. Figure 11 gives a picture of the clinical situation. Beside a space consuming sublingual mass with deviation of the lingual frenulum, a small erosive lesion lingual from the left lower anterior teeth (region: teeth 31 to 34) with subtle perifocal leukoplakia around the center of the lesion is shown. The examination revealed a solid tumor formation with its center mainly on the left floor of mouth. The tumor expanded from the left angle of the mandible with a midline crossing to the region of the first right lower incisor. Adherence to the bone was detectable in the region of the left lower canine and the first premolar. The oral hygiene status was moderate. Investigation of periodontal pockets revealed depths up to 4 mm and bleeding on probing. The patient smoked 10 cigarettes per day for ten years and occasionally drank a glass of wine. The OPTG (Figure 12) revealed a generalized horizontal type of bone loss within both jaws, with additional vertical bony defects and translucency as radiologic finding for an erosive process in the left anterior lower jaw. The radical intended surgery consisted of a bloc resection including parts of the mandible, tongue, floor of mouth, and hyoid with complete bilateral selective functional neck dissection [13]. The split-resection specimen (Figure 13) shows a periradicular tumor formation along the root of the canine with infiltration of the neighboring cancellous bone. HPV status by p16 immunostaining was positive, as shown in Figure 14.

A brief summary of all cases is given in Table 1.

3. Discussion

Our study presents four thoroughly documented cases with alveolar squamous cell carcinomas being directly associated

TABLE 1: Summary of the presented cases.

Patient	1	2	3	4
Gender	Female	Male	Male	Male
Age	59	48	50	53
Smoking	Never	Never	60 py	5 py
Alcohol	Never	Occasionally	Regularly	Occasionally
Oral hygiene	Sufficient	Sufficient	Worse	Moderate
Tumor localization	36	37	46	32
Radiologic signs of periodontal disease	Yes	Yes	Yes	Yes
Probing depths	5 mm	2 mm	7 mm	5 mm
TNM classification	pT2 pN2b pMx G2 R0	pT4 pN0 pM0 G2 R1	pT4a pN2b pM0 G2 pR0	pT4a pN2c pM0 G3 R2
Bleeding upon probing	Yes	No	Yes	Yes
Periodontal marker bacteria	Red complex	Orange and green complex	Orange and orange-associated complex	Not identified
HPV status (p16)	Negative	Negative	Negative	Positive

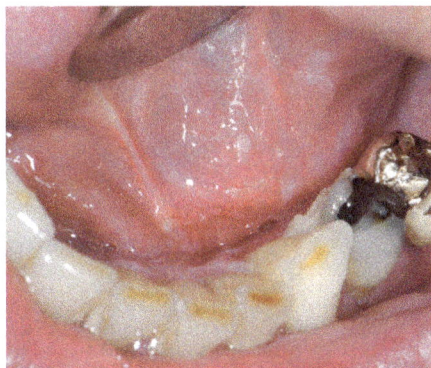

FIGURE 11: Case 4—a superficial ulcerous lesion atop of a mass at the left sublingual space with extension to the lingual aspect of the alveolar crest comprising the teeth 31 to 34 and surrounding leukoplakia.

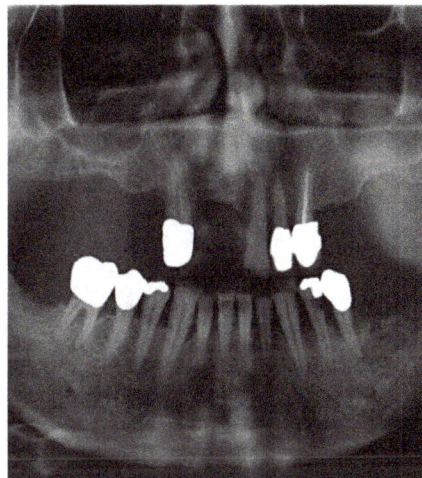

FIGURE 12: Case 4—preoperative OPTG. A general horizontal loss of bone in both jaws with additional vertical translucencies in the front aspect of the mandible and signs of erosion of the alveolar crest at the left lower quadrant.

to teeth that show considerable signs of chronic periodontitis. Chronic periodontitis represents the most common infection worldwide with high clinical relevance for the dentist. In front of this clinical setting, four different models of chronic periodontitis with alveolar squamous cell carcinomas are discussed as follows. The first patient had no precursor lesions, and no other risk factors had been identified except clinical signs of chronic periodontitis. In this patient, a de novo development caused by genomic instability as consequence of chronic inflammation caused by gram-negative bacteria as postulated by Guerra et al. appears possible [14]. In this model, chronic periodontitis itself would trigger the development of oral squamous cell carcinoma. Recently, there is improving interest in the development of various types of cancer and their association to inflammation as also the underlying pathophysiological mechanisms that lead to malignant transformation [15]. One important factor in cancer-related inflammation is the transcription factor NF-κB. Beside its function as key coordinator of innate inflammation and immunity by activated expression of inflammatory cytokines, adhesion molecules, and angiogenic factors, it has also been identified as endogenous tumour promoter [16]. Moreover, it is substantially involved in the inflammatory process of chronic periodontitis [17]. In addition, an association between oral cancer and chronic mechanical trauma was also described [18], suggesting that inflammation independent of its cause may predispose to cancer. Hereby, malignant transformation of oral epithelium would be a consequence of the immune response like macrophage and T-cell activation and cytokine release (e.g., IL-1, IL-8, and TNF-α) [19]. Aside malignant transformation as sequel of unspecific inflammation, a specific bacterial, or viral agent may also promote malignancies. This sequence is supposed for gastric lymphomas [20], H. pylori infection and gastric

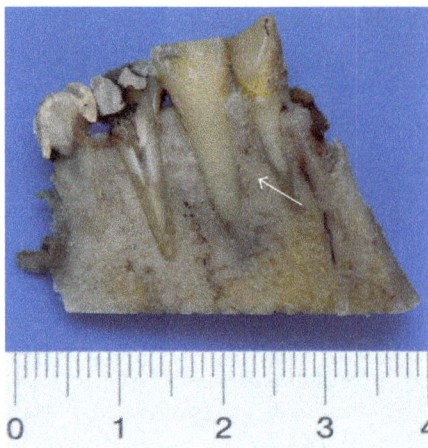

FIGURE 13: Case 4—the split resection specimen from a lingual view demonstrates the association of tumor formation along the root of the left lower canine (white arrows) as also further invasion of the cancellous bone.

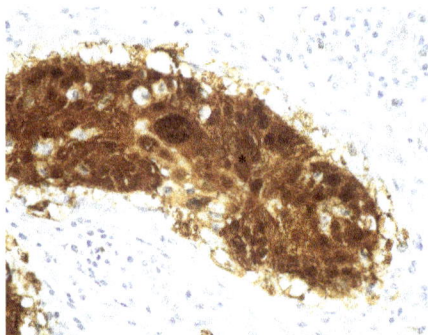

FIGURE 14: Case 4—histological view of the tumor after immune-histochemical staining against p16. The brown signal (∗) proves the infection with HPV.

cancer [21], Hepatitis B Virus (HBV) and HCV infection in liver cancer [22] and HPV 16/18 infection in head and neck [23] or cervical cancer [24]. Herein, microbial activation of inflammatory cells leads to a respiratory burst and release of free radicals, which can contribute transformation to malignancy by DNA damage, peroxidation of lipids, or disturbance of physiological posttranslational modification of proteins [25]. Taken together, either genomic instability directly induced by the bacterial agent itself or as consequence of immunological response to chronic inflammation, both are main characteristics of chronic periodontitis. The clinical relevance of chronic periodontitis for the development of OSCC was investigated by Tezal et al. In a case control model, the loss of bone as clinical sign for chronic periodontitis was an independent risk factor for tongue carcinomas and was still of significance in a multiple regression model [12]. Particularly, these patients would benefit from periodontal therapy in terms of primary prevention. The second case offers another possible scenario. Here, chronic periodontitis acts as promoter for the invasion of tumor cells into the bone.

During the course of chronic periodontitis, the loss of clinical attachment level and the underlying bone is substantially triggered. The periodontal-localized inflammation macerates the cancellous bone by enhanced osteoclastic activity which may constitute a potential route for invasion of an adjacent carcinoma. Osteoclastic activity is enhanced by proinflammatory molecules like IL-1 or LPS [26], which can be found in gingival crevicular fluid (GCF) during chronic periodontitis [27]. Furthermore, seven potential routes for invasion of the mandible by OSCC have been reviewed by Brown [28]. Beside the occlusal route, neural foramina, attached gingiva, cortical bone defects in the edentulous ridge, or infiltration by secondary tumors in the neck through the lower border, the periodontal membrane in the dentate mandible was hypothesized as a possible way for tumor invasion by Bhattathiri and Nair in 1991 [29]. Supposing the periodontal space a weak point for tumor invasion, the instance of periodontal inflammation may promote an invasion of the mandible by a neighbored tumor [15, 19]. The cross-sectional specimen of the second case underlines this possible scenario with a tumor infiltrating the periodontal space, the surrounding adjacent cancellous bone, and the neighbored floor of the mouth.

The third case is an example for chronic periodontitis being a well-known comorbidity in oral cancer patients. The patient was a heavy smoker and drinker with insufficient oral hygiene. All these habits are for themselves potential risk factors for the development of oral cancer and chronic periodontitis [5, 30–32]. In this patient, chronic periodontitis and OSCC seem to be a coincidence without an option to uncover cause and effect.

An accredited model for the development of OSCC is the multistep theory [33]. Herein, the oral mucosa undergoes different developmental stages from hyperkeratosis over different degrees of dysplasia to invasive cancer, while each level shows consecutive accompanying alterations within the genetic profile [34]. Accordingly, it appears possible, that chronic periodontitis may trigger the pathogenesis of precancerous lesions. In case four, the clinical inspection of the oral cavity revealed a vast field of leukoplakia at the anterior floor of mouth. Besides, the clinical manifest OSCC and multiple teeth were affected by chronic periodontitis. A cross-interaction between the special inflammatory milieu with enhanced levels of proinflammatory cytokines and a change in the bacterial environment may induce the development and progression of precancerous lesions in the alveolar mucosa. This thesis was reinforced recently by Meisel et al., who identified chronic periodontitis as a risk factor for the development of leukoplakia predisposing for oral cancer [35].

4. Conclusion

We presented four clinical scenarios of OSCC in the neighbourhood of teeth affected by chronic periodontitis for discussion of the clinical relevance. Clinical experience characterizes most OSCC as coincidence since chronic periodontitis and the oral malignancy share multiple risk factors impeding a definition of cause and effect. On the other hand, we found clinical hints for an interaction of OSCC and chronic periodontitis by means of invasion route preformation or a promotive effect on present precursor lesions. Finally, we give an example for a possible de novo synthesis of the OSCC in a patient without other risk factors. These patients, in particular, would greatly benefit from early therapy of the underlying chronic periodontitis in terms of a primary prevention.

Conflict of Interests

The authors declare that they have no conflict of interests. There are no financial or personal relationships with other people or organisations inappropriately influencing our work. Furthermore, the authors state that there were no sources of funding.

References

[1] S. H. Landis, T. Murray, S. Bolden, and P. A. Wingo, "Cancer Statistics, 1999," *CA: A Cancer Journal for Clinicians*, vol. 49, no. 1, pp. 8–31, 1999.

[2] D. M. Parkin, F. Bray, J. Ferlay, and P. Pisani, "Global cancer statistics, 2002," *CA: A Cancer Journal for Clinicians*, vol. 55, no. 2, pp. 74–108, 2005.

[3] P. Rusin, L. Markiewicz, and I. Majsterek, "Genetic predeterminations of head and neck cancer," *Postępy Higieny i Medycyny Doświadczalnej*, vol. 62, pp. 490–501, 2008.

[4] P.-O. Rödström, M. Jontell, U. Mattsson, and E. Holmberg, "Cancer and oral lichen planus in a Swedish population," *Oral Oncology*, vol. 40, no. 2, pp. 131–138, 2004.

[5] C. Pelucchi, S. Gallus, W. Garavello, C. Bosetti, and C. L. Vecchia, "Alcohol and tobacco use, and cancer risk for upper aerodigestive tract and liver," *European Journal of Cancer Prevention*, vol. 17, no. 4, pp. 340–344, 2008.

[6] M. Tezal, M. S. Nasca, D. L. Stoler et al., "Chronic periodontitis-human papillomavirus synergy in base of tongue cancers," *Archives of Otolaryngology*, vol. 135, no. 4, pp. 391–396, 2009.

[7] C. Fakhry, W. H. Westra, S. Li et al., "Improved survival of patients with human papillomavirus—positive head and neck squamous cell carcinoma in a prospective clinical trial," *Journal of the National Cancer Institute*, vol. 100, no. 4, pp. 261–269, 2008.

[8] S. Marur, G. D'Souza, W. H. Westra, and A. A. Forastiere, "HPV-associated head and neck cancer: a virus-related cancer epidemic," *The Lancet Oncology*, vol. 11, no. 8, pp. 781–789, 2010.

[9] M. S. Meyer, K. Joshipura, E. Giovannucci, and D. S. Michaud, "A review of the relationship between tooth loss, periodontal disease, and cancer," *Cancer Causes and Control*, vol. 19, no. 9, pp. 895–907, 2008.

[10] D. S. Michaud, K. Joshipura, E. Giovannucci, and C. S. Fuchs, "A prospective study of periodontal disease and pancreatic cancer in US male health professionals," *Journal of the National Cancer Institute*, vol. 99, no. 2, pp. 171–175, 2007.

[11] B. Burt and Research, Science and Therapy Committee of the American Academy of Periodontology., "Position paper: epidemiology of periodontal diseases," *Journal of Periodontology*, vol. 76, no. 8, pp. 1406–1419, 2005.

[12] M. Tezal, M. A. Sullivan, A. Hyland et al., "Chronic periodontitis and the incidence of head and neck squamous cell carcinoma," *Cancer Epidemiology Biomarkers and Prevention*, vol. 18, no. 9, pp. 2406–2412, 2009.

[13] K. T. Robbins, G. Clayman, P. A. Levine et al., "Neck dissection classification update: revisions proposed by the American Head and Neck Society and the American Academy of Otolaryngology-Head and Neck Surgery," *Archives of Otolaryngology*, vol. 128, no. 7, pp. 751–758, 2002.

[14] L. Guerra, R. Guidi, and T. Frisan, "Do bacterial genotoxins contribute to chronic inflammation, genomic instability and tumor progression?" *FEBS Journal*, vol. 278, no. 23, pp. 4577–4588, 2011.

[15] S. F. Moss and M. J. Blaser, "Mechanisms of disease: inflammation and the origins of cancer," *Nature Clinical Practice Oncology*, vol. 2, no. 2, pp. 90–97, 2005.

[16] M. Karin, "Nuclear factor-κB in cancer development and progression," *Nature*, vol. 441, no. 7092, pp. 431–436, 2006.

[17] Y. Nagahama, T. Obama, M. Usui et al., "Oxidized low-density lipoprotein-induced periodontal inflammation is associated with the up-regulation of cyclooxygenase-2 and microsomal prostaglandin synthase 1 in human gingival epithelial cells," *Biochemical and Biophysical Research Communications*, vol. 413, no. 4, pp. 566–571, 2011.

[18] E. D. Piemonte, J. P. Lazos, and M. Brunotto, "Relationship between chronic trauma of the oral mucosa, oral potentially malignant disorders and oral cancer," *Journal of Oral Pathology and Medicine*, vol. 39, no. 7, pp. 513–517, 2010.

[19] A. Mantovani, P. Allavena, A. Sica, and F. Balkwill, "Cancer-related inflammation," *Nature*, vol. 454, no. 7203, pp. 436–444, 2008.

[20] M. Lecuit, M. C. Peterson, F. Suarez, and O. Lortholary, "Immunoproliferative small intestinal disease associated with *Campylobacter jejuni*," *The New England Journal of Medicine*, vol. 350, no. 3, pp. 239–248, 2004.

[21] N. Uemura, S. Okamoto, S. Yamamoto et al., "Helicobacter pylori infection and the development of gastric cancer," *The New England Journal of Medicine*, vol. 345, no. 11, pp. 784–789, 2001.

[22] D. M. Parkin, "Global cancer statistics in the year 2000," *The Lancet Oncology*, vol. 2, no. 9, pp. 533–543, 2001.

[23] M. L. Gillison and K. V. Shah, "Human papillomavirus-associated head and neck squamous cell carcinoma: mounting evidence for an etiologic role for human papillomavirus in a subset of head and neck cancers," *Current Opinion in Oncology*, vol. 13, no. 3, pp. 183–188, 2001.

[24] H. zur Hausen, "Papillomaviruses and cancer: from basic studies to clinical application," *Nature Reviews Cancer*, vol. 2, no. 5, pp. 342–350, 2002.

[25] S. P. Hussain, L. J. Hofseth, and C. C. Harris, "Radical causes of cancer," *Nature Reviews Cancer*, vol. 3, no. 4, pp. 276–285, 2003.

[26] T. Katagiri and N. Takahashi, "Regulatory mechanisms of osteoblast and osteoclast differentiation," *Oral Diseases*, vol. 8, no. 3, pp. 147–159, 2002.

[27] C. M. E. Champagne, W. Buchanan, M. S. Reddy, J. S. Preisser, J. D. Beck, and S. Offenbacher, "Potential for gingival crevice fluid measures as predictors of risk for periodontal diseases," *Periodontology 2000*, vol. 31, pp. 167–180, 2003.

[28] J. Brown, "Mechanisms of cancer invasion of the mandible," *Current Opinion in Otolaryngology & Head and Neck Surgery*, vol. 11, no. 2, pp. 96–102, 2003.

[29] V. N. Bhattathiri and M. K. Nair, "Periodontal space: a major route to bone involvement in oral cancer," *Medical Hypotheses*, vol. 34, no. 1, pp. 58–59, 1991.

[30] D. Kademani, "Oral cancer," *Mayo Clinic Proceedings*, vol. 82, no. 7, pp. 878–887, 2007.

[31] D. M. Laronde, T. G. Hislop, J. M. Elwood, and M. P. Rosin, "Oral cancer: just the facts," *Journal of the Canadian Dental Association*, vol. 74, no. 3, pp. 269–272, 2008.

[32] K. Rosenquist, J. Wennerberg, E.-B. Schildt, A. Bladström, B. G. Hansson, and G. Andersson, "Oral status, oral infections and some lifestyle factors as risk factors for oral and oropharyngeal squamous cell carcinoma. A population-based case-control study in southern Sweden," *Acta Oto-Laryngologica*, vol. 125, no. 12, pp. 1327–1336, 2005.

[33] A. Argiris, M. V. Karamouzis, D. Raben, and R. L. Ferris, "Head and neck cancer," *The Lancet*, vol. 371, no. 9625, pp. 1695–1709, 2008.

[34] J. Califano, P. van der Riet, W. Westra et al., "Genetic progression model for head and neck cancer: implications for field cancerization," *Cancer Research*, vol. 56, no. 11, pp. 2488–2492, 1996.

[35] P. Meisel, B. Holtfreter, R. Biffar, W. Suemnig, and T. Kocher, "Association of periodontitis with the risk of oral leukoplakia," *Oral Oncology*, vol. 48, no. 9, pp. 859–863, 2012.

24

Rapidly Progressing Osteomyelitis of the Mandible

Yukiko Kusuyama,[1] **Ken Matsumoto,**[2] **Shino Okada,**[1] **Ken Wakabayashi,**[1]
Noritami Takeuchi,[1] **and Yoshiaki Yura**[2]

[1] *Department of Dentistry and Oral Surgery, Matsubara Tokushukai Hospital, 7-13-26 Amamihigashi, Matsubara-shi,*
 Osaka 580-0032, Japan
[2] *Department of Oral and Maxillofacial Surgery II, Osaka University, Graduate School of Dentistry, Osaka 565-0871, Japan*

Correspondence should be addressed to Yukiko Kusuyama; kusu.yukiko@gmail.com

Academic Editors: P. G. Arduino, M. B. D. Gaviao, and M. J. Wahl

Acute osteomyelitis exists as a refractory disease even now, which usually exhibits systemic symptoms such as fever or malaise and local redness or swelling. The present paper describes a case of acute osteomyelitis of the mandible that was rapidly progressing without typical symptoms. The patient had liver cirrhosis, which should be one of the systemic factors that affect immune surveillance and metabolism. Actinomycotic druses and filaments were detected from the sequestrum. These were considered to play a role in the rapid progression of osteomyelitis without typical symptoms. There has been no evidence of local recurrence 24 months after surgery.

1. Introduction

Acute osteomyelitis of the jaws is not commonly seen in modern oral and maxillofacial surgery practice. Generally speaking, this can be related to our society having become more health conscious, resulting in an increased awareness of nutrition, as well as earlier and better access to health care than in the past [1, 2]. However, acute osteomyelitis exists as a refractory disease even now, which usually exhibits systemic symptoms such as fever, malaise or high levels of CRP and local redness, swelling, or pus discharge. It is known that osteomyelitis can be attributed to one or more of the predisposing systemic diseases [3]. In immune-compromised patients, it is easy to expect that acute inflammatory reactions are poor. Few case reports such as osteomyelitis of the jaws with poor acute inflammatory reactions and rapid progression have been documented. The present paper describes a case of acute osteomyelitis of the mandible, with liver cirrhosis, that was rapidly progressing without typical symptoms.

2. Case Report

A 77-year-old man was referred to our hospital for postextraction hemorrhage and spontaneous pain in the socket of the left mandibular first molar. The patient had a 1-month history of spontaneous pain of the left mandibular first molar. At a nearby dental clinic, restorative treatment was performed. However, as the pain continued, the tooth was finally extracted on January 19, 2011. Next day he visited our hospital.

When first examined, he had neither swelling in his cheek nor paresthesia in his lower lip. Postextraction hemorrhage of the mandibular first molar had already arrested. Instead, the clot was absent and the socket made the pale alveolar bone expose (Figure 1(a)). There was no redness or swelling in the regional gum and no mobility and percussion pain of the adjacent teeth. Panoramic radiograph showed neither abnormal consolidation nor ill-defined trabecular bone structure around the socket (Figure 1(b)). The clinical diagnosis was delayed healing of postextraction wound. White blood cell counts (WBC) were in normal range, and C-reactive protein (CRP) level slightly increased to 1.41 mg/dL. There was poor clinical evidence of acute inflammation (Figure 2). The information that the patient had been suffering from nonviral liver cirrhosis for 6 years and unremedied was not given at that time. Aspartate aminotransferase (AST) and alanine aminotransferase (ALT) were also in normal range. Clarithromycin

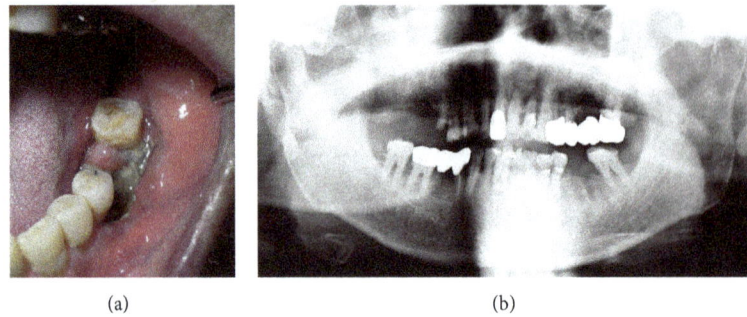

(a)   (b)

FIGURE 1: Clinical findings at the initial visit. (a) Close-up view of the socket in the left mandibular first molar region. (b) Panoramic radiograph showing neither abnormal consolidation nor ill-defined trabecular bone structure around the socket and clear running of the inferior alveolar arteries.

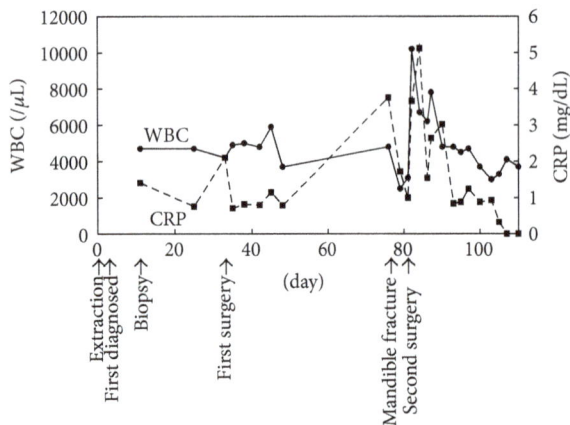

FIGURE 2: Overview of the clinical events and laboratory data.

(CAM) was administered for a week, but his spontaneous pain did not diminish. Mobility of the adjacent teeth and necrosis of the gum around the socket was present at 10 days after the first visit. We performed biopsy of the socket and extraction of the left mandibular second premolar, the results of which revealed no malignancy. CAM was administered for 10 more days. Computed tomography (CT) scans at 14 days after the first visit showed absorption of the cortical bone in the left mandibular molar region (Figure 3). Twenty-nine days after the first visit, the sequestrectomy and corticectomy of the left mandibular molar region and the extraction of the left mandibular first premolar and second molar were performed under general anesthesia. The surgical site was filled with gauze with pasta of dimethyl isopropyl azulene and clindamycin. Next day hyperbaric oxygen (HBO) utilization (2 atmosphere absolute, 90 minutes per day) begun for a total of 20 times. The patient was treated with intravenous penicillin for a week. After the sequestrectomy, spontaneous pain became bearable, and there was little clinical evidence of inflammation such as gum swelling or drainage. Fourty-two days after the surgery, he had swelling in his cheek. The patient was treated with intravenous piperacillin and clindamycin. Fourty-five days after the surgery, the mandible was

fractured at the surgical site, and CT scans showed the bone resorption at the mandibular anterior teeth. Actinomycotic druses and filaments were detected from the sequestrum of the fracture site (Figure 4). Segmental resection and reconstruction were performed at 49 days after the first surgery. Actinomyces it was not detected any more from the resected mandible.

There has been no evidence of local recurrence 24 months after the treatment.

3. Discussion

Osteomyelitis of the jaws is caused in association with hematogenous germ spread, drug- or radiation-related, or local odontogenic or nonodontogenic processes [1]. Schafer states that dental infection is the most frequent cause of osteomyelitis of the jaws [4]. In the present case, panoramic radiograph at the time of preextraction of the left mandibular first molar showed neither abnormal consolidation nor ill-defined trabecular bone structure around the tooth, and the running of the inferior alveolar artery was clear. Osteomyelitis was esteemed to occur after the extraction, but the reason of the spontaneous pain which was the cause of the extraction was unclear.

Panoramic radiograph at the initial visit to our hospital also showed no abnormal findings. Because of the clinical findings without mobility of the adjacent teeth, paresthesia in the left lower lip or swollen gums around the socket, the first diagnosis was just a delayed healing of the extraction wound as dry socket. However, the inflammation progressed rapidly, so we rediagnosed it as an acute osteomyelitis of the mandible. In the acute osteomyelitis, vascular compromise caused by the infective process occurs early in the course of the disease, making a cure unlikely unless medical management with the appropriate antibiotic is instituted within the first 3 days after the onset of the symptoms [1]. Early diagnosis is the key to prevent the disease from progressing.

Acute osteomyelitis of the jaw is often accompanied by symptoms as fever, malaise, facial cellulitis, trismus, and significant leukocytosis. In our case, although it had begun as an acute osteomyelitis, WBC was not remarkable and CRP

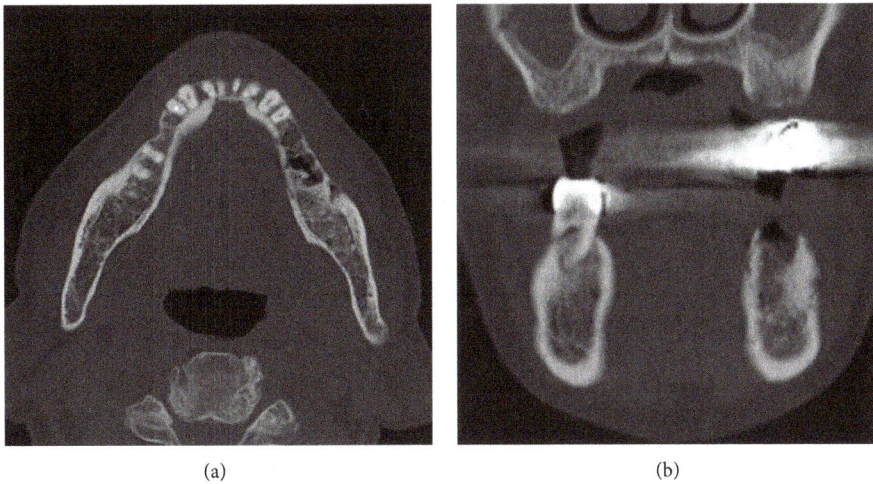

FIGURE 3: CT scans at 14 days after the initial visit showing remarkable absorption of the cortical bone in the left mandibular molar region. (a) Axial section. (b) Coronal section.

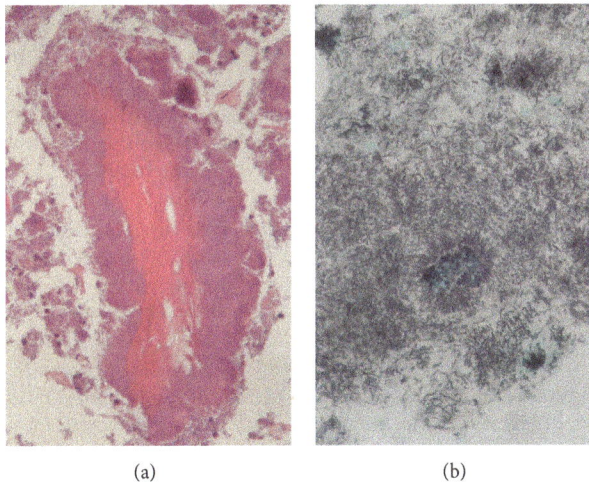

FIGURE 4: Actinomycotic druses (A, H.E. stain, 200x) and filaments (B, Grocott stain, 400x) detected from the sequestrum of the fracture site.

level increased only slightly (Figure 2), and there was neither pus discharge nor swelling of the cheek until just before the fracture of the mandible. Rapidly progressing osteomyelitis which was highly resistant to treatments without typical symptoms like this case is extremely rare [5]. Osteomyelitis without typical symptoms made the final diagnosis delay and might bring the inflammation to progress. Systemic factors such as diabetes mellitus, agranulocytosis, leukemia, severe anemia, malnutrition, or alcohol abuse affect immune surveillance and lead to impairing the osteomyelitis [1]. The Cierny-Mader classification of long-bone osteomyelitis is based on the anatomy of bone infection and the physiology of the host [3]. Cierny described that not only the anatomic classification but also the condition of the host, regional vascularity, local milieu, and extent of necrosis would influence the natural history of the disease. In the present case, the patient had liver cirrhosis. Liver cirrhosis

is one of the systemic factors in the classification that affect immune surveillance and metabolism. This patient's Child-Pugh score [6] was 8 points and the grade was B, significant functional compromise at the first surgery (Table 1). Child-Pugh grade can be used in patients with liver cirrhosis to assess the severity of the clinical condition [7]. Therefore, it was considered that impaired immunity introduced poor acute inflammatory reactions and the systemic compromise played a role in the asymptomatic and rapid progression of osteomyelitis.

Identification of responsible microorganisms can be extremely difficult. Simply swabbing a suspected area is not appropriate. The process of obtaining suitable material for culture is fraught with potential danger of contamination from nearby oral site. In our case, actinomycotic druses and filaments were detected from the sequestrum of the fracture site, while they were not from the resected mandibular

TABLE 1: Child-Pugh score in our case.

Measure	1 point	2 points	3 points	This case
Bilirubin (mg/dL)	<2	2-3	>3	2.1
Albumin (g/dL)	>3.5	2.8–3.5	<2.8	4
Prothrombin time (seconds)	1–3	4–6	>6	14.6
Ascites	None	Slight	Moderate	None
Encephalopathy (grade)	None	I-II	III-IV	None
Grade A = 5-6 points; well-compensated disease				8 points
Grade B = 7–9 points; significant functional compromise				
Grade C = 10–15 points; decompensated disease				

specimen. It was unclear whether their presence contributed to osteomyelitis development or they represented a secondary infection to the necrotic bone. However, it could not be denied to contribute to osteomyelitis development like in BRONJ [8–10]. Marx identified *Actinomyces* and other fastidious organisms such as *Eikenella* and *Arachnia* as pathogens in some of the more refractory forms of osteomyelitis of the jaws [11]. These organisms, in all likelihood, were contaminants with the original odontogenic microorganism invasion, but only became established after suboptimal therapeutics failed to eradicate all potential pathogens [2]. Robinson et al. [12] described that in the pediatric actinomycotic osteomyelitis the clinical manifestations are often subtle. Involvement by *Actinomyces* may be one of the causes that osteomyelitis progressed without typical symptoms in our case.

In this paper, we report the case of the asymptomatic and rapid progression of osteomyelitis of the mandible. Depending on the predisposing factors, osteomyelitis progresses rapidly without typical symptoms. Correction of the underlying predisposing factors, early diagnosis and evaluating the therapeutic response of a multimodality treatment approach as needed would offer the best course of the disease.

Conflict of Interests

This paper has neither been published nor has been under consideration for publication elsewhere. All the authors have read the paper and have approved this submission. The authors report no conflict of interest. Disclosure or financial support.

References

[1] L. G. Mercuri, "Acute osteomyelitis of the jaws," *Oral and Maxillofacial Surgery Clinics of North America—Infections of the Head and Neck*, vol. 3, no. 2, pp. 355–365, 1991.

[2] J. W. Hudson, "Osteomyelitis of the jaws: a 50-year perspective," *Journal of Oral and Maxillofacial Surgery*, vol. 51, no. 12, pp. 1294–1301, 1993.

[3] G. Cierny III, J. T. Mader, and J. J. Penninck, "A clinical staging system for adult osteomyelitis," *Clinical Orthopaedics and Related Research*, no. 414, pp. 7–24, 2003.

[4] W. G. Scafer, "Osteomyelitis," in *A Textbook of Oral Pathology*, p. 453, Elsevier Saunders, Philadelphia, Pa, USA, 3rd edition, 1974.

[5] D. J. Krutchkoff and L. Runstad, "Unusually aggressive osteomyelitis of the jaws. A report of two cases," *Oral Surgery Oral Medicine and Oral Pathology*, vol. 67, no. 5, pp. 499–507, 1989.

[6] M. Schwartz, S. Roayaie, and M. Konstadoulakis, "Strategies for the management of hepatocellular carcinoma," *Nature Clinical Practice Oncology*, vol. 4, no. 7, pp. 424–432, 2007.

[7] F. Durand and D. Valla, "Assessment of the prognosis of cirrhosis: child-pugh versus MELD," *Journal of Hepatology*, vol. 42, no. 1, pp. S100–S107, 2005.

[8] T. Mücke, J. Koschinski, H. Deppe et al., "Outcome of treatment and parameters influencing recurrence in patients with bisphosphonate-related osteonecrosis of the jaws," *Journal of Cancer Research and Clinical Oncology*, vol. 137, no. 5, pp. 907–913, 2011.

[9] T. Hansen, M. Kunkel, A. Weber, and C. James Kirkpatrick, "Osteonecrosis of the jaws in patients treated with bisphosphonates—Histomorphologic analysis in comparison with infected osteoradionecrosis," *Journal of Oral Pathology and Medicine*, vol. 35, no. 3, pp. 155–160, 2006.

[10] V. Thumbigere-Math, M. C. Sabino, R. Gopalakrishnan et al., "Bisphosphonate-related Osteonecrosis of the Jaw: clinical features, risk factors, management, and treatment outcomes of 26 patients," *Journal of Oral and Maxillofacial Surgery*, vol. 67, no. 9, pp. 1904–1913, 2009.

[11] R. E. Marx, "Chronic osteomyelitis of the jaws," *Oral and Maxillofacial Surgery Clinics of North America—Infections of the Head and Neck*, vol. 3, no. 2, pp. 367–381, 1991.

[12] J. L. Robinson, W. L. Vaudry, and W. Dobrovolsky, "Actinomycosis presenting as osteomyelitis in the pediatric population," *Pediatric Infectious Disease Journal*, vol. 24, no. 4, pp. 365–369, 2005.

25

Anchoretic Infection

S. Gokkulakrishnan,[1] Ashish Sharma,[2] Satish Kumaran,[1] and P. L. Vasundhar[3]

[1] *Department of OMFS, Institute of Dental Science Bareilly, Bareilly 243006, India*
[2] *Department of OMFS, Kothiwal Dental College & Research Centre, Moradabad, India*
[3] *Department of OMFS, Sri Sai College of Dental Surgery, Srikakulam, India*

Correspondence should be addressed to S. Gokkulakrishnan, drgokkul@gmail.com

Academic Editors: P. G. Arduino and Y. Nakagawa

Active and passive mouth opening exercises are a very common practice in oral and maxillofacial surgery especially for various conditions causing limited mouth opening like space infections, trauma, and ankylosis. But most of the practitioners do not follow basic principles while advocating these active mouth opening exercises and also take it for granted that it would benefit the patient in the long run. Because of this, the mouth opening physiotherapy by itself can at times lead to unwanted complications. We report a case wherein due to active physiotherapy, the patient had complications leading to persistent temporal space infection which required surgical intervention and hospitalization. This could have been because of hematoma formation during physiotherapy which got infected due to anchoretic infection of unknown etiology and resulted in temporal space infection. Hence, our conclusion is that whenever mouth opening exercises are initiated, it should be done gradually under good antibiotic coverage to avoid any untoward complications and for optimum results. According to the current English literature, such a complication has not been documented before.

1. Introduction

The term "Trismus" is derived from a Greek word "Trismos" meaning squeaking, whistling, or whizzing [1]. The principal manifestation of trismus is restricted jaw movement that can severely affect nutrition, oral hygiene, and speech and in some cases can result in airway compromise. It is one of the most common complications which can occur due to infection, trauma, temporomandibular joint disorders, MPDS, submucous fibrosis, and so forth. This condition is usually managed conservatively with analgesics, muscle relaxants, hot fomentations, and mouth opening physiotherapy. But sometimes surgical intervention is required which will again be followed by aggressive mouth opening physiotherapy [2].

In children fibrous ankylosis especially following injury to temporomandibular joint can also manifest as trismus. The most common treatment employed by majority of practioners for this is vigorous mouth opening physiotherapy [3]. This form of treatment is slow but eventually successful, and one can easily achieve good mouth opening. We present an unusual case report of a patient who had

temporal space infection as a result of vigorous mouth opening physiotherapy for trismus due to fibrous ankylosis. According to our present knowledge such a case has not been documented anywhere in the literature.

2. Case Report

A seven-year-old male patient from lower socioeconomic strata reported to the Department of Oral and Maxillofacial Surgery with a chief complaint of restricted mouth opening from two and a half months before. The patient gave a history of fall and trauma to the right side of face while playing three months before. Following this, the patient noticed gradual decrease in mouth opening with development of trismus which was not associated with any swelling or pain. On examination, reduced interincisal distance (12 mm) with restricted condylar movement of the right side was noticed. Panoramic radiograph (OPG) was advised, but nothing significant was revealed from it apart from carious 74 (Figure 1). A diagnosis of fibrous ankylosis of the right temporomandibular joint was reached.

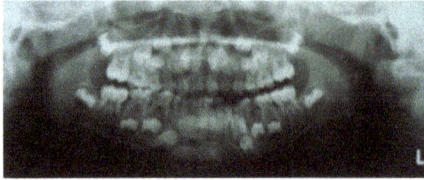

FIGURE 1: Preoperative OPG.

Considering the patient's age, diagnosis of fibrous anky-losis, application of force full mouth opening under general anesthesia followed by both active and passive vigorous physiotherapy was planned. Mouth opening of 32 mm was achieved after forceful mouth opening under general anesthesia. The patient was discharged on the next day, and the patient's parents were advised to continue mouth opening physiotherapy using Heister's mouth gag.

2 weeks later the patient reported back with complaint of restricted mouth opening associated with pain and swelling over the right temporoorbital region (Figure 2). Swelling was fluctuant, tender with rise in local temperature, and indicating towards infection of temporal region. No constitutional symptoms were noted and no correlation to any odontogenic cause for infection was found. The patient was further referred to an ophthalmologist, a neurologist, and an ENT surgeon for ruling out any eye, ear, nose, tonsil, cranial, or sinus infections which could be related to the infection over the temporal region.

The patient was treated with incision and drainage via extraoral approach under local anesthesia with empirical antibiotic coverage. Pus was sent for culture and sensitivity. Mild mouth opening physiotherapy was again initiated.

When the infection did not subside after 96 hours, another surgical exploration was planned under general anesthesia. A thorough exploration was carried out, the remaining pus, fat, hematoma, and necrosed fascia were removed, and the antibiotics were changed according to culture and sensitivity reports. The patient was advised mouth opening exercises after 24 hrs as his mouth opening had decreased considerably (Figure 3). As the condition of the patient improved, the patient was discharged with advice to continue mouth opening exercises under sensitive antibiotic coverage for two weeks. Subsequently the patient recovered completely and has been followed for last 14 months without any complication with a mouth opening of 38 mm. A final diagnosis of temporal space infection was established (Figure 4).

3. Discussion

Trismus, severely restricted mouth opening, may occur as a result of intracapsular pathology of the temporomandibular joint or as a result of extracapsular pathology. Intracap-sular causes of trismus are ankylosis, arthritis synovitis, meniscus pathology, and so forth. Extracapsular causes of trismus can be odontogenic (pulpal, periodontal), nonodon-togenic (peritonsillar abscess, brain abscess, tetanus), trauma

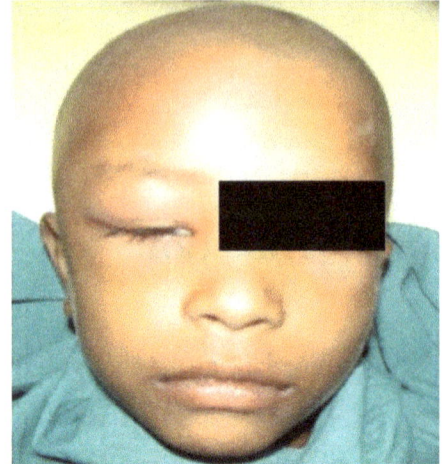

FIGURE 2: Swelling over the temporoorbital region.

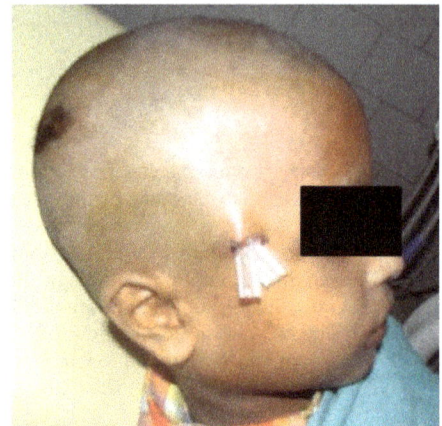

FIGURE 3: Postoperative picture after the second surgical interven-tion.

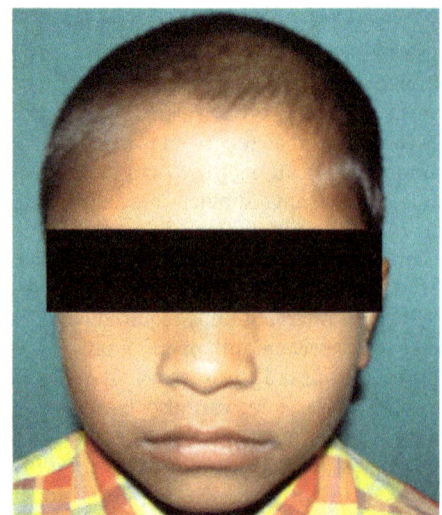

FIGURE 4: Two weeks postoperative picture of the patient.

(mandibular fracture, ZMC fracture), tumor and oral care, radiotherapy and chemotherapy, drug-related (phenothiazine, halothane), congenital (hypertrophy of coronoid) mandibular nerve blocks (postinjection trismus due to infection and hematoma) [4].

Sawhney [2] has classified TMJ ankylosis in children based on OPG findings and identified four types in which type 1 is described as fibrous adhesions [5]. Our diagnosis was also of fibrous ankylosis which was based on the history of trauma to the right side of jaw, gradual reduction in mouth opening, restricted movements of the right condyle with no pain, and swelling, and the OPG of the patient revealed slight reduced joint space of right side.

A variety of techniques for the treatment of TMJ ankylosis have been described including intraoral coronoidectomy, ramus osteotomy, high condylectomy, forceful opening of the jaw under general anesthesia, autogenous costochondral graft (CCG), and free vascularized whole-joint transplants [6]. Based on the diagnosis and age of the patient, it was decided to do a forceful mouth opening under general anesthesia, and the patient was further instructed to do aggressive physiotherapy following Kaban's seventh protocol.

The patient reported back with clinical signs and symptoms of right temporal space infection. We tried to rule out all probable causes of temporal space infections and came to the hypothesis that organized hematoma formation in the temporal muscle region due to recurrent trauma to temporalis muscle during aggressive physiotherapy may be the cause which got infected later.

Organized hematoma develops in several stages. Initially, blood accumulates and chronic hematoma changes to organized hematoma through angiogenesis and neovascularization, as has been reported for subdural hematoma. Fibrosis also occurs. The causes of initial bleeding are various, such as facial trauma, postoperative bleeding, and vessel injury [7]. For our patient also recurrent hematoma due to aggressive physiotherapy causing overstretching of temporalis muscle leading to intramuscular bleeding, injury, and inflammation of the muscle may be the cause.

We further try to find the cause due to which hematoma got infected. After ruling out all the probable reasons which may have leaded to infected hematoma, we hypothesized that anchoretic infection may be the cause. Anachoresis is defined as preferential collection or deposit of particles at a site, as of bacteria or metals that have localized out of the bloodstream in areas of inflammation [8]. Though the patient was free of any clinical infection, subclinical infections which are mostly present in pediatric age group may be the reason for the anachoresis leading to infection of the hematoma. We treated the patient with incision, drainage, and removal of infected and necrosed material, according to the principles of surgical and antimicrobial infection management.

The patient was further advised to continue physiotherapy but this time under antibiotic coverage, and subsequently the patient's mouth opening increased and no further infection was reported.

Thus the sequele was as follows:

trauma → hematoma → trismus due to fibrous ankylosis → forceful mouth opening and active physiotherapy → hematoma formation in temporal mucle region → hematoma getting organized and vascularized → anachoretic infection reaching hematoma due to increased vascularity → trismus due to temporal space infection → surgical intervention → active physiotherapy under antibiotic coverage → increased mouth opening.

4. Conclusion

The important factor that one needs to bear in mind with cases of trismus is that physiotherapy that includes unassisted and finger-assisted stretching exercises, and the Ferguson mouth gag when initiated should be gradual and of mild to moderate intensity with antibiotic cover to avoid any future unexpected complications. We advocate that further studies be done on complications of forceful mouth opening and active or passive physiotherapy. We also advocate that a standard protocol be formulated for the patients requiring mouth opening physiotherapy with emphasis on how much mouth opening to be done at what time and stage, to prevent any damage or complication to the surrounding structures involved during the physiotherapy.

Ethical Approval

This study did require an ethical approval.

Conflict of Interests

The authors have not declared any conflict of interests related to this paper.

References

[1] P. Poulsen, "Restricted mandibular opening (trismus)," *The Journal of Laryngology and Otology*, vol. 98, no. 11, pp. 1111–1114, l984.

[2] *Peterson's Principles of Oral and Maxillofacial Surgery*, vol. 2, 2nd edition, 2004.

[3] K. Abdel-Galil, R. Ananda, C. Pratt, B. Oeppen, and P. Brennan, "Trismus: an unconventional approach to treatment," *British Journal of Oral and Maxillofacial Surgery*, vol. 45, no. 4, pp. 339–340, 2007.

[4] P. J. Dhahrajani and O. Jonaidel, "Trismus: aetiology differential diagnosis and treatment," *Dental Update*, vol. 29, no. 2, pp. 88–94, 2002.

[5] M. A. Qudah, M. A. Qudeimat, and J. Al-Maaita, "Treatment of TMJ ankylosis in jordanian children—a comparison of two surgical techniques," *Journal of Cranio-Maxillo-Facial Surgery*, vol. 33, no. 1, pp. 30–36, 2005.

[6] U. M. Das, R. Keerthi, D. P. Ashwin, R. Venkata Subramaniam, D. Reddy, and N. Shiggaon, "Ankylosis of temporomandibular joint in children ," *Journal of Indian Society of Pedodontics and Preventive Dentistry*, vol. 27, no. 2, pp. 116–120, 2009.

[7] H. K. Lee, W. R. Smoker, B. J. Lee, S. J. Kim, and K. J. Cho, "Organized hematoma of the maxillary sinus: CT findings," *American Journal of Roentgenology*, vol. 188, no. 4, pp. W370–W373, 2007.

[8] *Saunders Comprehensive Veterinary Dictionary*, 3rd edition.

26

Keratocystic Odontogenic Tumor with an Ectopic Tooth in Maxilla

Basavaraj T. Bhagawati,[1] **Manish Gupta,**[1] **Gaurav Narang,**[1] **and Sharanamma Bhagawati**[2]

[1] *Department of Oral Medicine and Radiology, Shree Bankey Bihari Dental College, Masuri, Ghaziabad, Utta Pradesh-201302, India*
[2] *Department of Periodontology, Shree Bankey Bihari Dental College, NH-24, Masuri, Ghaziabad, Utta Pradesh-201302, India*

Correspondence should be addressed to Basavaraj T. Bhagawati; drbasavarajb@yahoo.com

Academic Editors: M. M. Kassab, S. Kourtis, and S. I. Ramoglu

The term odontogenic keratocyst was first used by Philipsen in the year 1956. The lesion was renamed by him as keratocystic odontogenic tumor (KCOT) and reclassified as odontogenic neoplasm in the World Health Organization's 2005 edition that occurs commonly in the jaws having a predilection for the angle and ascending ramus of mandible. In contrast, KCOTs arising in the maxillary premolar region are relatively rare. Here, we discuss a rare case of keratocystic odontogenic tumor occurring in the maxilla with an ectopic tooth position.

1. Introduction

Keratocystic odontogenic tumor (KCOT) is defined as "a benign uni- or multicystic, intraosseous tumor of odontogenic origin, with a characteristic lining of parakeratinized stratified squamous epithelium and potential for aggressive, infiltrative behavior."

In 2005, the World Health Organization redefined the odontogenic keratocyst as a result of its biological behavior as a benign tumor of odontogenic origin and named it as keratocystic odontogenic tumor.

KCOTs comprise approximately 11% of all cysts of the jaws. They occur most commonly in the mandible, especially in the posterior body and ramus regions. They almost always occur within bone, although a small number of cases of peripheral KCOT have been reported.

2. Case Report

A 17-year-old male patient came to the department with a chief complain of pus discharge from the right upper back teeth region 3-4 months ago with pain and swelling 15–20 days ago. Pain was gradual in onset, throbbing type, continuous, nonradiating, aggravates on mastication, and relieved on taking medication. Swelling was initially smaller in size and gradually increased to the present size associated with pus discharge from right upper back region 2-3 months ago. There was no history of trauma or fever. Patient also gave history of exfoliation of a tooth from right upper back tooth region on its own (Figure 1).

On general physical examination, patient was found to be moderately built and nourished. He was conscious, cooperative, and well oriented with time, place, and person. Extraoral examination showed no abnormality.

On intraoral examination, a localized, solitary swelling was present in the right upper back vestibular region measuring approximately 1–1.5 cm in diameter in relation to teeth 15, 16 with overlying mucosa slightly erythematous in appearance; however the surface appeared to be smooth and the surrounding area appeared normal. On palpations all inspectory findings were confirmed. The swelling was nontender, bony hard in consistency, nonfluctuant, nonpulsatile, noncompressible, and nonreducible. Hard tissue examination revealed missing 13, 14 and over retained 53. On percussions 15, 16 were tender. All other teeth were present in the oral cavity with no abnormality. On the basis of history and clinical examination, a provisional diagnosis of dentigerous cyst was given.

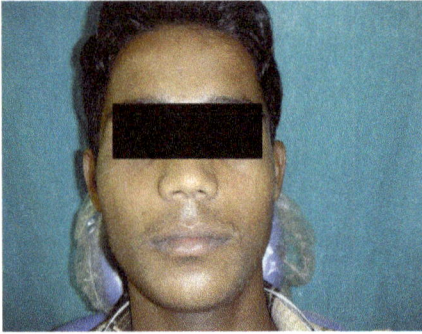

FIGURE 1: Profile photograph of the patient.

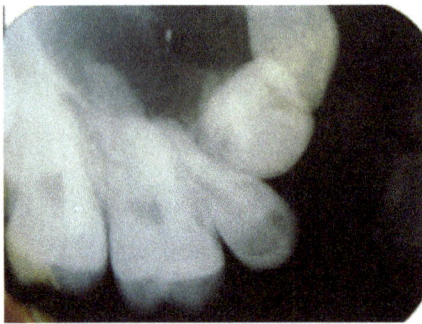

FIGURE 3: Maxillary cross-sectional occlusal radiograph showing radiolucency involving the right maxilla.

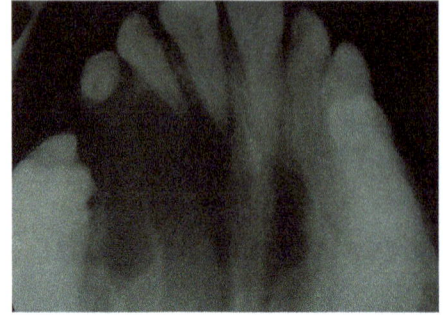

FIGURE 2: IOPA showing diffuse radiolucency in the region 15, 16, overretained 53 and crowns of 13, 14.

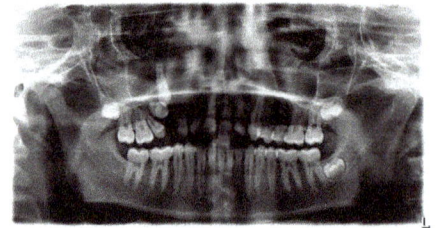

FIGURE 4: Panoramic radiograph showing impacted 13, 14.

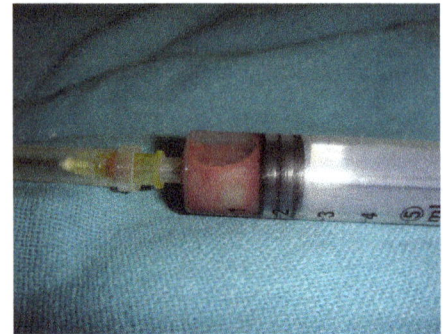

FIGURE 5: Fine needle aspiration cytology showing straw colored fluid intermixed with blood.

Patient was further subjected to radiographic investigation where intraoral periapical radiograph (Figure 2), occlusal maxillary cross-sectional (Figure 3), and panoramic radiograph (Figure 4) were done. IOPA revealed an ill-defined radiolucency around the apices of 15, 16 with poorly defined borders. Occlusal radiograph showed ill-defined radiolucency with intermittent septa involving the entire right maxilla and crossing the midline.

Panoramic radiograph revealed multilocular radiolucency separated with intermittent septa involving the right maxilla with impacted canine and first premolar. Displacement of second premolar is also seen.

Fine needle aspiration of the cyst was done which revealed straw colored fluid intermixed with blood (Figure 5). The sample was sent for protein estimation which revealed 3.2 gm/dL protein content.

Surgical excision of the lesion was done and was sent for histopathological confirmation. Histopathologic features reveal cystic lining with parakeratinized, corrugated stratified squamous epithelium exhibiting palisading basal cells, nuclear hyperchromatism, and flattened epithelial connective tissue junction at places. The underlying connective tissue capsule is fibrillar with admixed population of acute and chronic inflammatory cells at places, blood vessels, and peripheral bone. Features are suggestive of keratocystic odontogenic tumor (Figures 6(a) and 6(b)).

3. Discussion

Keratocystic odontogenic tumor (KCOT), formerly known as OKC, is a benign unicystic or multicystic intraosseous neoplasm of odontogenic origin which arises from the remnants of the dental lamina both in mandible and maxilla [1].

The discovery of increased mitotic activity in the cyst epithelium, the potential for epithelial budding from basal layer or daughter cysts in the cyst wall, the presence of chromosomal abnormalities, and the role of mutation of the PTCH gene in the etiology of KCOT resulted in its reclassification and renaming as keratocystic odontogenic tumor [1–6].

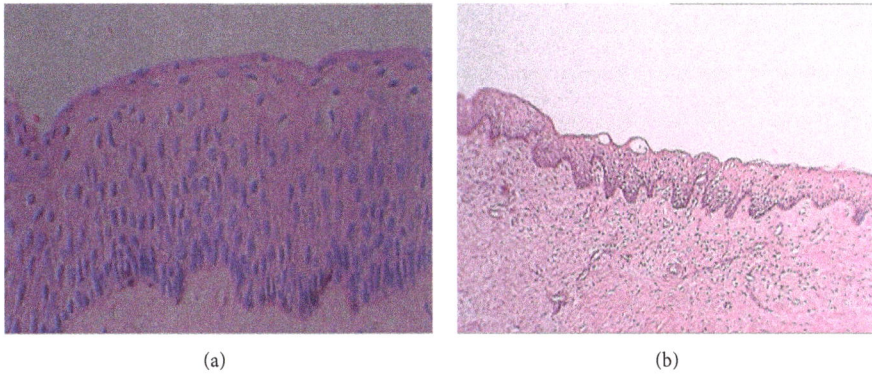

(a)   (b)

FIGURE 6: Photomicrograph of the histopathological slide.

Keratocystic odontogenic tumors are sometimes related to nevoid basal cell carcinoma syndrome, which is a rare inheritance disorder caused by mutations in the PTCH gene on chromosome 9 causing multiple odontogenic keratocyst of the jaws, basal cell carcinoma (BCC) of the skin, and vertebral anomalies [7].

According to Madras and Lapointe three factors led to the recharacterization of the keratocyst as KCOT. The KCOT exhibits locally destructive and highly recurrent behavior; the histopathology of the KCOT reveals budding of the basal layer into the connective tissue and frequent mitotic figures, and, finally, the KCOTs are associated with an inactivation of PCHT, the tumor suppressor gene [8].

KCOT has a predilection for occurring in the mandible (75.58%) as compared to maxilla [9–12]. In mandible, majority occur in third molar-ramus area, followed by first and second molar, and then followed by anterior mandible. In maxilla, the most common site is the third molar area followed by the cuspid region [9, 10, 13, 14].

KCOT when involving the maxilla sinus must be carefully assessed because the orbital damage and the spreading of associated infections could lead to local and systemic compromise to the patient, present with pain. Displacement of tooth and destruction of the floor of the orbit and proptosis of eyeball when it involves maxilla are most common features [15].

The ectopic eruption of teeth in the regions other than the oral cavity is rare, although there have been reports of teeth in unusual locations, one of them being the maxillary sinus. The etiology of ectopic eruption has not yet been completely clarified but may occur as a result of trauma, infection, developmental anomalies, and pathologic condition such as odontogenic cysts. As the growth of an odontogenic cyst continues, the cyst encroaches on the space of the sinus and displaces its borders: it may be that the displacement of teeth buds by this expansion of a cyst results in the ectopic eruption of a tooth [16].

KCOT is more common in males than females and occurs over a wide age range and is typically diagnosed during second to fourth decade [9].

On radiographic examination, KCOT cannot be distinguished from other intrabony cysts. In mandible, the epicenter is commonly located superior to the inferior alveolar nerve canal. It usually shows evidence of a cortical border with a scalloped outline which represents variation in the growth pattern of the cyst [13]. An important characteristic of KCOT is its propensity to grow along the internal aspect of jaws causing minimal expansion [9].

The keratocystic odontogenic tumor wall is usually thin unless there has been a superimposed inflammation [9, 10, 13, 14]. Characteristic features are

(i) a parakeratinized surface which is typically corrugated, rippled, or wrinkled;

(ii) uniformity of thickness of epithelium ranging from 6 to 10 cells thick;

(iii) a prominent palisaded, polarized basal cell layer of cells having "picket fence" or "tomb stone" appearance.

Numerous surgical modalities have been suggested for the treatment of KCOTs, including enucleation with primary closure, enucleation with open packing, and resection with or without loss of jaw continuity. The treatment depends on several factors, such as age, location, and size of lesion and whether the lesion is primary or recurrent. Total enucleation with or without "peripheral ostectomy" is the treatment of choice for most KCOTs unless lesion is recurrent or has significantly invaded soft tissue [9, 17].

4. Conclusion

The destructive, high recurrence potential of KCOTs and their ability to resemble other jaw cysts make it important to consider them in differential diagnosis of radiolucent lesions occurring in the maxilla. Also due to aggressive behavior and high recurrence rate of KCOT, all pathologic tissue should be properly excised and histopathologic confirmation should be made for a definitive diagnosis. The followup is advised for every six months for the next two years.

References

[1] A. Habibi, N. Saghravanian, M. Habibi, E. Mellati, and M. Habibi, "Keratocystic odontogenic tumor: a 10-year retrospective study of 83 cases in an Iranian population," *Journal of Oral Science*, vol. 49, no. 3, pp. 229–235, 2007.

[2] H. P. Phillpsen, "Keratocystic odontogenic tumour," in *WHO Classification of Tumors: Pathology and Genetics of Head and Neck Tumors*, L. Barnes, J. W. Eveson, P. Reichart, and D. Sidransky, Eds., pp. 306–307, IARC Press, Lyon, France, 3rd edition, 2005.

[3] D. M. G. Main, "Epithelial jaw cysts: a clinicopathological reappraisal," *British Journal of Oral Surgery*, vol. 8, no. 2, pp. 114–125, 1970.

[4] H. Myoung, S. Hong, S. Hong et al., "Odontogenic keratocyst: review of 256 cases for recurrence and clinicopathologic parameters," *Oral Surgery, Oral Medicine, Oral Pathology, Oral Radiology, and Endodontics*, vol. 91, no. 3, pp. 328–333, 2001.

[5] J. Henley, D. J. Summerlin, C. Tomich, S. Zhang, and L. Cheng, "Molecular evidence supporting the neoplastic nature of odontogenic keratocyst: a laser capture microdissection study of 15 cases," *Histopathology*, vol. 47, no. 6, pp. 582–586, 2005.

[6] D. C. Barreto, R. S. Gomez, A. E. Bale, W. L. Boson, and L. de Marco, "PTCH gene mutations in odontogenic keratocysts," *Journal of Dental Research*, vol. 79, no. 6, pp. 1418–1422, 2000.

[7] S. Seifi, S. Shafaie, and S. Ghadiri, "Microvessel density in follicular cysts, keratocystic odontogenic tumours and ameloblastomas," *Asian Pacific Journal of Cancer Prevention*, vol. 12, no. 2, pp. 351–356, 2011.

[8] D. S. MacDonald-Jankowski, "Keratocystic odontogenic tumour: systematic review," *Dentomaxillofacial Radiology*, vol. 40, no. 1, pp. 1–23, 2011.

[9] M. B. Motwani, S. S. Mishra, R. M. Anand et al., "Keratocystic odontogenic tumor: case reports and review of literature," *Journal of Indian Academy of Oral Medicine and Radiology*, vol. 23, no. 2, pp. 150–154, 2011.

[10] G. Shafer, K. Hine, and M. Levy, "Cysts and tumors of odontogenic origin," in *Shafer'S Textbook of Oral Pathology*, R. Rajendran, Ed., vol. 6, pp. 254–262, Elsevier, Noida, India, 2009.

[11] P. J. W. Stoelinga, "Long-term follow-up on keratocysts treated according to a defined protocol," *International Journal of Oral and Maxillofacial Surgery*, vol. 30, no. 1, pp. 14–25, 2001.

[12] H. Myoung, S. Hong, S. Hong et al., "Odontogenic keratocyst: review of 256 cases for recurrence and clinicopathologic parameters," *Oral Surgery, Oral Medicine, Oral Pathology, Oral Radiology, and Endodontics*, vol. 91, no. 3, pp. 328–333, 2001.

[13] N. K. Wood and P. W. Goaz, "Solitary cysts like radiolucencies and necessarily contacting teeth," in *Differential Diagnosis of Oral and Maxillofacial Lesions*, vol. 5, pp. 318–321, Mosby (Elsevier), Kundli, India, 2007.

[14] B. W. Neville, D. D. Damm, C. M. Allen et al., "Odontogenic cysts an tumors," in *Oral and Maxillofacial Pathology*, vol. 3, pp. 683–687, Saunders (Elsevier), Noida, India, 2009.

[15] K. Priya, P. Karthikeyan, and V. Nirmal Coumare, "Odontogenic keratocyst: a case series of five patients," *Indian Journal of Otolaryngology and Head and Neck Surgery*, 2012.

[16] H. Kwon, W. B. Lim, J. S. Kim et al., "odontogenic keratocyst associated with an actopic tooth in maxillary sinus- a report of two cases and a review of the literature," *The Korean Journal of Pathology*, vol. 45, supplement 1, pp. S5–S10, 2011.

[17] S. B. Blanchard, "Odontogenic keratocysts: review of the literature and report of a case," *Journal of Periodontology*, vol. 68, no. 3, pp. 306–311, 1997.

27

Bilateral Mesiodens in Monozygotic Twins: 3D Diagnostic and Management

Carla Vecchione Gurgel,[1] **Ana Lídia Soares Cota,**[1] **Tatiana Yuriko Kobayashi,**[1] **Salete Moura Bonifácio Silva,**[1] **Maria Aparecida Andrade Moreira Machado,**[1] **Daniela Rios,**[1] **Daniela Gamba Garib,**[1,2] **and Thais Marchini Oliveira**[1,2]

[1] *Department of Pediatric Dentistry, Orthodontics and Public Health, Bauru School of Dentistry,*
  University of São Paulo, São Paulo, Brazil
[2] *Hospital for the Rehabilitation of Craniofacial Anomalies, University of São Paulo, São Paulo, Brazil*

Correspondence should be addressed to Thais Marchini Oliveira; marchini@usp.br

Academic Editors: I. Anic, N. Brezniak, A. Epivatianos, C. S. Farah, L. J. Oesterle, and E. F. Wright

Mesiodens is the most frequent type of supernumerary tooth and may occur in several forms, causing different local disorders, such as impaction of the anterior permanent teeth. High-resolution three-dimensional (3D) images have improved the diagnosis and treatment plan of patients with impacted and supernumerary teeth. The purpose of this paper was to report a case of two mesiodens in monozygotic twin boys with appropriate 3D diagnostic and treatment plan.

1. Introduction

A supernumerary tooth is a development anomaly of number characterized by the presence of tooth in addition to the normal series [1]. The mesiodens is the most frequent supernumerary tooth and is located in the maxillary central incisor region [2, 3]. The prevalence of this anomaly varies between 0.15% and 1.9%, being more frequent in males than in females, with a 2 : 1 ratio [3].

Mesiodens could be discovered accidentally during radiological examination of the premaxillary area. The diagnostic commonly occurs between 7 and 9 years of age probably because permanent central incisors erupt at this stage and the complaint of noneruption induces a radiological examination that might reveal the presence of mesiodens [4]. Several studies have applied cone-beam-computed tomography (CBCT) to accurately diagnose supernumerary teeth with the potential to overcome most of the technical limitations of the plain film projection and the capability of providing a high-resolution three-dimensional (3D) representation of the maxillofacial tissues in a cost- and dose-efficient manner [5–8].

The occurrence of mesiodens in twins is unusual if not a rare event in the literature. Therefore, the purpose of this paper was to report a case of two mesiodens in monozygotic twin boys with appropriate 3D diagnostic and treatment plan.

2. Case Report

Two monozygotic twin boys were referred to the Pediatric Dentistry Clinic of our University when they were 9 years old for treatment of impacted permanent maxillary central incisors. Their past medical histories showed no systemic diseases, and the dental histories showed no facial trauma or other tooth abnormalities.

A clinical examination in twin A revealed the absence of the permanent maxillary central incisors and the presence of overretained primary maxillary central right incisor (Figure 1(a)). In twin B the clinical analysis showed the absence of the permanent maxillary central incisors and the presence of overretained primary maxillary central incisors (Figure 1(b)).

Panoramic and periapical radiographs were performed in both patients. The radiographs revealed impacted permanent

(a)

(b)

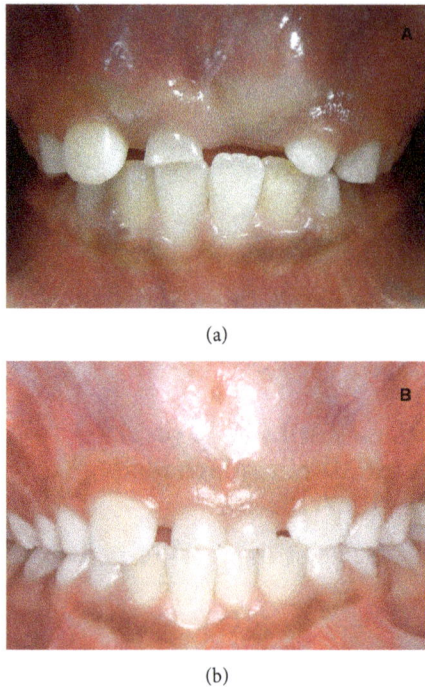

FIGURE 1: Initial intraoral view showing the absence of the permanent maxillary central incisors in both twins.

maxillary central incisors because of the presence of two mesiodens in the eruption path in both twins, being that in twin B the supernumerary teeth were in a higher position (Figures 2(a), 2(b), 3(a), and 3(b)). Then, both twins were submitted to CBCT exam of the maxilla to assist in localization and orientation of the two mesiodens. CBCT images were requested for diagnosing accurately the morphology and exact location of the two mesiodens and the radicular formation of the permanent maxillary central incisors. The images were created and viewed interactively using a dental computed tomography software program. Axial sections images revealed horizontal impaction of the permanent maxillary incisors, and cross-section oblique images revealed impacted permanent maxillary central incisors, as well as the relationship with the adjacent teeth and structures (Figures 4(a) and 4(b)).

After explaining the advantages and disadvantages of the therapeutic options for the patients and their family, the treatment plan was surgical extraction of the two mesiodens and waits for spontaneous eruption of the impacted permanent maxillary central incisors in both twins.

The surgical technique was performed under local anesthesia. Initially, the overretained primary teeth were extracted. Then, an incision was performed along the gingival margin, from the primary maxillary right canine to the permanent maxillary central left incisor, and a mucoperiosteal flap was elevated to the minimum necessary extent. The mucoperiosteal soft tissues underlying the permanent central incisors were removed. When necessary, the bone which covered the dental crowns was removed with surgical

round burs to expose the labial surface. The supernumerary teeth were extracted, and, after cleaning the area and getting hemostasis, the flap was repositioned and sutured. After 1 week, the sutures were removed in both twins (Figures 5(a) and 5(b)).

After 4 months of followup, the permanent maxillary central right incisor in twin a erupted in the oral cavity. In both twins, there were a lack of space for the eruption of the permanent maxillary central incisors, and a Hyrax-type palatal expansion appliance was installed (Figures 6(a) and 6(b)). The permanent maxillary central incisors completely erupted in twin A after 10 months of followup (Figure 7(a)). In twin B, the permanent maxillary central right incisor completely erupted after 12 months of the mesiodens removal (Figure 7(b)). However, the permanent maxillary central left incisor had not erupted in twin B after 18 months of followup. The soft tissue, periodontal attachment, gingival contour, and probing depth were normal after eruption in both twins. After 20 months of followup, both twins were referred to orthodontic treatment.

3. Discussion

The etiology of a mesiodens is still not clearly established in the literature. The pathogenesis of mesiodens has been attributed to various theories such as locally induced hyperactivity of the dental lamina, a phylogenetic relic of extinct ancestral tissue, a dichotomy of tooth buds [2, 9], heredity, and some environmental factors [10]. The familial pattern of occurrence of mesiodens in twins strongly supports a genetic influence, possibly inherited as an autosomal dominant inheritance [2, 11, 12]. The theory, involving hyperactivity of the dental lamina, is the most widely supported one. According to this theory, remnants of the dental lamina or palatal offshoots of active dental lamina are induced to develop into an extra tooth bud, which results in a supernumerary tooth [13]. Although no investigation proved the hereditary condition of mesiodens, genetics are also thought to contribute to its development, as such occurrence has been diagnosed in twins, siblings, and sequential generations of a single family [14]. Sedano and Gorlin [12] proposed a genetic theory in which mesiodens is an autosomal dominant trait with lack of penetrance in some generations. A sex-linked pattern has also been proposed, as males are affected twice as frequently as females [15].

The monozygotic twins presented here displayed similarly located supernumerary and impacted teeth suggesting the influence of genetic factors on the etiology of mesiodens. However, some differences observed in the twins dentition suggested that environmental factors may also affect the formation of the phenotype [16, 17]. Seddon et al. [11] concluded, after reviewing eight previous cases and one of their own, that mesiodens were likely to be concordant in monozygotic twins with respect to number, but they noted that minor variations in size, shape, and orientation were common. In the present case, the abovementioned traits are similar in both twins; however, in twin B mesiodens are located in a higher position when compared to twin A. There were some differences during the treatment, but the

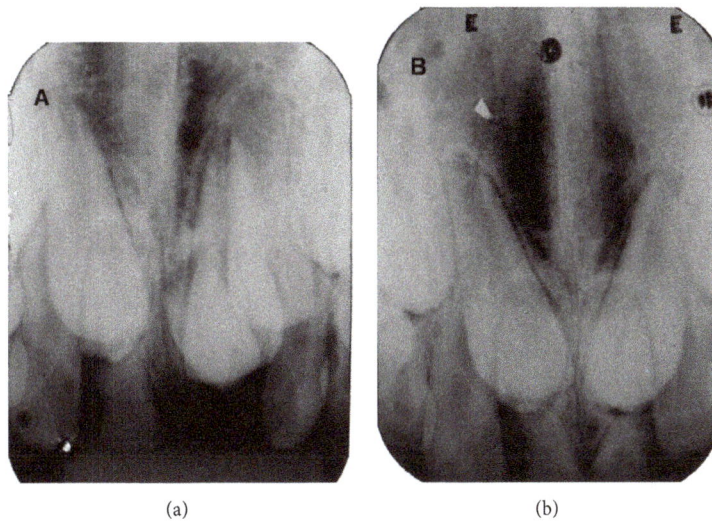

(a)   (b)

FIGURE 2: Periapical radiograph showing impacted permanent maxillary central incisors and the presence of two mesiodens in both twins.

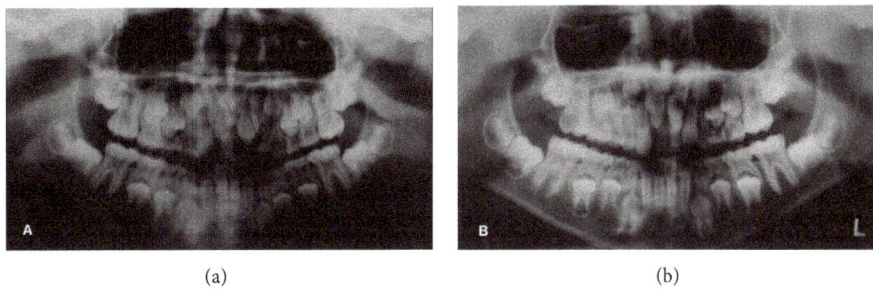

(a)   (b)

FIGURE 3: Panoramic radiograph showing impacted permanent maxillary central incisors and the presence of two mesiodens in both twins.

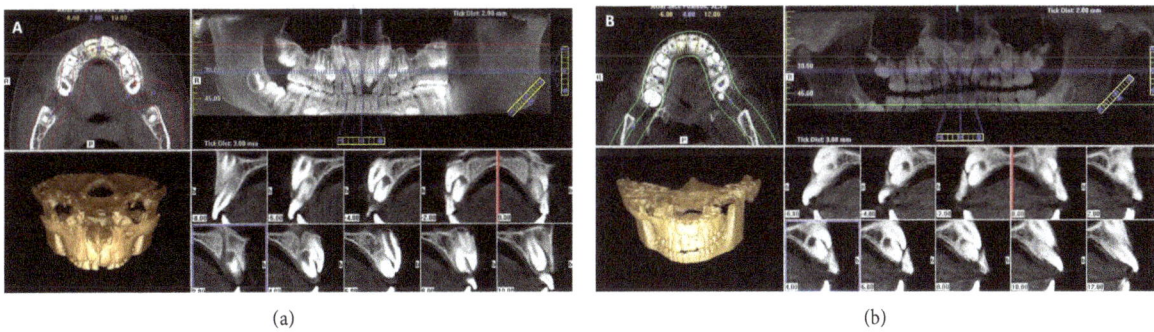

(a)   (b)

FIGURE 4: The cross-section oblique images showing impacted permanent maxillary central incisors and the relationship with two mesiodens in both twins.

treatment plan was the same for both twins. Also, in twin A both impacted teeth erupted spontaneously after 10 months while in twin B only the permanent maxillary central right incisor erupted after 12 months of the mesiodens removal. It also suggests an influence of phenotype factors on the occurrence of mesiodens.

The choice of the best treatment plan depends on the correct diagnosis. Oral surgeons require information on both the location and the shape of supernumerary and impacted teeth before performing an operation for extraction. Intraoral and/or panoramic radiography has conventionally been used for preoperative examination [8, 18]. However, panoramic radiography alone is not sufficient for determining the exact location of supernumerary and impacted teeth, due to the image superimposition [6, 19]. CBCT seems to be a good tool for the evaluation, accurate diagnosis, and determination of the location of mesiodens and impacted teeth [5–8]. In the present case, CBCT provided valuable information that

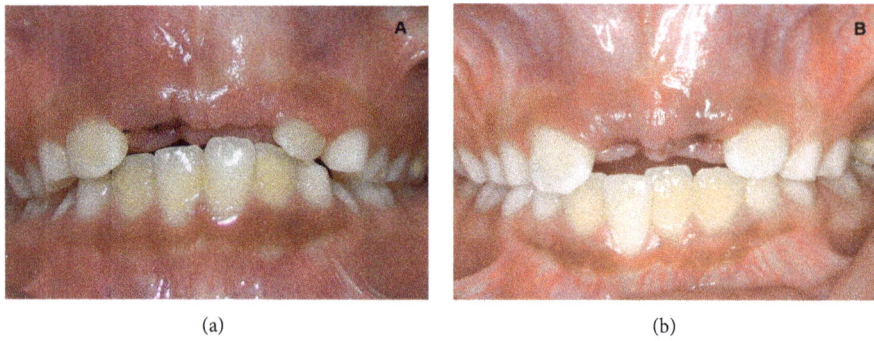

(a)   (b)

FIGURE 5: Intraoral view showing the intraoral aspect after 1 week of the mesiodens removal in both twins.

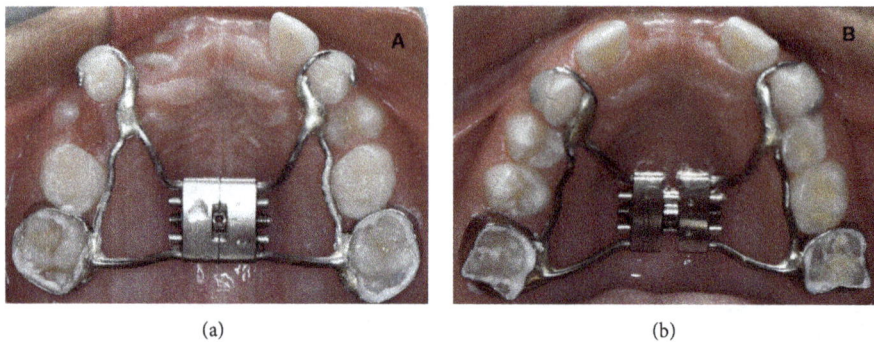

(a)   (b)

FIGURE 6: Palatal view of the Hyrax-type palatal expansion appliance in both twins.

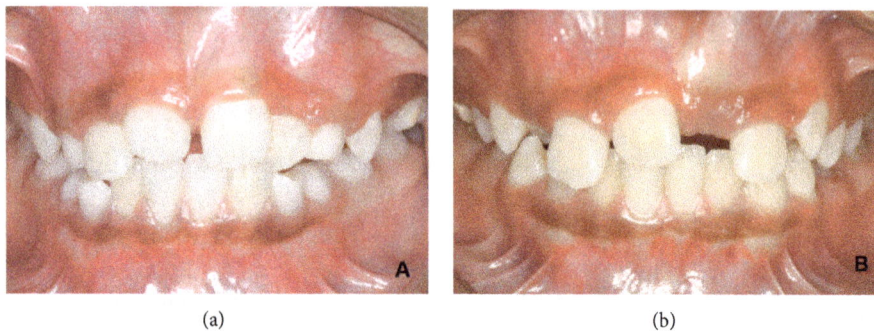

(a)   (b)

FIGURE 7: Intraoral view showing the permanent maxillary central incisors erupted in twin A and the permanent maxillary central right incisor erupted in twin B.

helped us to determine the morphology of the mesiodens and exact 3D positioning of the impacted permanent teeth.

There is no consensus on the literature about the best time for mesiodens removal. Studies have shown that the removal of a mesiodens during the early mixed dentition stage allows normal eruptive forces to promote spontaneous eruption of the impacted tooth after 6 to 24 months [2, 13, 16]. Some authors recommend postponement of surgical intervention until the age of 8–10 years, when unerupted apex of central incisor is almost mature [10]. However, the later the extraction of the mesiodens, the greater the chance that the permanent tooth either will not spontaneously erupt.

Unfortunately, by this time the forces that cause normal eruption of the incisors are diminished, and surgical exposure and subsequent orthodontic treatment are more frequently required. Also, space loss and a midline shift of the central incisors may have already occurred by this age, since the lateral incisors will have erupted and may have drifted mesially into the central space. Thus, a significant delay in treatment may create the need for more complex surgical and orthodontic management. In the case presented here, the option was immediately the removal of the mesiodens, and the spontaneous eruption of the maxillary central incisors occurred after 10 months in twin A and 12 months in twin

B. However, in Twin B the maxillary central left incisor did not erupt after 18 months of followup, and he was referred to orthodontic treatment.

4. Conclusion

It is necessary to emphasize the role of the dentistry in management of cases of mesiodens, principally, due to the possibility of early detecting of these abnormalities and could establish an adequate treatment plan. Also, CBCT may help in the correct 3D diagnostic and management of impacted and supernumerary teeth.

References

[1] J. F. Liu, "Characteristics of premaxillary supernumerary teeth: a survey of 112 cases," *Journal of Dentistry for Children*, vol. 62, no. 4, pp. 262–265, 1995.

[2] H. Babacan, F. Öztürk, and H. B. Polat, "Identical unerupted maxillary incisors in monozygotic twins," *American Journal of Orthodontics and Dentofacial Orthopedics*, vol. 138, no. 4, pp. 498–509, 2010.

[3] M. M. Gallas and A. García, "Retention of permanent incisors by mesiodens: a family affair," *British Dental Journal*, vol. 188, no. 2, pp. 63–64, 2000.

[4] S. Mukhopadhyay, "Mesiodens: a clinical and radiographic study in children," *Journal of Indian Society of Pedodontics and Preventive Dentistry*, vol. 29, no. 1, pp. 34–38, 2011.

[5] C. V. Gurgel, N. Lourenço Neto, T. Y. Kobayashi et al., "Management of a permanent tooth after trauma to deciduous predecessor: an evaluation by cone-beam computed tomography," *Dental Traumatology*, vol. 27, no. 5, pp. 408–412, 2011.

[6] D. G. Liu, W. L. Zhang, Z. Y. Zhang, Y. T. Wu, and X. C. Ma, "Three-dimensional evaluations of supernumerary teeth using cone-beam computed tomography for 487 cases," *Oral Surgery, Oral Medicine, Oral Pathology, Oral Radiology and Endodontology*, vol. 103, no. 3, pp. 403–411, 2007.

[7] K. D. Kim, A. Ruprecht, K. J. Jeon, and C. S. Park, "Personal computer-based three-dimensional computed tomographic images of the teeth for evaluating supernumerary or ectopically impacted teeth," *The Angle Orthodontist*, vol. 73, no. 5, pp. 614–621, 2003.

[8] C. V. Gurgel, A. L. S. Cota, T. Y. Kobayashi et al., "Cone beam computed tomography for diagnosis and treatment planning of supernumerary teeth," *General Dentistry*, vol. 60, no. 3, pp. 131–135, 2012.

[9] C. M. Marya and B. R. A. Kumar, "Familial occurrence of mesiodentes with unusual findings: case reports," *Quintessence International*, vol. 29, no. 1, pp. 49–51, 1998.

[10] V. K. Kulkarni, S. Reddy, M. Duddu, and D. Reddy, "Multidisciplinary management of multiple maxillary anterior supernumerary teeth: a case report," *Quintessence International*, vol. 41, no. 3, pp. 191–195, 2010.

[11] R. P. Seddon, S. C. Johnstone, and P. B. Smith, "Mesiodentes in twins: a case report and a review of the literature," *International Journal of Paediatric Dentistry*, vol. 7, no. 3, pp. 177–184, 1997.

[12] H. O. Sedano and R. J. Gorlin, "Familial occurrence of mesiodens," *Oral Surgery, Oral Medicine, Oral Pathology*, vol. 27, no. 3, pp. 360–362, 1969.

[13] K. A. Russell and M. A. Folwarczna, "Mesiodens—diagnosis and management of a common supernumerary tooth," *Journal Canadian Dental Association*, vol. 69, no. 6, pp. 362–366, 2003.

[14] A. H. Brook, "A unifying aetiological explanation for anomalies of human tooth number and size," *Archives of Oral Biology*, vol. 29, no. 5, pp. 373–378, 1984.

[15] F. N. Hattab, O. M. Yassin, and M. A. Rawashdeh, "Supernumerary teeth: report of three cases and review of the literature," *Journal of Dentistry for Children*, vol. 61, no. 5-6, pp. 382–393, 1994.

[16] H. Łangowska-Adamczyk and B. Karmańska, "Similar locations of impacted and supernumerary teeth in monozygotic twins: a report of 2 cases," *American Journal of Orthodontics and Dentofacial Orthopedics*, vol. 119, no. 1, pp. 67–70, 2001.

[17] G. C. Townsend, L. Richards, T. Hughes, S. Pinkerton, and W. Schwerdt, "Epigenetic influences may explain dental differences in monozygotic twin pairs," *Australian Dental Journal*, vol. 50, no. 2, pp. 95–100, 2005.

[18] S. Raupp, P. F. Kramer, H. W. de Oliveira, F. M. da Rosa, and I. M. Faraco Jr., "Application of computed tomography for supernumerary teeth location in pediatric dentistry," *Journal of Clinical Pediatric Dentistry*, vol. 32, no. 4, pp. 273–276, 2008.

[19] T. Sawamura, K. Minowa, and M. Nakamura, "Impacted teeth in the maxilla: usefulness of 3D Dental-CT for preoperative evaluation," *European Journal of Radiology*, vol. 47, no. 3, pp. 221–226, 2003.

28

Custom Metal Occlusal Surface for Acrylic Resin Denture Teeth to Enhance Wear Resistance

Rizwan Ali Shivji, Vaibhav D. Kamble, and Mohd. Atif Khan

Department of Prosthodontics, VSPM Dental College and Research Centre, Nagpur, India

Correspondence should be addressed to Vaibhav D. Kamble, vaibhavk056@gmail.com

Academic Editors: I. El-Hakim and E. F. Wright

Wear of the occlusal surface of the denture is a known fact which leads to subsequent changes in jaw relation, vertical dimension, loss of aesthetics, aged looks, and decrease in masticatory efficiency. Treatment modalities includes, change of denture set after a regular interval of 4-5 years, use of wear resistant denture teeth that includes wear resistant resin or porcelain teeth, teeth with cast metal occlusal surface, and altering occlusal contact areas of denture teeth by use of silver amalgam fillings. A case report of a patient who had increased tendency of occlusal wear was treated with custom made metal occlusal surface of denture teeth to enhance wear resistance and to improve the masticatory efficiency.

1. Introduction

Thought is the child of action and necessity is the mother of invention. This is the soul of newly based dentistry. A little diverse approach from traditional modalities available in dentistry can solve patient's problem to a greater extent, thereby adding to his well-being and comfort. Wear changes in the occlusal surface of the denture wearing patient is a known fact. But need to change the dentures on an increased frequency ask a call for lateral thinking. This calls the change in approach and technique. One such patient reported to VSPM Dental College and Research Centre, Nagpur, who had frequent need for change of his denture sets due to excessive wear, resulting in loss of masticatory efficiency, function, aesthetics, and comfort.

2. Case Report

A 58-years-old male patient reported in the Department of Prosthetic Dentistry, VSPM Dental College and Research Centre, Nagpur with the chief complaint of worn out denture occlusal surfaces and difficulty in mastication (Figure 1). Detailed medical and dental history revealed that the patient was suffering from neuromuscular disorder (differential diagnosis-trigeminal myoclonus) resulting in repetitive episodes of cyclic, involuntary, and uncoordinated brisk jaw movements. Oral manifestations showed severe wear of occlusal surface of prosthetic teeth (Figures 2(a) and 2(b)). Further it was found that it was his fourth denture set within a span of three years. Although the retention of the denture was satisfactory, he was forced to have his denture remade frequently. This forced the patient to undergo great physical and mental stress of dental procedures and frequent visits to dental operatory. To meet this vague problem and to reduce wear rate of prosthetic denture teeth, it was decided to fabricate the complete denture prostheses with cast metal occlusal surface.

Metal occlusal surface are used to construct denture that oppose natural dentition or for reconstruction of dental arch with metal occlusal surface. Wallace [1] used gold for occlusal surface. On comparing the wear of gold, porcelain, heat-cured, and light-cured resin in occlusal contact, Ekfeldt and Oilo [2] found that all materials had the greatest loss of substance when the opposing teeth were of porcelain. The heat-cured, unfilled resin was the least wear-resistant material, followed by light-cured resin, porcelain, and gold. The heat-cured resin showed a combined tribochemical and fatigue type of wear. The light-cured resin and porcelain

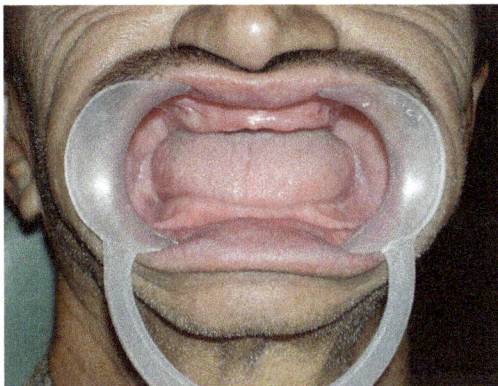

FIGURE 1: Preoperative view: complete edentulous arches.

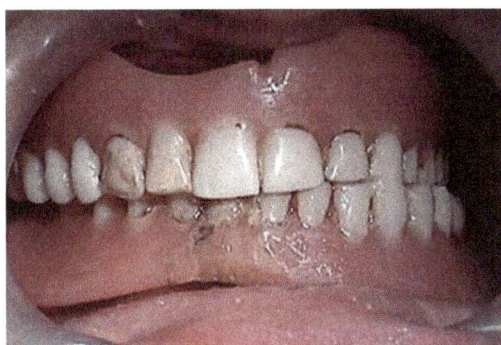

(a)

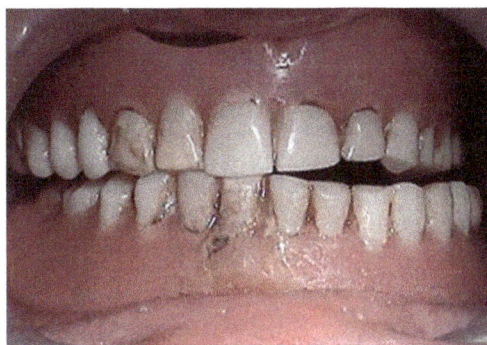

(b)

FIGURE 2: Wear of prosthetic denture teeth leading to difficulty in mastication.

showed mainly a fatigue type of wear, whereas gold showed a combined abrasive and fatigue type of wear. Tanaka et al. [3] stated that the traditional denture fabrication technique using resin teeth with metal occlusal surfaces is rather complicated and time consuming. The teeth are arranged on the wax denture and processed in the usual manner. The patient is allowed to use the completed denture for a period of time to harmonize the occlusal surfaces with oral function. The occlusal portions of the teeth are then separated from the base and invested as a resin pattern for casting. The new cast occlusal portions are reset on the base portions with a resin adhesive. Krantz et al. [4] described a simplified method for making esthetic cast metal occlusal surfaces. Posterior acrylic resin teeth casted in a nickel-chrome alloy are coated with silane and an esthetic composite resin veneer is applied to the buccal surface. These veneered posterior metal teeth are incorporated in the wax setup and the dentures are processed and finished. Ekfeldt et al. [5] conducted a study to compare a gravimetric method and an impression technique in the evaluation of occlusal substance loss. The wear of gold, porcelain, and microfilled resin was studied in vivo. The gravimetric method showed lower substance loss for porcelain than for gold, whereas the microfilled resin had the highest substance loss. The observed findings corroborated with previous findings of the wear mechanism of the

materials; that is, gold has mainly abrasive wear in contact with porcelain, whereas porcelain has a fatigue type and microfilled resin a tribochemical type of wear. After complete evaluation of the patient's problem and need, a modified technique of fabricating denture prosthesis with metal occlusal surface was planned. Standard technique using conventional clinical and laboratory steps were followed to fabricate the denture and essential modifications were made to attend anticipated results. Following satisfactory wax try-in appointment, Putty index impression of denture teeth were made for each quadrant separately with polyvinyl siloxane impression material (Aquasil Soft putty/Regular set, Dentsply, Germany). Wax pattern from the same were made using inlay casting wax (Harvard, Blauwachs, Berlin, Germany) with attention to get occlusal and lingual/palatal surface anatomy of each quadrant. Wax patterns were further refined and retentive tags and beads were added for retention of the tooth coloured acrylic facing and also for mechanical locking of the prosthetic tooth to denture base. Patterns were invested in phosphate bonded investment (Bellasun, Bego, Germany) and casted in nickel-chromium alloy (Ruby Dental Products Inc., Osaka, Japan). Castings were finished and polished using standard procedures. Acrylic resin facings were then added to the castings with appropriate tooth coloured heat polymerized acrylic resin (A3)

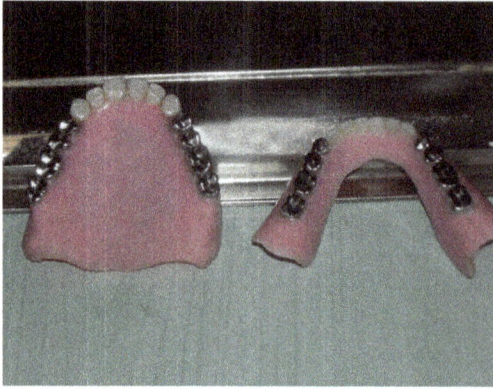

Figure 3: Custom metal occlusal surfaces for acrylic resin denture teeth.

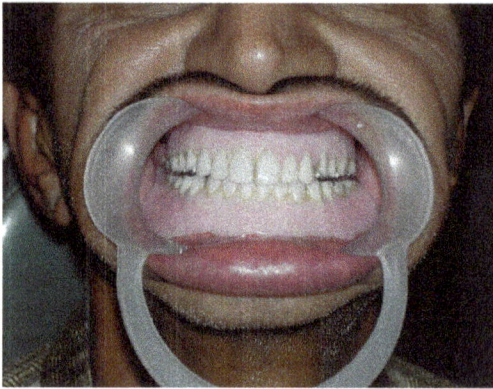

Figure 4: Postoperative intraoral view: denture insertion with metal occlusal surfaces on posterior teeth.

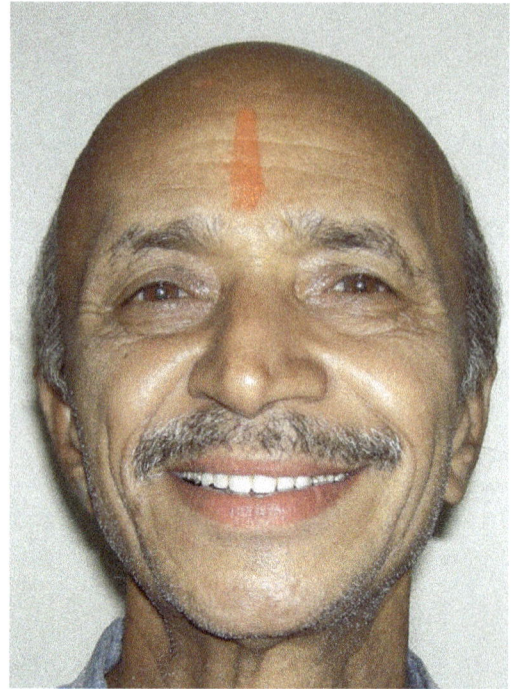

Figure 5: Postoperative extraoral view.

(DPI, Mumbai, India). Acrylic denture teeth were replaced with custom-made metal occlusal surface denture teeth in respective quadrants maintaining the verified jaw relation record on the articulator. Wax try-in was repeated for final evaluation of the jaw relation, phonetics, aesthetics, and occlusion. Prosthesis was processed, finished, and polished following laboratory remount procedure (Figure 3). Denture insertion was done following the necessary clinical remount procedure (Figure 4). Recall visits were scheduled after 24 hours, 1 week, 1 month, and then every subsequent 3 months initially. Patient was on regular yearly follow up thereafter. Denture provided the effective services to the patient satisfaction (Figure 5). Seeing the patient's compliance and complete satisfaction of denture prosthesis, new dentures were fabricated using the same procedure after six years.

3. Discussion

The use of standard technique with required indicated clinical and laboratory alterations may contribute to greater clinical success. With this technique there is increase in one clinical and laboratory step, but had contributed significantly in solving patient's long term problem. Metal occlusal surface has advantages of inherent physical property of metal, the

adaptability of the occlusal surface and a definite albeit subjective and psychological advantage. Disadvantages of metal occlusal surface include compromised aesthetics, mechanical method of locking of the acrylic resin and increased weight of prosthesis. Alternative to metal occlusal surface, porcelain teeth can be used but they contribute to maximum stress, brittle, expensive, and mechanical locking with denture base [2, 5]. Silver amalgam filling may be used but will cover only occlusal fossae, pit and fissure areas but not the complete occlusal surface. This will be mostly effective in cases with single complete denture but the advantages are economical and require less clinical and laboratory steps.

4. Conclusion

In a nut shell, the present approach towards the patient's diverse problem has served as a better treatment modality. The approach seemed to be best suited for the patients not too keen on posterior aesthetics. Patients opinion and compliance is been taken annually since 4 years of denture use. Patient seemed to be happy and satisfied with the denture service with no need for remake to be done since then.

References

[1] D. H. Wallace, "The use of gold occlusal surfaces in complete and partial dentures," *The Journal of Prosthetic Dentistry*, vol. 14, no. 2, pp. 326–333, 1964.

[2] A. Ekfeldt and G. Oilo, "Occlusal contact wear of prosthodontic materials. An in vivo study," *Acta Odontologica Scandinavica*, vol. 46, no. 3, pp. 159–169, 1988.

[3] Y. Tanaka, T. Sugimoto, S. Tanaka, and K. Hiranuma, "Development of a two-piece artificial resin tooth specially designed for a metal occlusal surface," *The International Journal of Prosthodontics*, vol. 3, no. 3, pp. 292–298, 1990.

[4] W. A. Krantz, J. R. Ivanhoe, and E. D. Adrian, "A simplified technique for fabricating esthetic cast metal occlusal surfaces for dentures," *The Journal of Prosthetic Dentistry*, vol. 63, no. 6, pp. 713–715, 1990.

[5] A. Ekfeldt, B. Fransson, B. Söderlund, and G. Oilo, "Wear resistance of some prosthodontic materials in vivo," *Acta Odontologica Scandinavica*, vol. 51, no. 2, pp. 99–107, 1993.

29

CT Images of a Severe TMJ Osteoarthritis and Differential Diagnosis with Other Joint Disorders

K. L. Ferrazzo,[1] L. B. Osório,[2] and V. A. Ferrazzo[2]

[1] School of Dentistry, Franciscan University Center, Andradas Street, 1614, 97010-032 Santa Maria, RS, Brazil
[2] Department of Stomatology, School of Dentistry, Federal University of Santa Maria, Floriano Peixoto Street, 1184, 97015-372 Santa Maria, RS, Brazil

Correspondence should be addressed to K. L. Ferrazzo; kivialinhares@uol.com.br

Academic Editors: R. A. de Mesquita and E. F. Wright

Osteoarthritis (OA) is the most common arthritis which affects the human body and can affect the temporomandibular joint (TMJ). The diagnosis of TMJ OA is essentially based on clinical examination. However, laboratory tests and radiographic exams are also useful to exclude other diseases. The diagnosis of OA may be difficult because of other TMJ pathologies that can have similar clinical and radiographic aspects. The purpose of this study was to describe an unusual case of bilateral TMJ OA in an advanced stage and discuss its most common clinical, laboratory, and radiographic findings, focusing on their importance in the differential diagnosis with other TMJ diseases. Erosion, sclerosis, osteophytes, flattening, subchondral cysts, and a reduced joint space were some of the radiographic findings in TMJ OA. We concluded that, for the correct differential diagnosis of TMJ OA, it is necessary to unite medical history, physical examination, laboratory tests, and radiographic findings. Computed tomography is the test of choice for evaluating bone involvement and for diagnosing and establishing the degree of the disease.

1. Introduction

Osteoarthritis (OA) is a chronic noninflammatory degenerative condition that is the most common form of arthritis affecting the human body [1, 2]. Osteoarthrosis, deforming arthritis, and degenerative joint disease are the most used synonymous terms of OA [3]. In the pathogenesis of OA, evidence is growing for the role of systemic and biomechanical factors [2]. OA can be broadly divided into two groups: (1) primary osteoarthritis, when there is no previous pathology and the cause is unknown; (2) secondary osteoarthritis, when it is secondary to some previous injury, stress, or pathology in the joint [4–6]. The disease can be defined as a gradual loss of articular cartilage primarily, associated with thickening of the subchondral bone. The bone undergoes reactive hypertrophy forming peripheral osteophytes. Secondly, there is a mild, chronic nonspecific synovial inflammation. It most commonly affects middle-aged and older people with a predilection for women after the age of 50 [6]. Women with osteoarthritis of the hands often develop bony lumps at the ends of their fingers called Heberden's nodes. They most frequently occur in women over forty and may run in families. These nodes may be confined to one or several fingers. They are painless, grow gradually, and are not progressive [6, 7]. Although OA occurs more frequently in the joints of the hips, knees, and spine, which support more weight, it also affects the neck, hands, and temporomandibular joint (TMJ). In the TMJ, the most common signs and symptoms of OA are swelling and palpable tenderness of the joint, crepitation, and limited mandibular movement. Joint pain is usually mild in the morning and gets worse in the evening after a day's activity [1, 6–11].

The diagnosis of TMJ OA is mainly based on medical history and clinical examination. There are no specific laboratory tests to make a definitive diagnosis of OA. Results of laboratory tests such as rheumatoid factor (RF), antinuclear antibody (ANA), and erythrocyte sedimentation rate (ESR) are normal and are, therefore, useful only to rule out other diagnoses [7]. For complete analyses, imaging examinations are required. Panoramic and conventional radiographs may identify rough TMJ changes, but these methods are restricted in diagnosis, because of the anatomical superposition that

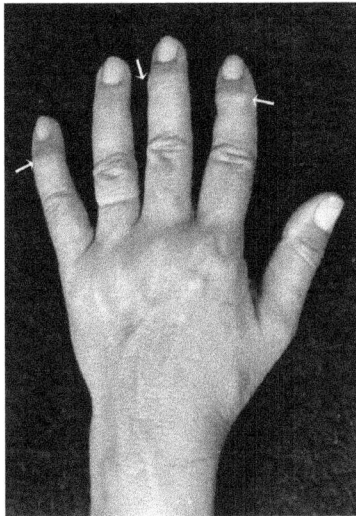

FIGURE 1: Bony growth spurs at the joint at the end of the fingers—Heberden's nodes (arrows).

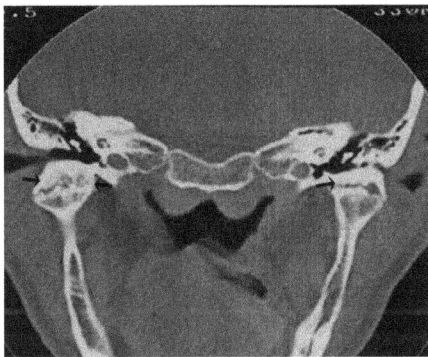

FIGURE 2: Coronal CT image demonstrating bilateral joint space narrowing, rough condylar surfaces, and sclerosis of the subchondral bone (arrows).

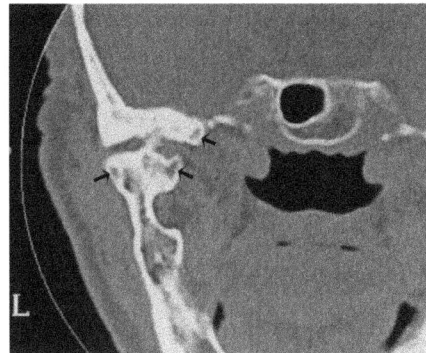

FIGURE 3: Subchondral cysts called Ely's cysts (arrows).

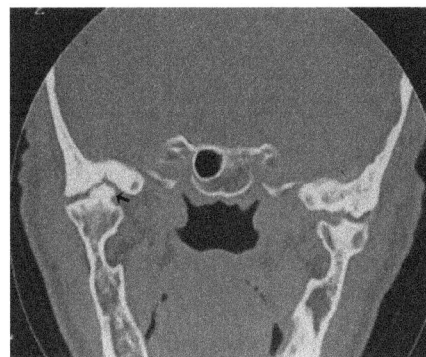

FIGURE 4: Large bone outgrowth (osteophyte) in the left TMJ (arrow) and bilateral subchondral cysts.

prevents accurate view of the bone components. In this way, computed tomography (CT) is a useful exam that helps to confirm the diagnosis of TMJ OA and also to grade its severity [7, 8].

In the current paper, we present an unusual case of bilateral TMJ OA in an advanced stage focusing on clinical, laboratory, and radiographic differential diagnosis of the disease.

2. Case Report

A 68-year-old white female presented with the main complaint of moderate pain in the TMJ (preauricular region), and a reduced opening of the mouth. Her medical history revealed good general health. Curiously, during anamnesis she reported she was involved in a car accident 10 years before and had a mandible injury, which caused only a chin laceration and local swelling. However, the patient associated the injury with the beginning of the symptoms—on occasion there was a severe bilateral pain in TMJ, with reduction on mandibular movements for about five weeks. At that time, she was treated with nonsteroidal anti-inflammatory drugs until the disappearance of the symptoms, when she recuperated the movement limitation.

At the present examination, intraoral investigation revealed a limitation of the vertical mouth opening (25 mm interincisally) and occlusion disorder with dental loss. The assessment of the other mandibular movements, such as lateral excursion or mandibular deflection, was not possible because of the pain and movements limitation. On physical examination, a characteristic enlargement at the distal interphalangeal joint, called Heberden's node (Figure 1), was seen. There was no familial history of arthrosis. Laboratory studies for evaluation were requested including complete blood count, erythrocyte sedimentation rate, rheumatoid factor, and antinuclear antibodies. All results were within normal limits.

Computed tomography of the TMJ was performed, and coronal segments showed erosion of the articular surface of the condyle, rough condylar surfaces with bilateral joint space narrowing, thickening of the subchondral bone, sclerosis areas (Figure 2), subchondral cysts (Figure 3), and bone outgrowths—osteophytes (Figure 4). Although evaluation of disc position is important, it was not possible to take it as there was no magnetic resonance equipment at the public

TABLE 1: Differential diagnosis among osteoarthritis (OA), rheumatoid arthritis (RA), and pain dysfunction syndrome (PDS) [3, 12, 13].

Findings	OA	RA	PDS
Pain	Localized	Diffuse	Irradiated
TMJ involvement	Symmetric or not	Symmetric	Symmetric or not
Subcutaneous nodes	Absent	Present (20%)	Absent
Type of hand swelling	Hard	Soft	Absent
Extra-articular findings	Absent	May be present	Absent
Morning stiffness	Absent	Present	Absent
Crepitation	Present	Rarely	Rarely
Clicking	Rarely	Absent	Present
Rheumatoid factor	Rarely present	Present	Absent
Erythrocyte sedimentation rate	Normal	Usually elevated	Normal
Synovial fluid	Normal	Inflammation	Normal
Radiographic findings	Erosive + exophytic (asymmetric cartilage loss)	Erosive (symmetric cartilage loss)	May be present

hospital, and also, the patient could not afford it at a private service.

On the basis of the clinical and tomographic findings and negative laboratory tests that excluded other articular diseases, final diagnosis was bilateral osteoarthritis of the TMJ.

Regarding the therapy, a nonsurgical treatment with load reduction in the TMJ by modifying the patient's diet (liquid diet initially and, after that, some soft food) was firstly proposed. Moreover, an analgesic with myorelaxing effect 3 times a day during two weeks (flupirtine maleate 100 mg—Katadolon, Asta Medica, Frankfurt, Germany) was prescribed in order to reduce joint pain. She was monitored for pain control for 1 month. The pain assessment tool was the verbal rating scale. She was asked to rate verbally the level of perceived pain by selecting the category that best described her pain: none, mild, moderate, or severe pain. After two weeks, TMJ pain on palpation and on movement had completely disappeared, but the vertical mouth opening had not been improved.

The second step would be the surgical treatment, because of the limitation of mouth opening. The patient was then informed about the indication of surgical treatment and prognosis. She was submitted to the clinical management, which temporarily relieved her pain, but refused any surgical procedure. Therefore, she was only treated for pain control until she was lost for follow-up.

3. Discussion

There are various conditions which are similar to TMJ OA and must be taken into account in the differential diagnosis. In this paper, the diagnosis of osteoarthritis was in accordance with the Research Diagnostic Criteria for temporomandibular disorders, regarding the physical signs and pain symptomatology [14]. Many patients with symptoms in the TMJ are frequently misdiagnosed as having myofascial pain dysfunction syndrome, and it is essential to consider

other pathologies of the joint, because some of these diseases have different treatment planning. Primarily, the differential diagnosis of OA of the TMJ should include the rheumatoid arthritis (RA) and its variants, pain dysfunction syndrome (PDS), and various forms of internal derangement (ID) [12, 15]. However, the major difficulty is to differentiate OA from early PDS and RA [3]. The main features to distinguish among them are listed on Table 1.

Osteoarthritis has been classified as primary when no precipitating cause is apparent, and as secondary when a related or preexisting condition may lead to its development [4, 5]. From this point of view, our clinical case is uncertain because the patient associated the beginning of the symptoms with a trauma (secondary OA). Despite this, the presence of Heberden's nodes showed that the OA was not localized. Although the relationship between acute joint trauma and development of posttraumatic OA remains poorly understood, it is clear that traumas increase the risk for later OA [2]. Both Heberden's (distal interphalangeal joint) and Bouchard's (proximal interphalangeal joint) deformities can be observed in the hand of rheumatoid patients, but the first usually is more frequent in OA [3, 13, 16]. Proximal interphalangeal and metacarpophalangeal involvement are more common in RA [3, 16]. OA of TMJ usually affects both mandibular condyle and articular eminence resulting in erosion, sclerosis, osteophytes, flattening, subchondral cysts, and a reduced joint space [11, 17–21]. Therefore, accurate image exams are important in detecting osseous and soft tissue changes [7, 8, 11, 20]. Several image techniques to TMJ examination have been described, as conventional tomography, magnetic resonance imaging, computed tomography, and, more recently, cone beam computed tomography [7, 8, 22].

Conventional radiographs of the joint are limited, and interpretation of these exams is difficult [5, 7, 17, 23]. The bone changes of TMJ are best showed in CT images [3, 7, 23, 24].

OA is a chronic disease, and so, as all chronic process, shows destructive and reparative features, both many times occurring simultaneously. As previously described, this case showed on TC scan erosion areas, rough condylar surfaces, sclerosis areas, and bone outgrowths (osteophytes). According some authors, erosion and rough condylar surfaces with the loss of contour reflect the destructive stage of the disease, whilst sclerosis areas and bone outgrowths would be related to tissue repair [17].

Specific changes in the architecture of the subchondral trabecular bone due to accelerated bone turnover can form subchondral cysts called pseudocysts or Ely's cysts [1], which corroborated with the findings presented in our case. In symptom-free individuals, radiographic evidence of OA of the TMJ occurs in 14% to 44%. However, clinical evidence of the disease occurs in only 8% to 16% of the population [3]. In accordance with previous studies [25], the clinical symptoms in the present case were not consistent with the CT findings that showed the disease in a late stage. It reveals that, in some patients, degenerative lesions can be present with few or without symptoms and they can only be visibly detected by CT scan [23, 24].

It is accepted that OA and internal derangement (ID) may coexist in about one-third of the cases [26]. ID is considered the most common cause of severe TMJ pain and dysfunction. de Leeuw et al. (1996) found a significant correlation between disc position and the severity of degenerative changes of TMJ in radiographs in symptomatic and asymptomatic TMJ [27]. The best way to assess changes of the articular disc, condyle, and the articular eminence is by magnetic resonance imaging (MRI) of the TMJ [28–32]. In this case, we did not evaluate our patient's disc position, but the diagnosis of TMJ OA is doubtlessly based on clinical findings. No radiographic criterion is pathognomonic for rheumatoid diseases. All of them can show erosion, sclerosis, osteophytes, flattening, subchondral cysts, and a reduced joint space. However, reduced joint space, flattening of the condyle, and osteophytes have been reported to be more common in OA, whereas erosions in the condyle are more frequently found in RA [20, 33].

There are in the literature different types of treatment for TMJ OA, but in general, they fall into two lines: nonsurgical and surgical procedures. The treatment may be initially performed using conservative therapies, being surgery reserved for those cases where nonsurgical approach was not effective, and pain and the loss of function were resistant to conservative measures [26, 34].

Based on the aspects discussed, we concluded that, for the correct differential diagnosis of TMJ OA, it is necessary to unite medical history, physical examination, laboratory tests, and image findings. For image study, CT scan is considered the main imaging modality for assessing the osseous components of the TMJ OA.

Conflict of Interests

The authors certify that they do not have any commercial or associate interest that represent a conflict of interests in connection with the submitted paper.

References

[1] B. W. Benson and L. L. Otis, "Disorders of the temporomandibular joint," *Dental Clinics of North America*, vol. 38, no. 1, pp. 167–185, 1994.

[2] D. T. Felson, R. C. Lawrence, P. A. Dieppe et al., "Osteoarthritis: new insights. Part 1: the disease and its risk factors," *Annals of Internal Medicine*, vol. 133, no. 8, pp. 635–646, 2000.

[3] A. O. Abubaker, "Temporomandibular disorders: an evidence-based approach to diagnosis and treatment," in *TMJ Arthritis*, D. M. Laskin, C. S. Greene, and W. L. Hylander, Eds., pp. 234–241, Quintessence Publishing, Hanover Park, Ill, USA, 2006.

[4] N. S. Mitchell and R. L. Cruess, "Classification of degenerative arthritis," *Canadian Medical Association Journal*, vol. 117, no. 7, pp. 763–765, 1977.

[5] A. O. Abubaker, "Differential diagnosis of arthritis of the temporomandibular joint," *Oral and Maxillofacial Surgery Clinics of North America*, vol. 7, pp. 1–21, 1995.

[6] R. E. Bates Jr., H. A. Gremillion, and C. M. Stewart, "Degenerative joint disease. Part II: symptoms and examination findings," *Cranio*, vol. 12, no. 2, pp. 88–92, 1994.

[7] A. Hunter and S. Kalathingal, "Diagnostic imaging for temporomandibular disorders and orofacial pain," *Dental Clinics of North America*, vol. 57, pp. 405–418, 2013.

[8] R. Boeddinghaus and A. Whyte, "Computed tomography of the temporomandibular joint," *Journal of Medical Imaging and Radiation Oncology*, vol. 57, pp. 448–454, 2013.

[9] P. A. Toller, "Osteoarthrosis of the mandibular condyle," *British Dental Journal*, vol. 134, no. 6, pp. 223–231, 1973.

[10] R. J. Gray, S. J. Davies, and A. A. Quayle, "A clinical approach to temporomandibular disorders. 1. Classification and functional anatomy," *British Dental Journal*, vol. 176, no. 11, pp. 429–435, 1994.

[11] S. B. Milan, "Temporom andibular disorders: an evidence-based approach to diagnosis and treatment," in *TMJ osteoarthritis*, D. M. Laskin, C. S. Greene, and W. L. Hylander, Eds., pp. 105–123, Quintessence Publishing, Hanover Park, ILL, USA, 2006.

[12] J. S. Broussard Jr., "Derangement, osteoarthritis, and rheumatoid arthritis of the temporomandibular joint: implications, diagnosis, and management," *Dental Clinics of North America*, vol. 49, no. 2, pp. 327–342, 2005.

[13] D. Caspi, G. Flusser, I. Farber et al., "Clinical, radiologic, demographic, and occupational aspects of hand osteoarthritis in the elderly," *Seminars in Arthritis and Rheumatism*, vol. 30, no. 5, pp. 321–331, 2001.

[14] S. F. Dworkin and L. LeResche, "Research diagnostic criteria for temporomandibular disorders: review, criteria, examinations and specifications, critique," *Journal of Craniomandibular Disorders*, vol. 6, no. 4, pp. 301–355, 1992.

[15] R. J. M. Gray, "Pain dysfunction syndrome and osteoarthrosis related to unilateral and bilateral temporomandibular joint symptoms," *Journal of Dentistry*, vol. 14, no. 4, pp. 156–159, 1986.

[16] M. F. Zide, D. M. Carlton, and J. N. Kent, "Rheumatoid disease and related arthropathies. I. Systemic findings, medical therapy, and peripheral joint surgery," *Oral Surgery Oral Medicine and Oral Pathology*, vol. 61, no. 2, pp. 119–125, 1986.

[17] R. D. Leeuw, G. Boering, B. Stegenga, and G. M. Lambert, "Radiographic signs of temporomandibular joint osteoarthrosis and internal derangement 30 years after nonsurgical treatment," *Oral Surgery, Oral Medicine, Oral Pathology, Oral Radiology and*, vol. 79, no. 3, pp. 382–392, 1995.

[18] A. B. Reiskin, "Temporomandibular joints," in *Advances in Oral Radiology*, pp. 201–222, PSG Publishing Company, 1980.

[19] J. McIvor, "Temporomandibular joint," in *Dental and Maxillofacial Radiology*, pp. 101–104, Churchill Livingstone, London, UK, 1986.

[20] G. W. Gynther, G. Tronje, and A. B. Holmlund, "Radiographic changes in the temporomandibular joint in patients with generalized osteoarthritis and rheumatoid arthritis," *Oral Surgery, Oral Medicine, Oral Pathology, Oral Radiology, and Endodontics*, vol. 81, no. 5, pp. 613–618, 1996.

[21] K. Yamada, I. Saito, K. Hanada, and T. Hayashi, "Observation of three cases of temporomandibular joint osteoarthritis and mandibular morphology during adolescence using helical CT," *Journal of Oral Rehabilitation*, vol. 31, no. 4, pp. 298–305, 2004.

[22] K. Tsiklakis, K. Syriopoulos, and H. C. Stamatakis, "Radiographic examination of the temporomandibular joint using cone beam computed tomography," *Dentomaxillofacial Radiology*, vol. 33, no. 3, pp. 196–201, 2004.

[23] L. G. M. de Bont, B. van der Kuijl, B. Stegenga, L. M. Vencken, and G. Boering, "Computed tomography in differential diagnosis of temporomandibular joint disorders," *International Journal of Oral and Maxillofacial Surgery*, vol. 22, no. 4, pp. 200–209, 1993.

[24] American Society of Temporomandibular Joint Surgeons, "Guidelines for diagnosis and management of disorders involving the temporomandibular joint and related musculoskeletal structures," *Cranio*, vol. 21, pp. 68–76, 2003.

[25] G. Palconet, J. B. Ludlow, D. A. Tyndall, and P. F. Lim, "Correlating cone beam CT results with temporomandibular joint pain of osteoarthritic origin," *Dentomaxillofacial Radiology*, vol. 41, no. 2, pp. 126–130, 2012.

[26] G. Dimitroulis, "The prevalence of osteoarthrosis in cases of advanced internal derangement of the Temporomandibular Joint: a clinical, surgical and histological study," *International Journal of Oral and Maxillofacial Surgery*, vol. 34, no. 4, pp. 345–349, 2005.

[27] R. de Leeuw, G. Boering, B. van der Kuijl, and B. Stegenga, "Hard and soft tissue imaging of the temporomandibular joint 30 years after diagnosis of osteoarthrosis and internal derangement," *Journal of Oral and Maxillofacial Surgery*, vol. 54, no. 11, pp. 1270–1281, 1996.

[28] R. E. Marguelles-Bonnet, P. Carpentier, J. P. Yung, D. Defrennes, and C. Pharaboz, "Clinical diagnosis compared with findings of magnetic resonance imaging in 242 patients with internal derangement of the TMJ," *Journal of orofacial pain*, vol. 9, no. 3, pp. 244–253, 1995.

[29] R. Emshoff, A. Rudisch, K. Innerhofer, R. Bösch, and S. Bertram, "Temporomandibular joint internal derangement type III: relationship to magnetic resonance imaging findings of internal derangement and osteoarthrosis. An intraindividual approach," *International Journal of Oral and Maxillofacial Surgery*, vol. 30, no. 5, pp. 390–396, 2001.

[30] R. Emshoff, K. Innerhofer, A. Rudisch, and S. Bertram, "The biological concept of "internal derangement and osteoarthrosis": a diagnostic approach in patients with temporomandibular joint pain?" *Oral Surgery, Oral Medicine, Oral Pathology, Oral Radiology, and Endodontics*, vol. 93, no. 1, pp. 39–44, 2002.

[31] R. Emshoff, I. Brandlmaier, S. Bertram, and A. Rudisch, "Relative odds of temporomandibular joint pain as a function of magnetic resonance imaging findings of internal derangement, osteoarthrosis, effusion, and bone marrow edema," *Oral Surgery, Oral Medicine, Oral Pathology, Oral Radiology, and Endodontics*, vol. 95, no. 4, pp. 437–445, 2003.

[32] R. Emshoff, S. Gerhard, T. Ennemoser, and A. Rudisch, "Magnetic resonance imaging findings of internal derangement, osteoarthrosis, effusion, and bone marrow edema before and after performance of arthrocentesis and hydraulic distension of the temporomandibular joint," *Oral Surgery, Oral Medicine, Oral Pathology, Oral Radiology and Endodontology*, vol. 101, no. 6, pp. 784–790, 2006.

[33] G. W. Gynther and G. Tronje, "Comparison of arthroscopy and radiography in patients with temporomandibular joint symptoms and generalized arthritis," *Dentomaxillofacial Radiology*, vol. 27, no. 2, pp. 107–112, 1998.

[34] M. F. Dolwick and G. Dimitroulis, "Is there a role for temporomandibular joint surgery?" *British Journal of Oral and Maxillofacial Surgery*, vol. 32, no. 5, pp. 307–313, 1994.

30

Association of Mesiodentes and Dens Invaginatus in a Child

A. N. Sulabha[1] and C. Sameer[2]

[1] Department of Oral Medicine and Radiology, Al-Ameen Dental College and Hospital, Athani Road, Karnataka, Bijapur 586108, India
[2] Department of Oral and Maxillofacial Surgery, Al-Ameen Dental College and Hospital, Karnataka, Bijapur 586108, India

Correspondence should be addressed to A. N. Sulabha, sulabha595@gmail.com

Academic Editors: Y.-K. Chen and Y. Nakagawa

Supernumerary teeth are defined as any teeth in excess of normal number. Mesiodens is a supernumerary tooth, in the central region of premaxilla between two central incisors. Dens invaginatus is a developmental anomaly resulting from invagination in the surface of tooth crown before calcification has occurred. Radiographically, it is observed as infolding of a radioopaque ribbon like structure, with equal density as enamel, extending from cingulum into a root canal and sometimes reaching the root apex. This paper aims to present a rare association of dens invaginatus with two mesiodentes in a child causing the eruption disturbance and unaesthetic appearance in anterior maxilla.

1. Introduction

Supernumerary teeth or hyperdontia is defined as excess number of teeth as compared to the normal dental formula [1]. The most common supernumerary tooth as indicated by Alberti is mesiodens. A mesiodens is a supernumerary tooth located in maxillary central incisor region. Mesiodens may occur as single, multiple, unilateral, or bilateral. Multiple mesiodens are called mesiodentes [2, 3]. Single supernumerary teeth account for 76–86%, in pair accounts for 12–23% and less than 1% cases with three or more extra teeth [4].

Dens invaginatus is a rare malformation of teeth showing a broad spectrum of morphological variation [5]. It is a developmental anomaly resulting from invagination of enamel organ into a dental papilla, beginning at the crown and sometimes extending into the root before calcification occurs [6]. Although a clinical examination reveals a deep pit or fissures on lingual surfaces of anterior teeth, the radiographic examination is the sine quo non for diagnosis of dens invaginatus [7].

Association of dens invaginatus with mesiodens is a very rare phenomenon. Extensive Pubmed search revealed only five case reports published in literature till date [8–10]. This paper aims to report a rare association of dens invaginatus in two unusual mesiodens in a child causing the eruption failure of permanent teeth and unaesthetic appearance.

2. Case Report

A 13-years-old child reported with complaint of abnormally erupted tooth in maxillary anterior region (Figure 1). Intraoral examination revealed partial horizontally erupted tooth in left central incisor region. Only incisal and part of middle one third of the abnormally erupted tooth was visible. The lingual surface appeared abnormal with infolding of mesial and distal edges towards centre creating a central depressed area (Figure 2).

Radiographically examination revealed unerupted left central incisor. Two supernumerary teeth were found in maxillary central incisor region. One of the supernumerary teeth was partially erupted in left central incisor region in horizontal manner and the other was impacted. Root appeared to be incomplete (Figure 3). Partial erupted mesiodens showed invagination of radioopaque line towards the pulp suggesting dens invaginatus. As these mesiodens caused

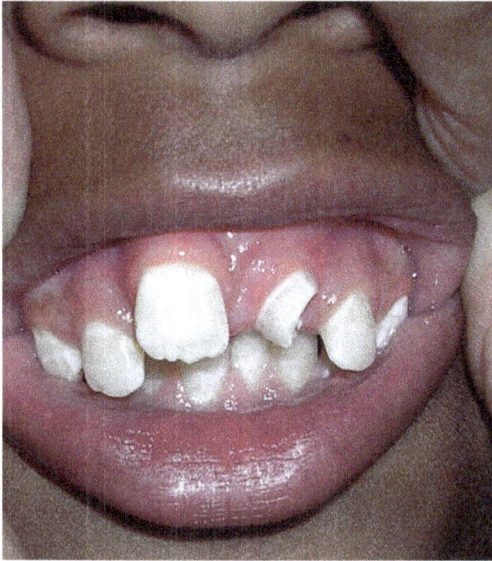

FIGURE 1: Clinical picture showing horizontal partial eruption on mesiodens.

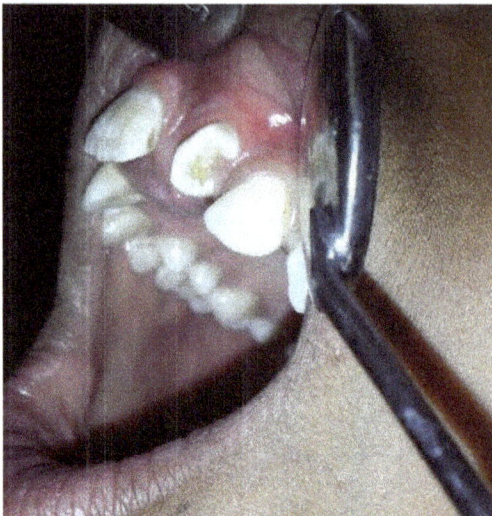

FIGURE 2: Clinical picture showing the lateral aspects of mesiodens.

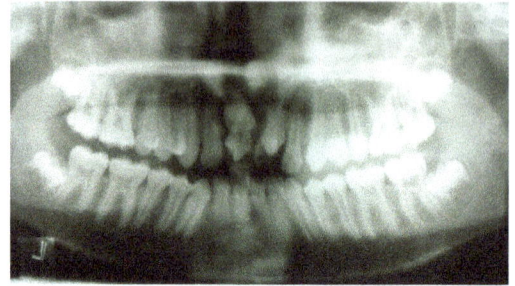

FIGURE 3: Panoramic view showing the two mesiodens in the anterior region of maxilla with unerupted left central incisor.

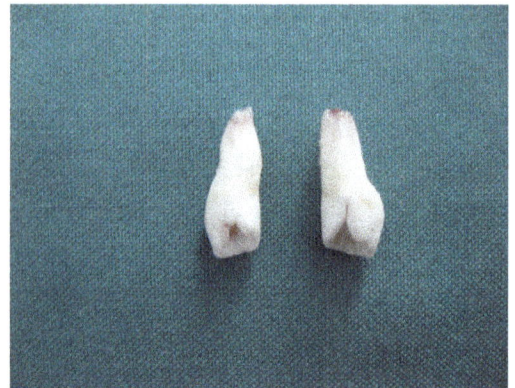

FIGURE 4: Lingual aspect of both mesiodens showing the dens invaginatus.

eruption failure of left central incisor and was esthetically unpleasant, extraction of both mesiodens was done. After extraction, patient was advised on wait and watch policy for eruption of the left central incisor.

Extracted mesiodentes were unusual (Figures 4 and 5). Partially erupted mesiodens was bigger with crown morphology resembling central incisor, other had smaller crown morphology resembling the lateral incisor. Root formation was incomplete with wide open apex with both mesiodentes. The labial surface showed some indentation. The lingual surface of both showed complete infolding of both mesial and distal edges till midline giving a central depressed area and extended till cervical part of root, bifurcating the pulp without invading it (Figure 6). Both mesiodentes

showed dilacerations, smaller mesiodens in root portion, and bigger in the crown portion. Based on these a diagnosis of mesiodens with dens invaginatus and dilaceration was made.

3. Discussion

Supernumerary teeth are developmental disturbances occurring during the odontogenesis resulting in the formation of teeth in excess of the normal number. Mesiodens refers to supernumerary tooth in the premaxilla between the two central incisor and these are more common in the permanent dentition than in primary dentition [11].

Mesiodentes can be classified on basis of their occurrence in permanent dentition (rudimentary) and according to their morphology as conical, tuberculate, molariform, or supplemental. Most commonly mesiodens presents in conical shape. Tuberculate mesiodentes are barrel shaped with several cusp or tubercles and have incomplete roots or abnormal root formation. They rarely erupt into the oral cavity. The rare form is molariform mesiodens. Supplemental mesiodens resembles natural teeth in both size and shapes are usually seen at end of tooth series. Supplemental maxillary incisors are much less common than conical or tuberculate supernumerary teeth in an anterior maxilla. Supplementary lateral incisor is more common than supplemental central incisor [12, 13]. In the present case the crown resembled supplemental central and lateral incisor but had incomplete

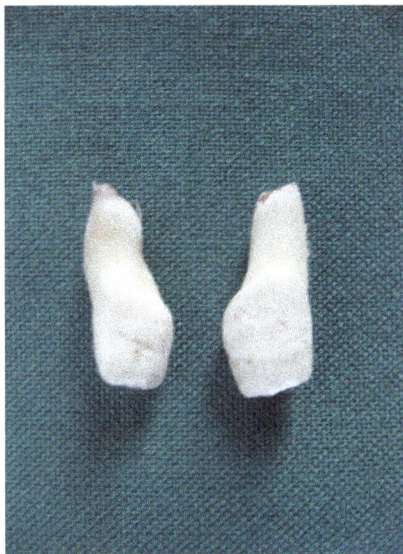

FIGURE 5: Labial aspect of mesiodens showing the dilaceration and indentation on crown of mesiodens.

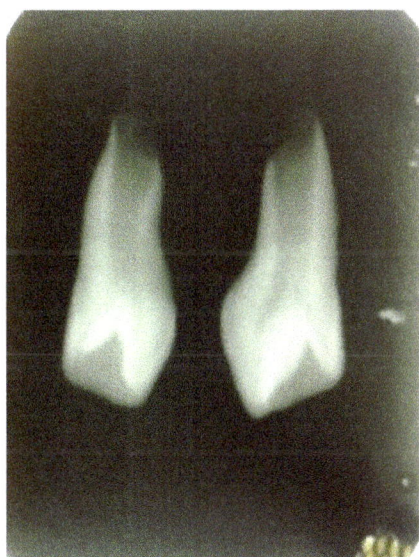

FIGURE 6: Postoperative X-ray showing incomplete root formation of mesiodens.

root. Both mesiodentes showed the dilaceration with dens invaginatus.

Dens invaginatus is a developmental malformation resulting from invagination of the tooth crown or root before calcification has occurred [6]. The etiology of this is unknown and controversial. In most cases it is detected by chance on radiograph. Clinically an unusual crown (dilated, peg shaped, barrel shaped) or deep foramen coecum may be an important hint [5]. Radiographically it is observed as infolding of a radioopaque ribbon like structure with equal density as enamel extending from cingulum into root canal and sometimes reaching the root apex, assigning the appearance of a small tooth within the coronal pulp cavity [8].

Oehlers classification is most commonly used for the dens invaginatus [5].

Type 1: an enamel lined minor form occurs in the crown of the tooth and not extending beyond the cemento enamel junction.

Type 2: an enamel lined form which invades the root but remains confined as blind sac. It may or may not communicate with dental pulp.

Type 3: a form which penetrates through the root perforating at the apical area showing a second foramen in the apical or in the periodontal area. There is no immediate communication with the pulp. In the present case both mesiodentes had a blind sac extending to pulp and dividing it without communicating.

This anomaly occurs frequently in lateral incisors followed by central incisor, premolars canines, and molars [7]. Association of this anomaly with the mesiodens is extremely rare and its occurrence in two mesiodentes is even a rarer phenomenon. Review of English language literature only showed five case reports of dens invaginatus in mesiodens and among them involvement of two mesiodentes is limited to only two case reports [8–10]. Sannomiya et al. [8] presented two cases of mesiodens and dens invaginatus of which one case presented with two mesiodentes associated with dens invaginatus. Archer and Silverman [10] presented dens invaginatus in bilateral rudimentary supernumerary teeth. In the present case dens invaginatus was noted with different types of mesiodens having supplemental crown morphology of central and lateral incisor with incomplete root and dilaceration which is very rare and unusual.

Various complications might occur as a result of the presence of supernumerary teeth and dens invaginatus. Delayed eruption, crowding, spacing, impaction, diastema, cystic lesion, root resorption, and so forth are complications associated with supernumerary teeth. The dens invaginatus in dens in dente allows entry of irritants into an area which is separated from pulpal tissue by only a thin layer of enamel and dentine and presents a predisposition for development of caries. Pulpal necrosis, abscess formation, cyst, and internal resorption are other complications [3, 5]. In the present case partial erupted mesiodens in horizontal manner gave unaesthetic appearance along with eruption failure of the left central incisor.

Supernumerary teeth either can be managed by removal, endodontic treatment or can be monitored without its removal [13, 14]. In this case as it was associated with unaesthetic appearance and eruption failure of permanent teeth, surgical removal of both mesiodentes was done.

To conclude as mesiodentes are associated with various complications, early diagnosis and treatment are very important to prevent physiological, esthetics, and functional problems especially in children.

References

[1] V. Verma, A. Goel, and M. Sabir, "Supernumerary eumorphic mandibular incisor in association with aggressive periodontitis," *Journal of Indian Society of Periodontology*, vol. 14, no. 3, pp. 136–138, 2010.

[2] V. Khandelwal, A. V. Nayak, R. B. Navan, N. Ninawe, P. A. Nayak, and S. V. Saiprasad, "Prevalence of mesiodens among six to seventeen year old school going children of Indore," *Journal of Indian Society of Pedodontics and Preventive Dentistry*, vol. 29, no. 4, pp. 288–293, 2011.

[3] G. Meighani and A. Pakdaman, "Diagnosis and management of supernumerary (mesiodens). A review of the literature," *Journal of Dentistry Tehran University of Medical Sciences*, vol. 7, pp. 41–49, 2010.

[4] S. A. Sharma, "Mandibular midline supernumerary tooth: a case report," *Journal of the Indian Society of Pedodontics and Preventive Dentistry*, vol. 19, no. 4, pp. 143–144, 2001.

[5] M. Hülsmann, "Dens invaginatus: aetiology, classification, prevalence, diagnosis, and treatment considerations," *International Endodontic Journal*, vol. 30, no. 2, pp. 79–90, 1997.

[6] A. Z. Zengin, A. P. Sumer, and P. Celenk, "Double dens invaginatus: report of three cases," *European Journal of Dentistry*, vol. 3, pp. 67–70, 2009.

[7] M. Mupparapu and S. R. Singer, "A rare presentation of dens invaginatus in a mandibular lateral incisor occurring concurrently with bilateral maxillary dens invaginatus: case report and review of literature," *Australian Dental Journal*, vol. 49, no. 2, pp. 90–93, 2004.

[8] E. K. Sannomiya, J. I. Asaumi, K. Kishi, and G. S. Dalben, "Rare associations of dens invaginatus and mesiodens," *Oral Surgery, Oral Medicine, Oral Pathology, Oral Radiology and Endodontology*, vol. 104, no. 2, pp. e41–e44, 2007.

[9] J. V Serrano, "Triple dens invaginatus in a mesiodens," *Oral Surgery Oral Medicine and Oral Pathology*, vol. 71, no. 5, pp. 648–649, 1991.

[10] W. H. Archer and L. M. Silverman, "Double dens in dente in bilateral rudimentary supernumerary central incisors (mesiodens). Report of a case," *Oral Surgery, Oral Medicine, Oral Pathology*, vol. 3, no. 6, pp. 722–726, 1950.

[11] P. Srivatsan and N. Aravind, "Mesiodens with an unusual morphology and multiple impacted supernumerary teeth in a non-syndromic patient," *Indian Journal of Dental Research*, vol. 18, no. 3, pp. 138–140, 2007.

[12] S. Nuvvula, M. Kiranmayi, G. Shilpa, and S. V. S. G. Nirmala, "Hypohyperdontia: agenesis of three third molars and mandibular centrals associated with midline supernumerary tooth in midline," *Contemporary Clinical Dentistry*, vol. 1, no. 3, pp. 136–140, 2010.

[13] M. T. Garvey, H. J. Barry, and M. Blake, "Supernumerary teeth—an overview of classification, diagnosis and management," *Journal of the Canadian Dental Association*, vol. 65, no. 11, pp. 612–616, 1999.

[14] A. Parolia, M. Kundabala, M. Dahal, M. Mohan, and M. S. Thomas, "Management of supernumerary teeth," *Journal of Conservative Dentistry*, vol. 14, pp. 221–224, 2011.

31

Removal of a Dental Implant Displaced into the Maxillary Sinus by Means of the Bone Lid Technique

Pietro Fusari, Matteo Doto, and Matteo Chiapasco

Unit of Oral Surgery, Department of Health Sciences, San Paolo Hospital, University of Milan, Via Beldiletto 1/3, 20142 Milan, Italy

Correspondence should be addressed to Matteo Doto; matteo.doto@fastwebnet.it

Academic Editors: R. A. de Mesquita, L. N. De Souza, I. El-Hakim, and S. R. Watt-Smith

Background. Rehabilitation of edentulous jaws with implant-supported prosthesis has become a common practice among oral surgeons in the last three decades. This therapy presents a very low incidence of complications. One of them is the displacement of dental implants into the maxillary sinus. Dental implants, such as any other foreign body into the maxillary sinus, should be removed in order to prevent sinusitis. *Methods.* In this paper, we report a case of dental implant migrated in the maxillary sinus and removed by means of the bone lid technique. *Results and Conclusion.* The migration of dental implants into the maxillary sinus is rarely reported. Migrated implants should be considered for removal in order to prevent possible sinusal diseases. The implant has been removed without any complications, confirming the bone lid technique to be safe and reliable.

1. Introduction

Rehabilitation of edentulous jaws with implant-supported prosthesis has become a common practice among oral surgeons and dentists in the last three decades [1].

The resorption of the alveolar ridges in the posterior maxilla and/or the maxillary sinus pneumatization often limits the available bone for positioning dental implants. To overcome these problems, the use of short implants or maxillary sinus floor lifting in association with dental implants is well documented and proved as successful procedures [2–5].

Implant displacement/migration in the paranasal sinuses, resulting from wrong planning or surgical inexperience, have been reported sporadically in the literature [6–11].

Implant migration into the sinuses may be followed by no relevant signs and symptoms of infection, but it can be associated with oroantral communication and/or infection that may involve the maxillary sinus and the ethmoidal, frontal, and sphenoid sinuses. These displaced foreign bodies should be removed as soon as possible to prevent such complications [12].

The major complication due to a foreign body in the maxillary sinus reported in the literature is sinusitis, that may bring more serious conditions such as pansinusitis, panophthalmitis, and orbital cellulitis [11, 13, 14].

Two main treatment modalities have been proposed for the removal of displaced implants in the sinuses and to treat the associated infectious complications: an intraoral approach with the creation of a window in the anterior-lateral wall of the maxillary sinus and a transnasal approach with functional endoscopic sinus surgery (FESS) [7–12].

2. Case Report

A 47-year-old man was referred to our department for treatment of a displaced dental implant, installed by an oral surgeon in a private dental office 30 days before, and migrated immediately after surgery into the maxillary sinus.

The CBCT scans showed a dental implant displaced in the maxillary sinus roof, with no evidence of sinusitis (Figures 1-2).

2.1. Surgical Procedure. An intraoral approach consisting im the elevation of a mucoperiosteal flap and the creation of a bony window pedicled to the Schneiderian membrane was adopted.

The patient was operated under local anesthesia. An oral antibiotic prophylaxis (amoxicillin + clavulanate, 2 g) was administered one hour prior to the start of the procedure.

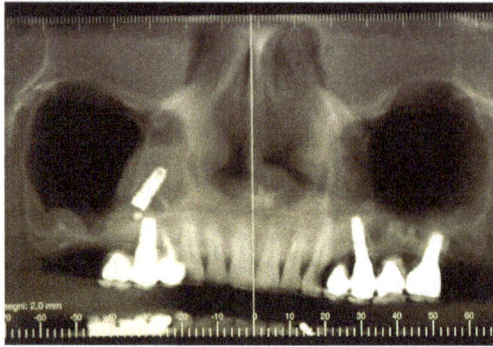

FIGURE 1: CBCT scans showing a dental implant displaced into the maxillary sinus.

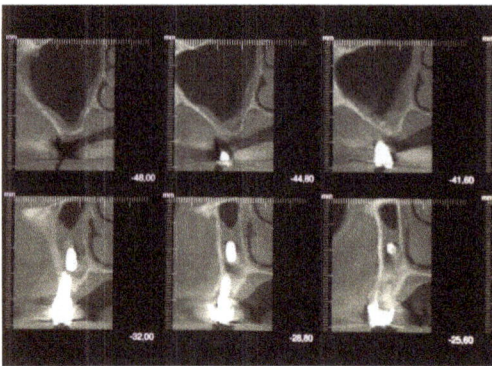

FIGURE 2: CBCT scans showing a dental implant displaced into the maxillary sinus.

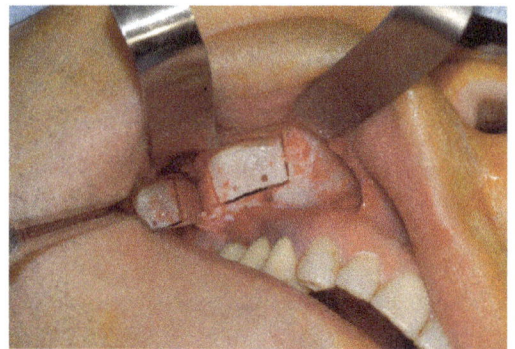

FIGURE 4: The osteotomy is performed by means of a piezoelectric instrument.

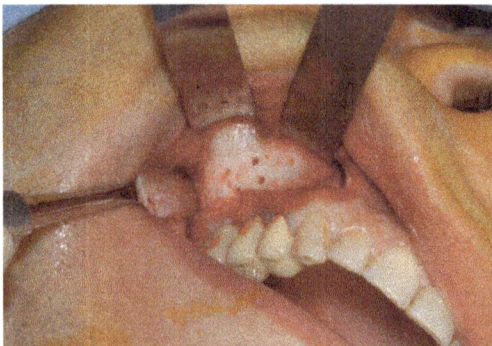

FIGURE 3: Four holes are performed after the elevation of a full-thickness flap.

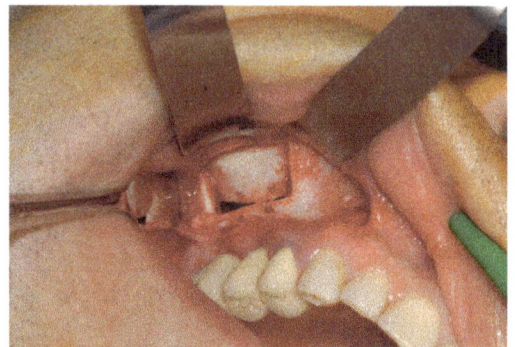

FIGURE 5: The bony window is left pedicled to the Schneiderian membrane.

The surgical intervention began with the elevation of a trapezoidal full-thickness mucoperiosteal flap. The buccal aspect of the flap was then retracted with the aid of Langenbeck's retractor to improve the access and visibility of the maxillary sinus bony wall. A traditional rotary instrument (low-speed straight handpiece and fissure bur) was used to drill the maxillary bone with four holes (Figure 3). At this point, a rectangular osteotomy was performed using piezoelectric instruments (Figure 4). The integrity of the mucosa was maintained only along the superior side of the lid to create a pedicled window as described by Biglioli and Goisis [15] (Figure 5).

The bone lid was then rotated upward; the implant was identified and removed with a surgical aspirator (Figures 6-7). The bony segment was repositioned and secured with an absorbable suture (Figure 8). After irrigation of the surgical field with sterile saline, the surgical flap was sutured, and compression with a sterile gauze was applied for a few minutes. To reduce postoperative swelling, dexamethasone (8 mg) was administered perioperatively via IM injection.

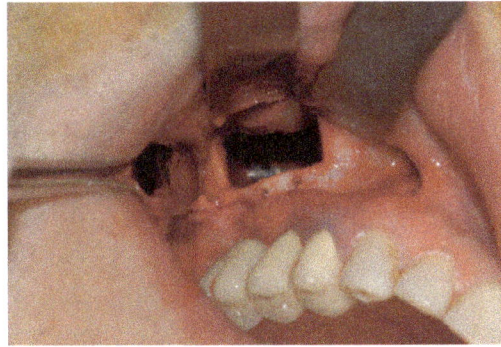

FIGURE 6: The implant is perfectly visible lying on the sinus floor.

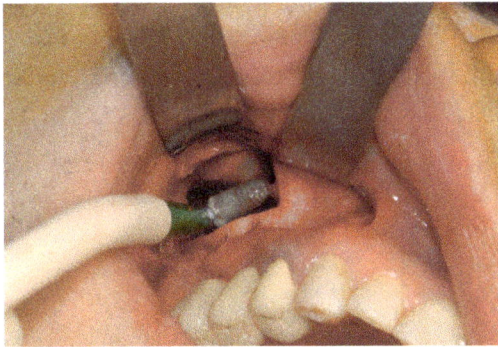

FIGURE 7: The implant is removed with a surgical aspirator.

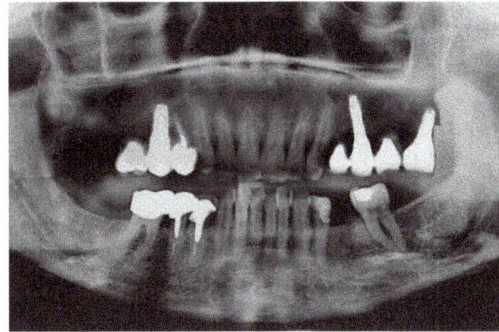

FIGURE 9: Panoramic X-ray after the intervention.

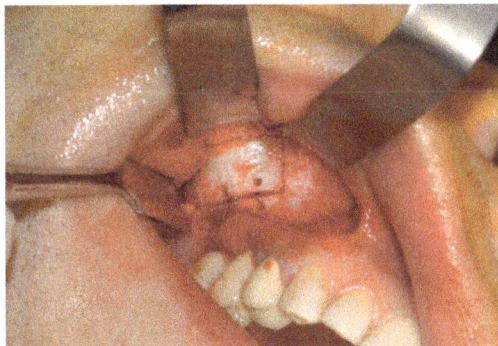

FIGURE 8: The bony segment is repositioned and secured with absorbable sutures.

Antibiotic therapy with amoxicillin and clavulanate (1 g) was prescribed in association with nonsteroidal anti-inflammatory drugs. Chlorhexidine mouth-washes were associated to the usual oral hygiene manoeuvres for seven days. Postoperative recovery was uneventful. After seven days, the patient went through an examination and the sutures were removed. At this time, a panoramic X-ray was taken (Figure 9).

3. Discussion

Surgical removal of dental implants from the maxillary sinus is not a very common oral surgery intervention. The approach proposed in this study (intraoral) is limited to the cases that do not need treatment of an obstructed maxillary sinus ostium and concomitant sinusitis of other paranasal sinuses.

Osteotomies for the bony window creation can be performed with traditional rotary instruments, or with piezoelectric instrumentation. The first method is widely used and very well documented, and it allows a fast and effective osteotomic path design. Piezoelectric instruments have been recently introduced, and they use microvibration of the surgical inserts at ultrasonic (27 to 29 kHz) frequencies to perform cutting of the hard tissues. These instruments demonstrated good cutting properties on cortical bone, allowing at the same time the preservation of soft tissues from damage in case of accidental contact [16, 17].

There are few works reported in the literature about implant migrations into the paranasal sinuses (Table 1).

Regev et al. [6] reported three cases of implant migration, and two of them were displaced into the maxillary sinus. One occurred at the time of abutment connection due to nonosseointegration. The other was observed two months after implant placement in the anterior maxilla, where an autogenous onlay bone graft had been performed. The authors suggested that the underlying osteopenia and

TABLE 1: Treatment options proposed by different authors.

Author	Implants displaced	Anatomic structures involved	Symptomatology	Treatment applied
Kluppel et al., 2010 [18]	2	Maxillary sinus	Absent	One removal, one followup
Felisati et al., 2007 [11]	1	Maxillary and sphenoid sinuses	Absent	Removal (endoscopy)
Galindo et al., 2005 [10]	2	Maxillary sinus	Absent	One removal, one followup
Kitamura, 2007 [9]	1	Maxillary sinus	Present	Removal (endoscopy)
Raghoebar and Vissink, 2003 [8]	1	Maxillary sinus	Absent	Removal + bone graft
Iida et al., 2000 [7]	1	Maxillary sinus	Absent	Removal
Regev et al., 1995 [6]	3	Maxillary sinus	Absent	Removal

the occlusal forces from the maxillary denture might have contributed to the displacement in the latter case.

Iida et al. [7] reported a case of a patient who underwent dental implant installation to replace a second upper molar. Five years later, the patient noticed mobility of the implant: the prosthesis was removed from the implant, but the implant was left in position, and he underwent occlusal reconstruction of the area with an extension bridge. Eleven years later, a panoramic radiograph revealed displacement of the implant into the right maxillary sinus, and the implant was removed under local anesthesia.

Raghoebar and Vissink [8] reported a case of a man who went through three implants installation. After three months, the migration of an implant into the maxillary sinus was discovered after a panoramic radiograph. The implant was removed in association with a sinus graft under general anesthesia.

Kitamura [9] reported a case of a woman with discomfort in the right maxilla and a discharge of pus from the nose. Panoramic radiographs and computed tomograms showed the presence of an implant in the right maxillary sinus. The patient underwent endoscopic removal of the implant under general anesthesia.

Galindo et al. [10] reported two asymptomatic cases of implant migration: one implant was kept in place after the patient refusal to undergo the operation; in the second case, the patient consented to surgical intervention, and the removal was performed 3 years later. Felisati et al. [11] reported a case of a woman who received one oral implant for the substitution of the left first upper molar, but during the surgical procedure the implant was displaced in the maxillary sinus. Owing to a delay in treatment, a spontaneous migration of the implant in the sphenoid sinus occurred. The implant was removed endoscopically through the nasal cavity.

Kluppel et al. [18] reported two cases of dental implants displaced in the maxillary sinus. One of them was removed and sinus lift performed; the other one has been kept in place with no complications after a 5-year followup.

In the literature, we can find three possible explanations of the implant migration:

(1) bone resorption caused by wrong distribution of occlusal forces;

(2) changes in nasal air pressure;

(3) inflammatory reaction around the implant (peri-implantitis).

The majority of the authors seem to agree that the removal of a displaced implant from the sinus should be performed to avoid the possibility of development of sinus infections.

4. Conclusion

The migration of dental implants into the maxillary sinus is rarely reported. Migrated implants should be considered for removal in order to prevent possible sinusal diseases. The removal of displaced implants in the maxillary sinus with a buccal approach by means of a bony window creation proved to be a safe and reliable technique.

References

[1] M. Esposito, L. Murray-Curtis, M. G. Grusovin, P. Coulthard, and H. V. Worthington, "Interventions for replacing missing teeth: different types of dental implants," *Cochrane Database of Systematic Reviews*, no. 1, Article ID CD003815, 2007.

[2] M. L. Arlin, "Short dental implants as a treatment option: results from an observational study in a single private practice," *International Journal of Oral and Maxillofacial Implants*, vol. 21, no. 5, pp. 769–776, 2006.

[3] M. Chiapasco, M. Zaniboni, and L. Rimondini, "Dental implants placed in grafted maxillary sinuses: a retrospective analysis of clinical outcome according to the initial clinical situation and a proposal of defect classification," *Clinical Oral Implants Research*, vol. 19, no. 4, pp. 416–428, 2008.

[4] M. Del Fabbro, T. Testori, L. Francetti, and R. Weinstein, "Systematic review of survival rates for implants placed in the grafted maxillary sinus," *International Journal of Periodontics and Restorative Dentistry*, vol. 24, no. 6, pp. 565–577, 2004.

[5] S. Taschieri, S. Corbella, R. Molinari, M. Saita, and M. Del Fabbro, "Short implants in maxillary and mandibular rehabilitations: interim results (6 to 42 months) of a prospective study," *Journal of Oral Implantology*, 2013.

[6] E. Regev, R. A. Smith, D. H. Perrott, and M. A. Pogrel, "Maxillary sinus complications related to endosseous implants," *The International Journal of Oral & Maxillofacial Implants*, vol. 10, no. 4, pp. 451–461, 1995.

[7] S. Iida, N. Tanaka, M. Kogo, and T. Matsuya, "Migration of a dental implant into the maxillary sinus: a case report," *International Journal of Oral and Maxillofacial Surgery*, vol. 29, no. 5, pp. 358–359, 2000.

[8] G. M. Raghoebar and A. Vissink, "Treatment for an endosseous implant migrated into the maxillary sinus not causing maxillary sinusitis: case report," *International Journal of Oral and Maxillofacial Implants*, vol. 18, no. 5, pp. 745–749, 2003.

[9] A. Kitamura, "Removal of a migrated dental implant from a maxillary sinus by transnasal endoscopy," *British Journal of Oral and Maxillofacial Surgery*, vol. 45, no. 5, pp. 410–411, 2007.

[10] P. Galindo, E. Sánchez-Fernández, G. Avila, A. Cutando, and J. E. Fernandez, "Migration of implants into the maxillary sinus: two clinical cases," *International Journal of Oral and Maxillofacial Implants*, vol. 20, no. 2, pp. 291–295, 2005.

[11] G. Felisati, P. Lozza, M. Chiapasco, and R. Borloni, "Endoscopic removal of an unusual foreign body in the sphenoid sinus: an oral implant: case report," *Clinical Oral Implants Research*, vol. 18, no. 6, pp. 776–780, 2007.

[12] M. Chiapasco, G. Felisati, A. Maccari, R. Borloni, F. Gatti, and F. Di Leo, "The management of complications following displacement of oral implants in the paranasal sinuses: a multicenter clinical report and proposed treatment protocols," *International Journal of Oral and Maxillofacial Surgery*, vol. 38, no. 12, pp. 1273–1278, 2009.

[13] N. Sugiura, K. Ochi, and Y. Komatsuzaki, "Endoscopic extraction of a foreign body from the maxillary sinus," *Otolaryngology—Head and Neck Surgery*, vol. 130, no. 2, pp. 279–280, 2004.

[14] G. Wilk, M. Modrzejewska, E. Lachowicz et al., "From ophthalmologist to dentist via radiology," *Polish Journal of Radiology*, vol. 77, no. 1, pp. 21–27, 2012.

[15] F. Biglioli and M. Goisis, "Access to the maxillary sinus using a bone flap on a mucosal pedicle: preliminary report," *Journal of Cranio-Maxillofacial Surgery*, vol. 30, no. 4, pp. 255–259, 2002.

[16] S. Stübinger, J. Kuttenberger, A. Filippi, R. Sader, and H. F. Zeilhofer, "Intraoral piezosurgery: preliminary results of a new technique," *Journal of Oral and Maxillofacial Surgery*, vol. 63, no. 9, pp. 1283–1287, 2005.

[17] T. Vercellotti, "Technological characteristics and clinical indications of piezoelectric bone surgery," *Minerva Stomatologica*, vol. 53, no. 5, pp. 207–214, 2004.

[18] L. E. Kluppel, S. E. Santos, S. Olate, F. W. V. F. Filho, R. W. F. Moreira, and M. de Moraes, "Implant migration into maxillary sinus: description of two asymptomatic cases," *Oral and Maxillofacial Surgery*, vol. 14, no. 1, pp. 63–66, 2010.

32

Restoration of Endodontically Treated Molars Using All Ceramic Endocrowns

Roopak Bose Carlos,[1] **Mohan Thomas Nainan,**[1] **Shamina Pradhan,**[1] **Roshni Sharma,**[1] **Shiny Benjamin,**[1] **and Rajani Rose**[2]

[1] Department of Conservative Dentistry and Endodontics, Vydehi Institute of Dental Sciences and Research Centre, No. 82, EPIP Area, Whitefield, Bangalore 560066, India
[2] Dental Solutions, 157, 4th Main, BEML layout, Off ITPL Road, Thubarahalli, Bangalore 560066, India

Correspondence should be addressed to Roopak Bose Carlos; carlosroop@gmail.com

Academic Editors: D. W. Boston and K. Seymour

Clinical success of endodontically treated posterior teeth is determined by the postendodontic restoration. Several options have been proposed to restore endodontically treated teeth. Endocrowns represent a conservative and esthetic restorative alternative to full coverage crowns. The preparation consists of a circular equigingival butt-joint margin and central retention cavity into the entire pulp chamber constructing both the crown and the core as a single unit. The case reports discussed here are moderately damaged endodontically treated molars restored using all ceramic endocrowns fabricated using two different systems, namely, CAD/CAM and pressed ceramic.

1. Introduction

Postendodontic restoration should preserve and protect the existing tooth structure, while restoring satisfactory esthetics, form, and function. The goal is to achieve minimally invasive preparations with maximal tissue conservation for restoring endodontically treated teeth. This will help to mechanically stabilize the tooth-restoration complex and increase surfaces available for adhesion.

A number of options are available in every clinical situation. The choice depends on the structural integrity of the tooth, esthetic, and protective requirements [1]. In this perspective, endocrowns can be considered as a feasible alternative to full crowns for restoration of nonvital posterior teeth, especially those with minimal crown height but sufficient tissue available for stable and durable adhesive cementation [2].

The evolution of ceramic technology especially dental CAD/CAM systems have enhanced the options to produce single all ceramic endocrowns with high biocompatibility and optimal mechanical properties [3].

In the present paper two ceramic endocrowns fabricated by different methods are presented as case reports.

2. Case 1

A 32-year-old female patient reported for the filling of her lower 1st molar. On clinical examination tooth number 36 was root canal treated one month back (Figure 1). It was asymptomatic and the occlusogingival height of the remaining crown structure was approximately 4 mm. The radiographic findings revealed well obturated canals with no periapical changes.

A conservative approach of restoring the tooth with an endocrown was decided as the treatment option, as more than half the residual tooth structure was remaining and there were no occlusal wear facets. On additional request by the patient for an advanced and a prompt restoration, CAD/CAM ceramic was chosen.

After removal of the provisional restoration, preparation for endocrown was initiated. Resin modified glass ionomer cement (Fuji II LC GC Corporation, Tokyo, Japan) was used

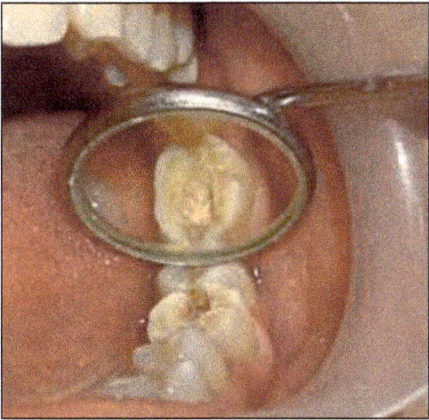

FIGURE 1: Postobturation occlusal view showing the amount of residual tooth structure.

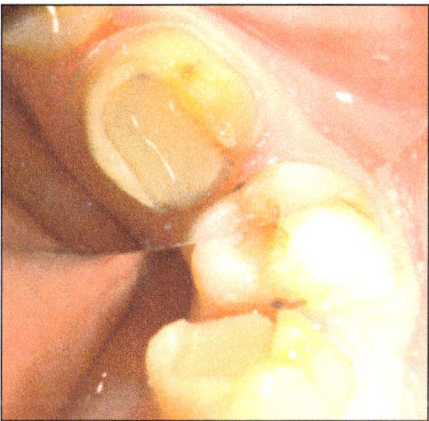

FIGURE 3: CAD/CAM image.

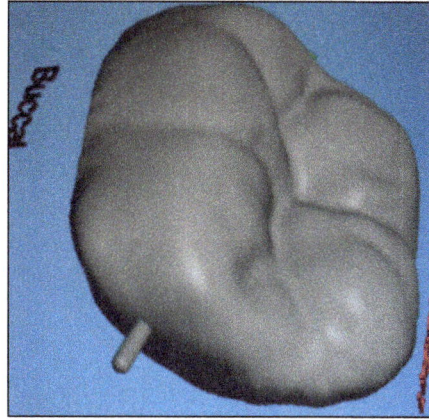

FIGURE 2: Tooth preparation for endocrown.

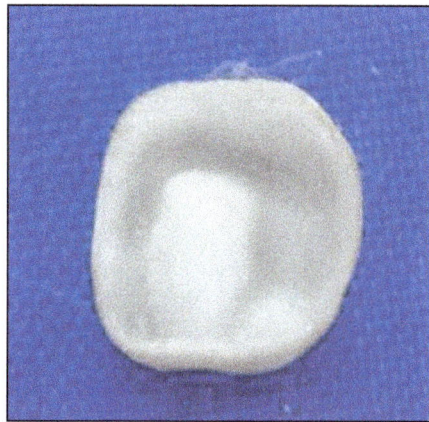

FIGURE 4: Tissue surface depicting the core and crown fabricated as a single unit.

to achieve a flat pulpal floor and to block the undercuts. The preparation consisted of a circular equigingival butt-joint margin and central retention cavity into the entire pulp chamber constructing both the crown and the core as a single unit. The appropriate reduction of the buccal and lingual walls was done (Figure 2).

Interocclusal space was carefully evaluated and occlusal reduction done to achieve a clearance of 2 mm. Shade-B_1 was selected (VITAPAN Zahnfabrik, Germany). Retraction cord was placed and impressions made with polyvinyl siloxane impression material (Aquasil LV, Putty/Light Body, Dentsply DeTrey, Germany) using putty wash technique. Die stone model was fabricated.

CAD/CAM Processing. The three-dimensional reconstruction of the preparation was done using the Yenadent D40 milling machine (Yenadent, Istanbul, Turkey) and DWOS scanner (Dental Wings Inc., Montreal, Canada). The 3D scanning of the individual die and the antagonist arch for occlusal function (virtual articulation) were done. The milling was then initiated on a monolithic solid zirconia block (Metoxit AG, Thayngen, Switzerland) (Figures 3 and 4).

The finished endocrown was checked for shade, fit, and occlusion in the patient's mouth and then cemented using dual cure resin luting agent (Variolink, Ivoclar/Vivadent, Schaan/Liechtenstein).

Clinical and radiographic evaluation was done and follow up after 28 months showed no secondary caries, fracture, discoloration or loosening/decementation of the crown (Figures 5 and 6).

3. Case 2

A 26-year-old female patient reported with a chief complaint of pain since 2 days. On radiographic examination radiolucency involving pulp of tooth 36 was seen. Based on the clinical and radiographic examination tooth 36 was diagnosed with acute irreversible pulpitis. Root canal treatment was performed. Based on the remaining tooth structure, that is, approximately 4-5 mm, occlusal evaluation, and patients esthetic demands, IPS E.max Press endocrown was decided as the treatment option. The endocrown preparation and the impression technique were performed as described in the previous case. IPS E.max Press HO

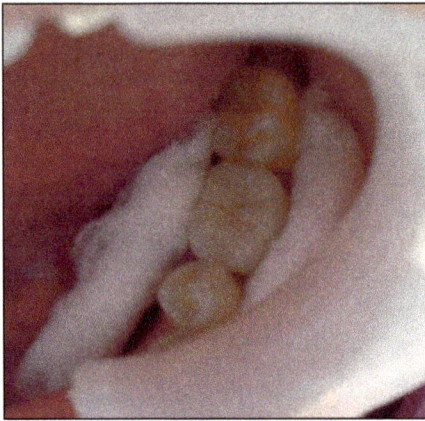

Figure 5: Occlusal view following final cementation.

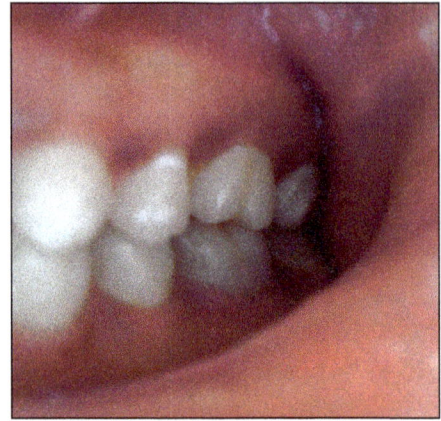

Figure 6: Buccal view of tooth 36 depicting the occlusion and imperceptible margins.

Lithium-disilicate glass ceramic ingots (Ivoclar/Vivadent, Schaan/Liechtenstein) were used for the press technology. The restoration was fabricated according to the lost wax technique of investing and wax pattern burnout followed by pressing of the ceramic ingot in the pressable furnace at a press temperature of 915–920°C. It was then finished and polished with Proxyt pink polishing paste (Ivoclar/Vivadent, Schaan/Liechtenstein). The endocrown was cemented using a dual cure resin luting agent (Variolink, Ivoclar/Vivadent, Schaan/Liechtenstein). Clinical and radiographic evaluation was done and a 28-month followup showed no secondary caries, fracture, discoloration or loosening/decementation of the crown (Figures 7, 8, 9, 10, 11, and 12).

4. Discussion

A successful endodontic treatment has to be complemented with an appropriate postendodontic restoration to integrate the pulpless tooth with the masticatory apparatus [4]. When up to one half of the coronal tooth structure is missing, complete occlusal coverage is achieved conservatively using endocrown [5].

The concept of a conservative protective restoration for posterior endodontically treated teeth is not new. Amalcore, inlays, and onlays are based on this principle. The amalcore harnessed, the large and retentive contours of the root canal orifices, and the pulp chamber to provide a monoblock foundation. Inlays and onlays promoted the concept of a supragingival finish line and conservative preparations. The endocrown is an esthetic and conservative addition to this continuum.

All ceramic systems have gained popularity in recent times as they offer both esthetics and function [6]. The development of CAD/CAM systems and software offers several advantages in clinical practice. Custom shaping and precise milling of ceramic restorations is now a reality; furthermore, the adaptation of the inner surface of the restoration and the replication of the occlusal morphology are better. Restorations can be produced chairside and seated in one appointment. Inaccuracies are minimal and cross-contamination due to impression making and laboratory procedures is reduced. The net result is better patient compliance and satisfaction [6, 7].

On the other hand, pressable ceramic systems yield good functionality, retention, esthetics, and durability [2]. The main advantage of endocrown fabricated using the pressing method is the greater depth of the root extension and the option of using an articulator [3].

The 28-month followup of both types of endocrowns showed no esthetic and functional degradation. These results are in agreement with the previous studies [2, 8, 9].

Bindl and Mörmann demonstrated similar results in a clinical study of Cerec endocrowns cemented adhesively. 19 endocrowns were checked (4 premolars and 15 molars) in 13 patients over 28 months. Only one molar endocrown failed because of recurrent caries [9].

Similar results were reported by Lander and Dietschi where a three-year followup of two Empress II endocrowns showed satisfactory behavior in terms of esthetics, restoration stability, and tissue preservation [2].

Endocrowns have several advantages over conventional crowns like reduced number of interfaces in the restorative system. Stress concentration is less because of the reduction in the nonhomogenous material present [10, 11]. The preparation design is conservative compared to the traditional crown [5]. Involvement of the biological width is minimal [12]. In comparison to the post and core restorations, bonding surface offered by the pulpal chamber of the endocrown is often equal or even superior to that obtained from the bonding of a radicular post of 8 mm depth. The application and polymerization of resins is also better controlled [13].

As presented in the case reports, instead of modifying the existing tooth structure to suit the restorative needs, resin modified glass ionomer cement was used to block the undercuts, thereby further conserving sound tooth structure. The endocrown is luted with resin cement. The adhesive monoblock system achieved reduces the need for macroretentive geometry and provides more efficient outcome and better esthetics [7].

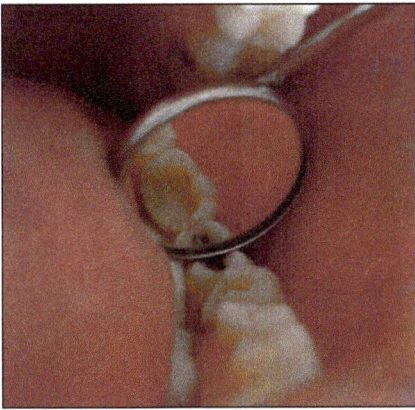

FIGURE 7: Occlusal view showing the amount of residual tooth structure postobturation.

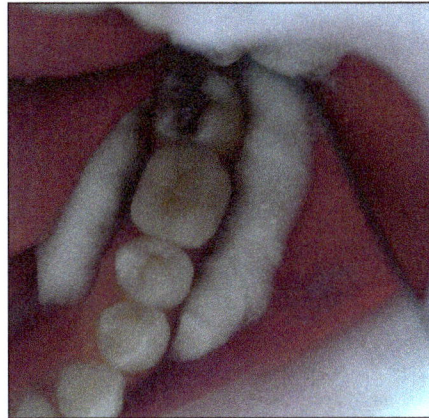

FIGURE 8: Tooth preparation for pressable ceramic endocrown.

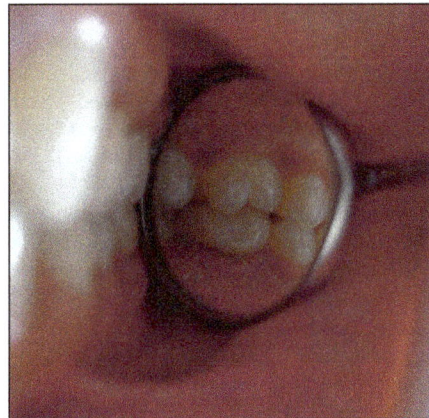

FIGURE 9: Tissue surface of pressed endocrown.

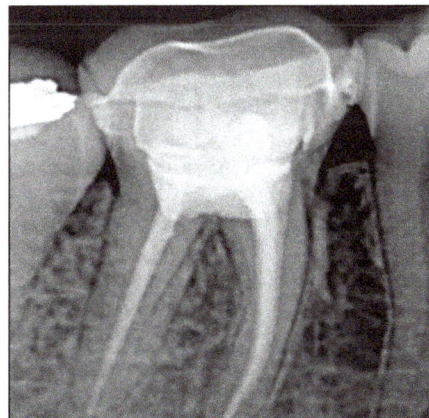

FIGURE 10: Occlusal view following final cementation.

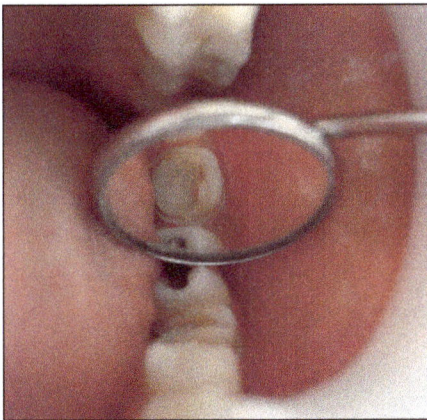

FIGURE 11: Buccal view of tooth 36 highlighting the excellent shade match and finish.

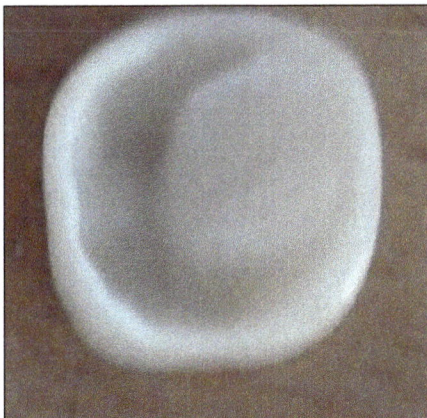

FIGURE 12: Radiographic view, postcementation. The supragingival finish line is clearly visible.

Endocrowns have their own disadvantages like, debonding and risk of root fracture because of the difference in the modulus of elasticity between the harder ceramic and softer dentin [3]. Hence case selection is critical for ensuring clinical success with endocrowns [14]. Endocrowns are indicated in cases where there are minimal functional and lateral stresses. When there is evidence of increased functional and lateral stresses as evident with steep occlusal anatomy, wear facets or parafunction, full coverage crown with or without post is the treatment of choice [12].

Based on current evidence, endocrowns fabricated using CAD/CAM and pressable ceramic technology can be considered as a reliable option for the restoration of moderately mutilated endodontically treated posterior teeth. However, long-term followup and longitudinal clinical studies are needed to ensure their overall success.

References

[1] K. Gulabivala, "Restoration of the root treated tooth," in *Endodontics*, C. J. R. Stock, K. Gulabivala, and R. Walker, Eds., pp. 279–305, Elsevier, 3rd edition, 2004.

[2] E. Lander and D. Dietschi, "Endocrowns: a clinical report," *Quintessence International*, vol. 39, no. 2, pp. 99–106, 2008.

[3] V. Veselinovic, A. Todorovic, D. Lisjak, and V. Lazic, "Restoring endodontically treated teeth with all ceramic endo-crowns case report," *Stomatoloski Glasnik Srbije*, vol. 55, pp. 54–64, 2008.

[4] B. Suresh Chandra and V. Gopi Krishna, *Grossman's Endodontic Practice*, Wolters Kluwer, New Delhi, India, 12th edition, 2010.

[5] D. Dietschi, O. Duc, I. Krejci, and A. Sadan, "Biomechanical considerations for the restoration of endodontically treated teeth: a systematic review of the literature—part 2 (Evaluation of fatigue behavior, interfaces, and in vivo studies)," *Quintessence International*, vol. 39, no. 2, pp. 117–129, 2008.

[6] T. S. Vinothkumar, D. Kandaswamy, and P. Chanana, "CAD/CAM fabricated single unit all ceramic post core crown restoration," *Journal of Conservative Dentistry*, vol. 14, no. 1, pp. 86–89, 2011.

[7] C.-Y. Chang, J.-S. Kuo, Y.-S. Lin, and Y.-H. Chang, "Fracture resistance and failure modes of CEREC endo-crowns and conventional post and core-supported CEREC crowns," *Journal of Dental Sciences*, vol. 4, no. 3, pp. 110–117, 2009.

[8] J. Bernhart, A. Bräuning, M. J. Altenburger, and K.-T. Wrbas, "Cerec3D endocrowns—two-year clinical examination of CAD/CAM crowns for restoring endodontically treated molars," *International Journal of Computerized Dentistry*, vol. 13, no. 2, pp. 141–154, 2010.

[9] A. Bindl and W. H. Mörmann, "Clinical evaluation of adhesively placed cerec endo-crowns after 2 years—preliminary results," *Journal of Adhesive Dentistry*, vol. 1, no. 3, pp. 255–265, 1999.

[10] F. Zarone, R. Sorrentino, D. Apicella et al., "Evaluation of the biomechanical behavior of maxillary central incisors restored by means of endocrowns compared to a natural tooth: a 3D static linear finite elements analysis," *Dental Materials*, vol. 22, no. 11, pp. 1035–1044, 2006.

[11] C.-L. Lin, Y.-H. Chang, and C.-A. Pai, "Evaluation of failure risks in ceramic restorations for endodontically treated premolar with MOD preparation," *Dental Materials*, vol. 27, no. 5, pp. 431–438, 2011.

[12] D. Dietschi, S. Bouillaguet, and A. Sadan, "Restoration of the endodontically treated tooth," in *Cohen's Pathways of the Pulp*, K. M. Hargreaves and S. Cohen, Eds., pp. 777–807, Elsevier Mosby, 10th edition, 2011.

[13] G. T. Rocca and B. Serge, "Alternative treatments for the restoration of non vital teeth," *Revue d'Odonto Stomatologie*, vol. 37, pp. 259–272, 2008.

[14] G. T. Rocca and I. Krejci, "Crown and post- free adhesive restorations for endodontically treated posterior teeth: from direct composite to endocrowns," *European Journal of Esthetic Dentistry*, vol. 8, pp. 156–179, 2013.

33

SEM Analysis and Management of Fracture Dental Implant

**Archana Singh, Ankita Singh, Rajul Vivek, T. P. Chaturvedi,
Pankaj Chauhan, and Shruti Gupta**

*Department of Prosthodontics, Faculty of Dental Sciences, Institute of Medical Sciences,
Banaras Hindu University, Varanasi 221005, India*

Correspondence should be addressed to Archana Singh; archanasingh.bhu26@gmail.com

Academic Editors: R. S. Brown, R. A. de Mesquita, Y. S. Khader, P. Lopez Jornet, and S. R. Watt-Smith

Implant fracture is one of the important biomechanical complications which can present with a considerable problem to the patient as well as the dental surgeon. The aim of this case report is to describe the management of a case of fractured endosseous dental implant in premolar region and microscopic evaluation of the fractured implant segment using scanning electron microscopy. In most of such cases, complete removal of the fractured implant has been a preferred treatment option. In the present case, fractured implant segment was successfully removed and rehabilitated immediately with larger diameter implant. It was found that retrieved fracture segment had a diameter of 3.3 mm, and SEM analysis shows fatigue fractures which may be the result of excessive overloading and use of small diameter implant which enhances fatigue failure.

1. Introduction

Dental implants have been a preferred treatment option for rehabilitation of completely and partially edentulous patients. A major concern for dentist and patient is the durability of the dental implantation. Although the success rate of this treatment is more than 90% [1], the incidence of implant fracture has been reported in 0.16–1.5 percent of the cases [2].

One of the major causes of implant fracture is biomechanical overloading which occur due to various parafunctional activities like bruxism, inadequate occlusion, the presence of distal extensions or cantilevers, and lack of prosthetic passive fit over the implants resulting in metal fatigue [3–7]. Other causes may be peri-implant vertical bone loss [8, 9] due to peri-implantitis and occlusal trauma; galvanic corrosion may be an additional causative factor contributing to implant fracture [10]. Management of a case of implant fracture may pose a challenge to the clinician because of its surgical, rehabilitative, and emotional implications.

The aim of this case report is to describe the management of a case of fractured endosseous dental implant and microscopic evaluation of the fractured implant segment using scanning electron microscopy (SEM).

2. Case Report

A 45-year-old female patient reported to the department with loss of coronal part of implant-supported prosthesis in the lower left premolar region. Detailed history revealed successful implant placement 3 years back in mandibular left second premolar region. Medical history of the patient was found to be noncontributory. Development of pain and mobility of the prosthesis started since the last few months with loss of mobile segment one week back. On radiographic examination, Dentascan revealed remaining part of the implant fixture to be still embedded in the bone (Figure 1).

Treatment plan for the removal of remaining implant fixture, the placement of a new implant of a larger diameter immediately, and consecutive prosthetic rehabilitation was discussed. After obtaining patient consent, the surgical phase was initiated. Under local anesthesia, a mucoperiosteal flap was elevated exposing the fractured implant which was removed by a trephine bur (Figure 2). This was followed by preparing the osteotomy site for placement of a new implant of larger diameter of 5 × 11.5 mm (Hi-tech tapered, self-threaded, Life Care Device private limited, Israel). The

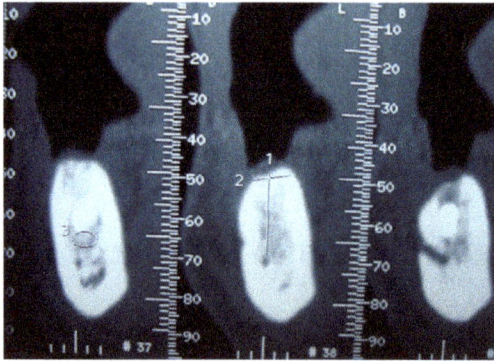

FIGURE 1: Preoperative Dentascan.

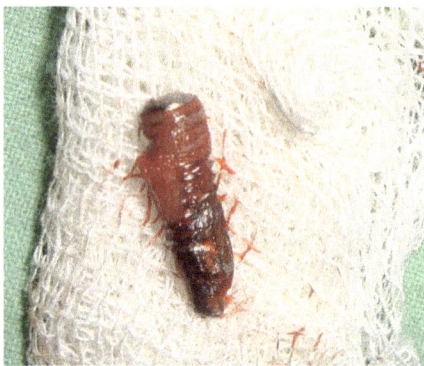

FIGURE 2: Surgically retrieved implant fragment.

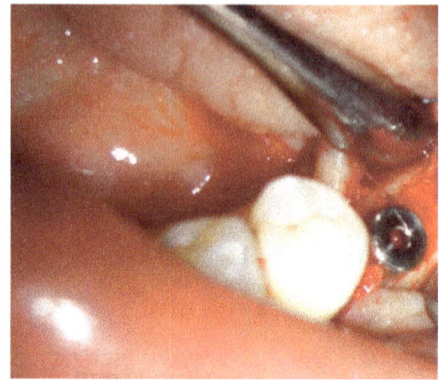

FIGURE 3: Implant placed at mandibular left second bicuspid region.

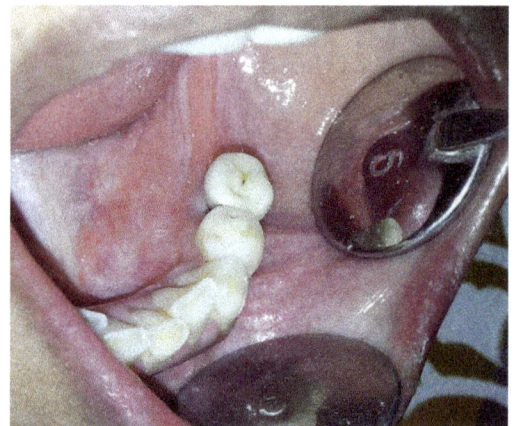

FIGURE 4: Fixed ceramometal prosthesis is placed (occlusal view).

recommended drills were used in required sequence, the endosseous implant was placed immediately after removing the fracture segment (Figure 3) with initial stability of 40 N, and mucoperiosteal flap was approximated with interrupted sutures. The patient was put on antibiotics, anti-inflammatory analgesics, and oral rinses for a week.

Second stage surgery was done after 4 months. The prosthetic phase was initiated by impression making use of open window technique with polyvinyl silicone impression material (Aquasil Dentsply/Caulk, Milford, DE, USA). Abutment preparation and try-in were done, and working cast was sent to the laboratory for fabrication of ceramometal prosthesis (Dentsply, Ceramco, York, PA, USA). Consecutively, the implant was loaded with cement-retained metal-ceramic crown (Figure 4). Reports of 36-month followup at every 3, 6, and 12 months interval have shown successful results so far (Figures 5 and 6).

The retrieved part of implant fixture (Figure 2) was sent for SEM analysis (Figure 7) for the probable cause of the fracture. Scanning electron micrograph of fracture implant surface shows an extent evidence of intergranular fracture. A large dimple at the centre of the implant surface was found which consists of various wavy lines or striations.

3. Discussion

Success and survival rates of osseointegrated dental implant have been reported close to 90–95% [1]. Although the success rate is high, one of the infrequent yet important causes of failure of dental implant is fracture. The incidences of implant fracture reported by Pylant et al. and Goodacre et al. are 0.98%, and 1.5%, respectively [4, 11].

A number of factors should be considered while analyzing the reasons of fractured dental implants. This may include an excessive occlusal load, location of the implant, an insufficient number of implants supporting the prosthesis, the material from which the prosthetic screws are made, and an implant diameter of under 3.75 mm [12].

Rangert et al. [3] reported that 90% of fractured implants are located in the region of molars and premolars. Balshi [13] found that all implant fractures occur in the area of premolars and molars, and no distinction has been made between the upper and lower jaws. Gargallo et al. [14] reported similar results with 80.9% fractured implants located in the molar and premolar region within 3-4 years after loading. This result is in agreement with our case where implant fracture was reported 3 years after implant placement in the mandibular second premolar region. In the present case report, the diameter of the retrieved implant was found to be 3.3 mm. Small diameter of implant <3.75 mm may be another factor contributing to the failure as reported by various studies [13, 15, 16]. According to Shemtov-Yona et al. 3.3 mm diameter implants did not exhibit a typical fatigue behavior like 5

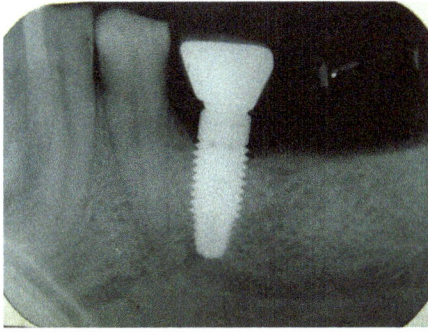

FIGURE 5: IOPA radiograph 3 months after prosthetic rehabilitation.

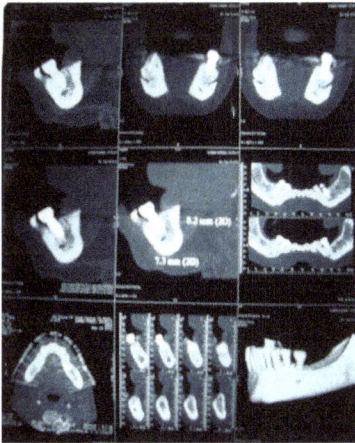

FIGURE 6: Dentascan 12 months after prosthetic rehabilitation.

and 3.75 mm implants; that is, implants were fractured at the abutment neck and screw region. In 3.3 mm implants, 52% of the fractured implants were fractured at the implants second thread and 48% were fracture at the implants third thread. This result is in agreement with our case [17].

Three options for management of implant fracture have been reported in literature [4, 13, 18].

(1) Complete removal of the fractured implant using explanation trephines.

(2) Removal of the coronal portion of fractured implant with the purpose of placing a new prosthetic post.

(3) Removal of the coronal portion of the fractured implant, leaving the remaining apical part integrated in bone.

Complete removal of fractured implant was the preferred treatment option for this patient. In this case complete removal the fractured implant was done, placing a newer larger diameter implant immediately in same surgical bed. External diameter of the trephine bur used for the removal of fractured implant was also kept in mind while selecting the diameter of new implant to ensure primary stability. The retrieved fractured implant was further sent for SEM analysis to study the microscopic features and to investigate the cause of implant fracture.

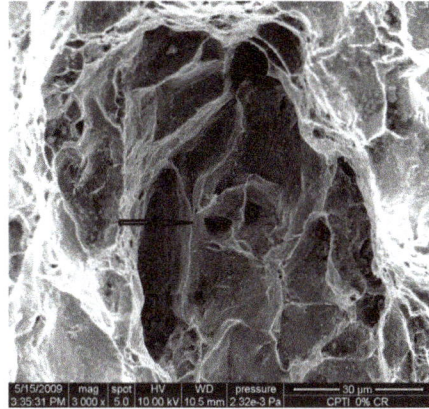

FIGURE 7: Scanning electron micrograph shows intergranular fracture of implant (large dimple at the center of implant surface is shown by arrow).

4. SEM Analysis of Fractured Implant Fragment

SEM image of fractured implant surface was shown in Figure 7. Although the fractured surface is rather complex, the surface shows to an extent evidence of intergranular fracture. A large dimple at the centre of the implant surface was found which consists of various wavy lines. These lines are considered to be the slip bands formed by repeated loading in the mouth. Excessive overloading produces increase in number of dislocation, which, by virtue of their interactions and stress field, gives rise to higher state of internal stresses and consequently leads to fatigue fracture. Shemtov-Yona et al. [19] also proposed that the nontypical fatigue behavior observed for 3.3 mm implant diameter is probably the result of stress concentrations generated along the structure's surface.

5. Conclusion

Dental implant fracture is an infrequent yet important cause of implant therapy failure, and adequate measures should be adopted to prevent it. In this case, it was concluded that cause of implant fracture was found to be metal fatigue due to repeated overloading and use of small diameter implant.

References

[1] T. Albrektsson, G. Zarb, P. Worthington, and A. R. Eriksson, "The long-term efficacy of currently used dental implants: a review and proposed criteria of success," *The International Journal of Oral & Maxillofacial Implants*, vol. 1, no. 1, pp. 11–25, 1986.

[2] T. Berglundh, L. Persson, and B. Klinge, "A systematic review of the incidence of biological and technical complications in implant dentistry reported in prospective longitudinal studies of at least 5 years," *Journal of Clinical Periodontology*, vol. 29, no. 3, pp. 197–212, 2002.

[3] B. Rangert, P. H. Krogh, B. Langer, and N. van Roekel, "Bending overload and implant fracture: a retrospective clinical analysis,"

The International Journal of Oral & Maxillofacial Implants, vol. 10, no. 3, pp. 326–334, 1995.

[4] C. J. Goodacre, J. Y. Kan, and K. Rungcharassaeng, "Clinical complications of osseointegrated implants," *The Journal of Prosthetic Dentistry*, vol. 81, no. 5, pp. 537–552, 1999.

[5] A. Piattelli, A. Scarano, M. Piattelli, E. Vaia, and S. Matarasso, "Hollow implants retrieved for fracture: a light and scanning electron microscope analysis of 4 cases," *Journal of Periodontology*, vol. 69, no. 2, pp. 185–189, 1998.

[6] G. Brunel, S. Armand, N. Miller, and J. Rue, "Histologic analysis of a fractured implant: a case report," *International Journal of Periodontics and Restorative Dentistry*, vol. 20, pp. 520–526, 2000.

[7] D. Flanagan, "External and occlusal trauma to dental implants and a case report," *Dental Traumatology*, vol. 19, no. 3, pp. 160–164, 2003.

[8] M. A. Sánchez-Gárces and C. Gay-Escoda, "Periimplantitis," *Medicina Oral Patologia Oral y Cirugia Bucal*, vol. 9, pp. 63–69, 2004.

[9] R. Uribe, M. Peñarrocha, J. M. Sanchis, and O. García, "Marginal peri-implantitis due to occlusal overload. A case report," *Medicina Oral*, vol. 9, no. 2, pp. 159–162, 2004.

[10] A. Sánchez-Pérez, M. J. Moya-Villaescusa, A. Jornet-García, and S. Gomez, "Etiology, risk factors and management of implant fractures," *Medicina Oral, Patologia Oral y Cirugia Bucal*, vol. 15, no. 3, pp. e504–e508, 2010.

[11] T. Pylant, R. G. Triplett, M. C. Key, and M. A. Brunsvold, "A retrospective evaluation of endosseous titanium implants in the partially edentulous patient," *The International Journal of Oral & Maxillofacial Implants*, vol. 7, no. 2, pp. 195–202, 1992.

[12] N. E. McDermott, S. K. Chuang, V. V. Woo, and T. B. Dodson, "Complications of dental implants: identification, frequency, and associated risk factors," *International Journal of Oral and Maxillofacial Implants*, vol. 18, no. 6, pp. 848–855, 2003.

[13] T. J. Balshi, "analysis and management of fractured implants: a clinical report," *International Journal of Oral and Maxillofacial Implants*, vol. 11, no. 5, pp. 660–666, 1996.

[14] J. Gargallo Albiol, M. Satorres Nieto, J. L. Puyuelo Capablo, M. A. Sánchez Garcés, J. Pi Urgell, and C. Gay-Escoda, "Endosseous dental implant fractures an analysis of 21 cases," *Medicina Oral, Patologia Oral y Cirugia Bucal*, vol. 13, no. 2, pp. 124–128, 2008.

[15] S. E. Eckert, S. J. Meraw, E. Cal, and R. K. Ow, "Analysis of incidence and associated factors with fractured implants: a retrospective study," *International Journal of Oral and Maxillofacial Implants*, vol. 15, no. 5, pp. 662–667, 2000.

[16] S. E. Eckert and P. C. Wollan, "Retrospective review of 1170 endosseous implants placed in partially edentulous jaws," *Journal of Prosthetic Dentistry*, vol. 79, no. 4, pp. 415–421, 1998.

[17] K. Shemtov-Yona, D. Rittel, E. Machtei, and L. Levin, "Effect of dental implant diameter on fatigue performance, part II: failure analysis," *Clinical Implant Dentistry and Related Research*, pp. 1–7, 2012.

[18] A. Piattelli, A. Scarano, M. Piattelli, E. Vaia, and S. Matarasso, "Hollow implants retrieved for fracture: a light and scanning electron microscope analysis of 4 cases," *Journal of Periodontology*, vol. 69, no. 2, pp. 185–189, 1998.

[19] K. Shemtov-Yona, D. Rittel, L. Levin, and E. Machtei, "Effect of dental implant diameter on fatigue performance, part I: failure analysis," *Clinical Implant Dentistry and Related Research*, 2012.

34

Cervical Necrotizing Fasciitis Caused by Dental Extraction

José Alcides Arruda,[1] Eugênia Figueiredo,[2] Pâmella Álvares,[1] Luciano Silva,[1] Leorik Silva,[3] Antônio Caubi,[1] Marcia Silveira,[1] and Ana Paula Sobral[1]

[1]Faculdade de Odontologia de Pernambuco, Universidade de Pernambuco, Avenida General Newton Cavalcante, 1650 Aldeia dos Camarás, 54753-020 Camaragibe, PE, Brazil
[2]Hospital da Restauração, Avenida Governador Agamenon Magalhães, S/N, Derby, 52010-040 Recife, PE, Brazil
[3]Universidade Federal do Rio Grande do Norte, Campus Universitário Lagoa Nova, P.O. Box 1524, 59078-970 Natal, RN, Brazil

Correspondence should be addressed to José Alcides Arruda; alcides_almeida@hotmail.com

Academic Editor: Alberto C. B. Delbem

Cervical necrotizing fasciitis is an unusual infection characterized by necrosis of the subcutaneous tissue and fascial layers. Risk factors for the development of necrotizing fasciitis include diabetes mellitus, chronic renal disease, peripheral vascular disease, malnutrition, advanced age, obesity, alcohol abuse, intravenous drug use, surgery, and ischemic ulcers. This report presents a case of necrotizing fasciitis in the cervical area caused by dental extraction in a 73-year-old woman. Cervical necrotizing fasciitis in geriatric patient is rare, and even when establishing the diagnosis and having it timely treated, the patient can suffer irreversible damage or even death. Clinical manifestations in the head and neck usually have an acute onset characterized by severe pain, swelling, redness, erythema, presence of necrotic tissue, and in severe cases obstruction of the upper airways. Therefore, the presentation of this clinical case can serve as guidance to dentists as a precaution to maintain an aseptic chain and be aware of the clinical condition of older patients and the systemic conditions that may increase the risk of infections.

1. Introduction

Necrotizing fasciitis (NF) is a potentially fatal infection generally characterized by a rapidly progressive process of necrosis of the subcutaneous tissues and muscle fascial layers. The most likely cause of the disease is a vascular obliteration with microthrombosis around the locus of infection, accompanied by acute inflammation of the subcutaneous tissue and swelling of the underlying tissues; with the progression there is no intravascular coagulation in place and the infected tissue becomes necrotic. Moreover, it is believed that the lack of specific antigens of group A streptococcus is a predisposing factor for the development of this disease [1]. NF in the cervical area caused by dental extraction in a geriatric patient is rare and only few cases in the medical literature in English are reported.

The primary sites of these infections in the head and neck are teeth, tonsils, or traumatic wounds [1]. To establish the diagnosis, areas of necrotic tissue surrounding the underlying fabric and the fascial spaces should be clinically observed. Clinical manifestations usually have acute onset and are characterized by intense algic pain, swelling, redness, erythema, the presence of necrotic tissue, presence of palpable crepitus due to subcutaneous gas, grey, foul-smelling "dishwater" exudate, and in severe cases obstruction of the upper airways [2, 3].

This report presents a case of NF in the cervical area caused by dental extraction in a 73-year-old woman.

2. Case Presentation

A 73-year-old woman attended at the emergency ward of Universidade de Pernambuco's Hospital da Restauração, Brazil, complaining of severe pain in the cervical area. During the anamnesis the patient reported extraction of the lower right lateral incisor six days priorly. The extraoral physical examination revealed extensive necrotic tissue in the cervical area, fetid odor, hyperemia, and edema (Figure 1). Respiratory rate

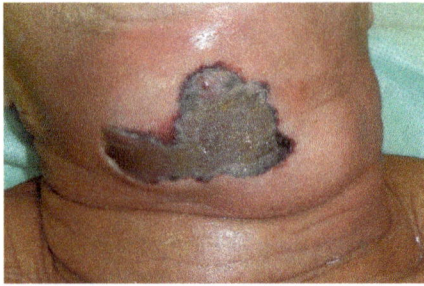

FIGURE 1: The extraoral physical examination revealed extensive necrotic tissue in the cervical area.

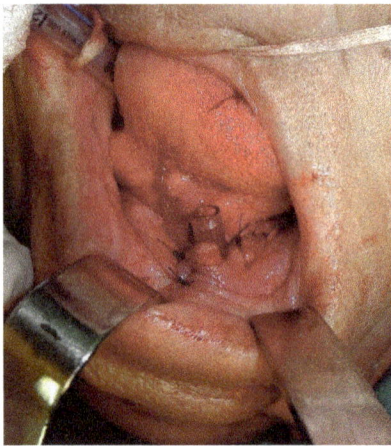

FIGURE 2: Installation of a Pen Rose irrigation drain.

anatomical site, tissue depth, type of bacteria, and general condition of the patient [4–6]. NF usually occurs secondarily to dental or gingival infections. Whitesides et al. [7] observed that the second and third molars were commonly the cause of this injury. However, any spread of microorganisms that causes some deep infection in the adjacent tissues of the neck can cause NF [8]. Extraction prior to the NF might be raised as a cause of breaking the aseptic chain during this surgical procedure and disrupting the systemic condition of the patient, and the infection in the present case may have begun this way, as the patient reported an extraction of the lower right lateral incisor six days priorly.

The age of the patient may have been triggering, despite the fact that NF can occur in all ages; however, Maria and Rajnikanth [8] claim that this is more common in patients in the fourth decade of life. We cannot discount the fact that the patient was 73 years old, and so the patient presents risk factors noted by Puvanendran et al. [2].

The diagnosis and treatment of NF should be established with the support of a multidisciplinary team before identifying the causative agent or the microbiota involved. Additionally, there is consensus that the elimination of the causative as well as the focus of the infection should be soon obtained to prevent further damage agent, since patients with NF are susceptible to rapid liquefaction in the progressive subcutaneous fat and connective tissue while the overlying skin is saved. Once the patient is not treated on time, the disease may progress rapidly to necrotizing mediastinitis and even death, which can occur in 10% to 40% of cases [9]. In the case reported the speed in establishing the diagnosis and initiating treatment resulted in the repair area having a decreased risk of sepsis and death.

Clinical and imaging findings can guide the dentist to the correct diagnosis of NF. The definitive diagnosis is made by surgical exploration, by the presence of necrosis of the fascia. However, the occurrence of local cyanosis and blistering yellowish or reddish dark content become present. Commonly, edema can be observed before other cutaneous signs appear. Other important aspects are palpable crepitation subcutaneous gas, as well as intense pain. The necrosis of the fascia is typically more extensive than suggested by the clinical aspect [10].

In the early stages, NF and cellulite are hardly distinguishable. In addition, NF and hemorrhaging blisters cellulite feature many other factors in common. Both are painful conditions, with potential to evolve quickly to necrosis and gangrene, which have the same predisposing factors and can have the same etiologic agents [10]. Clues to the diagnosis of NF include inelastic edema, cyanosis, pallor and hypoesthesia, crackling skin, muscle weakness, foul-smelling "dishwater" exudate, absence of lymphangitis, and rapid progression of the infection. Systemic manifestations of sepsis are usually present, including altered mental status, tachycardia, tachypnea, leukocytosis ($>12000\,mm^3$), fever, hypocalcemia, and metabolic acidosis. Bacteriological tests (direct and cultures) from the wound exudate, blister fluid, excised tissue, material aspirated tissue, and blood are essential for a proper diagnosis [11].

and blood pressure changes, however, were not observed. Culture was performed with antibiotic susceptibility of the affected region. Biochemical tests revealed a blood count showing leukocytosis ($22,000\,mm^3$) and a slightly increased glycemic index (144 mg/dL). Clinical diagnosis of NF was established. Preoperative antibiotic therapy was administered with Metronidazole 500 mg and Rocefin 1 g. The patient was submitted to surgical removal of necrotic tissue, debridement of the surrounding tissues, installation of a Pen Rose irrigation drain (physiologic solution 0.9%), and intravenous administration of Meropenem 500 mg for 10 days (Figure 2). After seven days, dehiscence of the wound edges was observed, a new surgical debridement was carried out, and occlusive dressing with silver alginate was applied and exchanged every 48 hours for 21 days (Figures 3(a) and 3(b)). After 30 days, the patient was discharged (Figure 4(a)), though complete repair of the surgical wound was not observed, as that only happened seven weeks after the operation by secondary intention (Figure 4(b)).

3. Discussion

The NF predominantly affects the tissues of the abdominal wall, the peritoneum, and extremities, being quite rare (approximately 3-4% of all NF cases) in the head and neck. The severity of this disease depends on the etiology,

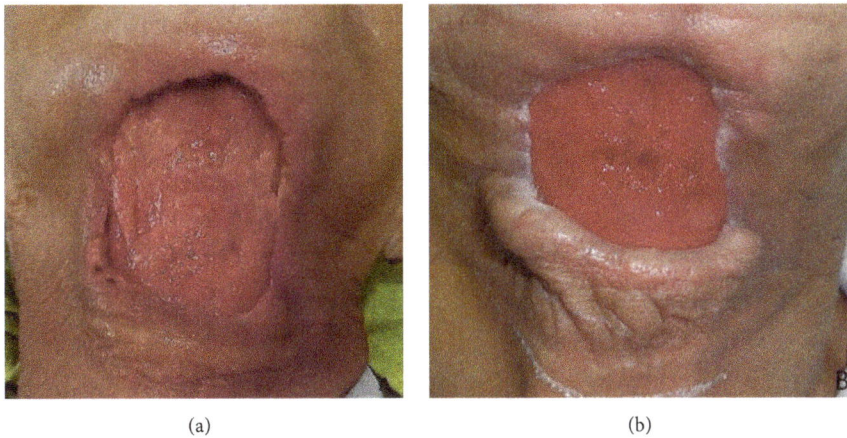

(a)   (b)

FIGURE 3: (a) After seven days and (b) after 21 days, dehiscence of the wound edges was observed.

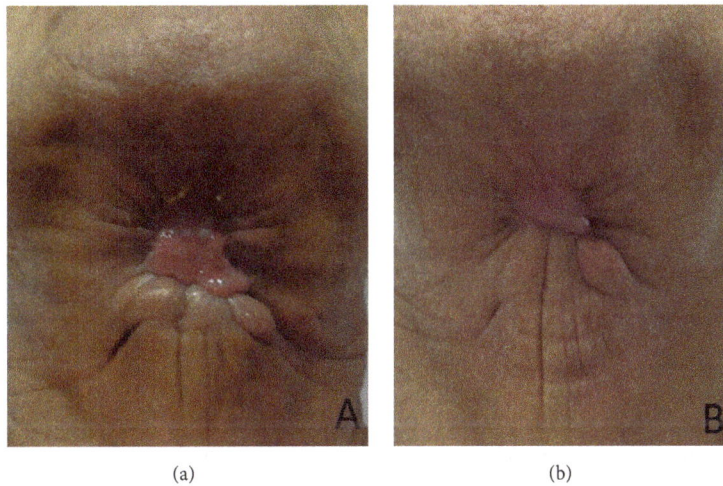

(a)   (b)

FIGURE 4: (a) After 30 days and (b) after seven weeks using silver alginate, a favorable healing was observed.

Disseminated intravascular coagulation and thrombocytopenia are common in any severe sepsis, and other hematological parameters should be interpreted with caution [12]. With a wide range of values reported in NF, the leucocyte count is less helpful for diagnosis. Acute renal failure is the norm in severe sepsis, and dosing of renal excreted antimicrobials should be adjusted accordingly. Bacterial infection, inflammation, thrombosis, and necrosis all increase serum C-reactive protein (CRP). Raised serum creatinine kinase (CK) indicates myositis or myonecrosis, as well as the effects of circulating toxins or ischemia [13, 14]. Involvement of adjacent muscle raises CK and is not present in all cases of NF, but CK levels of 600 U/L gave a sensitivity of 58% and a specificity of 95% for cases of NF. The most reliable indicators of underlying NF were found to be CRP, creatinine, hemoglobin, leucocyte count, sodium, and serum glucose [15].

X-ray is used to confirm the presence of gas in subcutaneous region as evidence of NF. However, unless the gas was confined more superficially, rarely could it be demonstrated

for this examination. In contrast, CT provides the presence and extent of abnormal gas, in addition, to show necrosis with asymmetric thickening of the fascia. Walshaw and Deans reviewed the scans of 20 patients with NF, and 11 (55%) of them had gas in subcutaneous region [16]. CT also helps in differential diagnosis for evidence of myonecrosis, which suggests muscle impairment and conditions other than NF, in that such involvement is late and secondary [17]. MRI can also provide early diagnosis of NF and demonstrate the need for surgery and also determine the extent of involvement, thus facilitating presurgery [18].

Surgical treatment is fundamental to increasing the chance of patient survival. Combining surgery with multiple broad-spectrum antibiotics may be performed to combat NF. In this case, the antibiotic, surgical debridement, electrolyte replacement, and the use of drains were effective in fighting this infection. Treatment also involved a surgical Pen Rose drain installation for removal of necrotic tissue, tissue debridement, and irrigation. An antibiogram culture was made, as recommended [8]. Hyperbaric oxygen (HBO) therapy was another studied approach to treatment in the late 20th century. This adjunctive therapy is thought to increase tissue partial pressure of oxygen up to four times the normal, thus increasing bacterial killing and facilitating wound healing [19]. However, the few studies that have investigated HBO therapy in NF show little outcome benefit [20–22]. HBO is also believed to increase the bactericidal action of neutrophils since at low oxygen tensions peroxide-dependent killing mechanisms are less efficient [23]. Nonetheless, the overall evidence of benefit in nonclostridial NF is weak. Despite reports of rapid amelioration of clinical and mental status after only one HBO session, there are few published data to support the use of HBO in NF [7, 9, 10, 24]. In this case report such therapy was not applied.

Early thorough debridement is essential and produces large areas that need covering [25, 26]. Negative pressure therapy, vacuum-assisted closure dressing, with a continuous pressure of 40–100 mmHg is useful for wound coverage and encourages granulation before and after skin grafting [27, 28]. Although debridement was performed by the conventional technique, modern techniques such as "bear claw" are used for this purpose.

Yadav et al. [29] state that, generally, recovery of the surgical wound may take up to 150 days; in the case described, the wound was completely repaired in 50 days, indicating that the therapy came to a proper resolution. In this case report, after cicatrization, the patient presents substance loss due to repair by second intention requiring plastic surgical correction, which was refused by the patient.

Cervical NF in geriatric patient is rare, and even when establishing the diagnosis and having it timely treated, patient can suffer irreversible damage or even death. Therefore, the presentation of this clinical case can serve as guidance to dentists in order to maintain an aseptic chain and be aware of the clinical condition of older patients and the systemic conditions that may increase the risk of infections.

Competing Interests

The authors declare that there is no conflict of interests regarding the publication of this paper.

References

[1] H. Wolf, M. Rusan, K. Lambertsen, and T. Ovesen, "Necrotizing fasciitis of the head and neck," *Head & Neck*, vol. 32, no. 12, pp. 1592–1596, 2010.

[2] R. Puvanendran, J. Huey, and S. Pasupathy, "Necrotizing fasciitis of the neck," *Indian Journal of Otolaryngology and Head & Neck Surgery*, vol. 54, no. 2, pp. 143–145, 2009.

[3] M. L. Shindo, V. P. Nalbone, and W. R. Dougherty, "Necrotizing fasciitis of the face," *Laryngoscope*, vol. 107, no. 8, pp. 1071–1079, 1997.

[4] C.-T. Hsiao, H.-H. Weng, Y.-D. Yuan, C.-T. Chen, and I.-C. Chen, "Predictors of mortality in patients with necrotizing fasciitis," *American Journal of Emergency Medicine*, vol. 26, no. 2, pp. 170–175, 2008.

[5] S. K. Lazow, "Orofacial infections in the 21st century," *The New York State Dental Journal*, vol. 71, no. 6, pp. 36–41, 2005.

[6] A. E. Obiechina, J. T. Arotiba, and A. O. Fasola, "Necrotizing fasciitis of odontogenic origin in Ibadan, Nigeria," *British Journal of Oral and Maxillofacial Surgery*, vol. 39, no. 2, pp. 122–126, 2001.

[7] L. Whitesides, C. Cotto-Cumba, and R. A. M. Myers, "Cervical necrotizing fasciitis of odontogenic origin: a case report and review of 12 cases," *Journal of Oral and Maxillofacial Surgery*, vol. 58, no. 2, pp. 144–151, 2000.

[8] A. Maria and K. Rajnikanth, "Cervical necrotizing fasciitis caused by dental infection: a review and case report," *National Journal of Maxillofacial Surgery*, vol. 1, no. 2, pp. 135–138, 2010.

[9] G. Dhaif, A. Al-Saati, M. Bassim, and A. Cabs, "Management dilemma of cervicofacial necrotizing fasciitis," *Journal of the Bahrain Medical Society*, vol. 21, no. 1, pp. 223–227, 2009.

[10] M. A. Gardam, D. E. Low, R. Saginur, and M. A. Miller, "Group B streptococcal necrotizing fasciitis and streptococcal toxic shock-like syndrome in adults," *Archives of Internal Medicine*, vol. 158, no. 15, pp. 1704–1708, 1998.

[11] M. C. Morantes and B. A. Lipsky, "'Flesh-eating bacteria': return of an old nemesis," *International Journal of Dermatology*, vol. 34, no. 7, pp. 461–463, 1995.

[12] D. B. Wall, C. de Virgilio, S. Black, and S. R. Klein, "Objective criteria may assist in distinguishing necrotizing fasciitis from non-necrotizing soft tissue infection," *The American Journal of Surgery*, vol. 179, no. 1, pp. 17–21, 2000.

[13] M. R. D. Barnham, N. C. Weightman, A. W. Anderson, and A. Tanna, "Streptoccocal toxic shock syndrome: a description of 14 cases from North Yorkshire, UK," *Clinical Microbiology and Infection*, vol. 8, no. 3, pp. 174–181, 2002.

[14] A. L. Bisno, F. R. Cockerill III, and C. T. Bermudez, "The initial outpatient-physician encounter in group A streptococcal necrotizing fasciitis," *Clinical Infectious Diseases*, vol. 31, no. 2, pp. 607–608, 2000.

[15] T. Simonart, J. M. Simonart, I. Derdelinckx et al., "Value of standard laboratory tests for the early recognition of group A β-hemolytic streptococcal necrotizing fasciitis," *Clinical Infectious Diseases*, vol. 32, no. 1, pp. e9–e12, 2001.

[16] C. F. Walshaw and H. Deans, "CT findings in necrotizing fasciitis- a report of four cases," *Clinical Radiology*, vol. 51, no. 6, pp. 429–432, 1996.

[17] S. Fink, T. K. Chaudhuri, and H. H. Davis, "Necrotizing fasciitis and malpractice claims," *Southern Medical Journal*, vol. 92, no. 8, pp. 770–774, 1999.

[18] T. E. Brothers, D. U. Tagge, J. E. Stutley, W. F. Conway, H. Del Schutte Jr., and T. K. Byrne, "Magnetic resonance imaging differentiates between necrotizing and non-necrotizing fasciitis of the lower extremity," *Journal of the American College of Surgeons*, vol. 187, no. 4, pp. 416–421, 1998.

[19] D. M. Aronoff and K. C. Bloch, "Assessing the relationship between the use of nonsteroidal antiinflammatory drugs and necrotizing fasciitis caused by group A streptococcus," *Medicine*, vol. 82, no. 4, pp. 225–235, 2003.

[20] Health Protection Agency. Group A Streptococcus Working Group, "Interim UK guidelines for management of close community contacts of invasive group A streptococcal disease," *Communicable Disease and Public Health*, vol. 7, pp. 364–371, 2004.

[21] A. Fustes-Morales, P. Gutierrez-Castrellon, C. Duran-McKinster, L. Orozco-Covarrubias, L. Tamayo-Sanchez, and R. Ruiz-Maldonado, "Necrotizing fasciitis: report of 39 pediatric cases," *Archives of Dermatology*, vol. 138, no. 7, pp. 893–899, 2002.

[22] S. Sakata, R. Das Gupta, J. F. Leditschke, and R. M. Kimble, "Extensive necrotising fasciitis in a 4-day-old neonate: a successful outcome from modern dressings, intensive care and early surgical intervention," *Pediatric Surgery International*, vol. 25, no. 1, pp. 117–119, 2009.

[23] S. J. Escobar, J. B. Slade Jr., T. K. Hunt, and P. Cianci, "Adjuvant hyperbaric oxygen therapy (HBO_2) for treatment of necrotizing fasciitis reduces mortality and amputation rate," *Undersea and Hyperbaric Medicine*, vol. 32, no. 6, pp. 437–443, 2005.

[24] D. R. Aitken, M. C. T. Mackett, and L. L. Smith, "The changing pattern of hemolytic streptococcal gangrene," *Archives of Surgery*, vol. 117, no. 5, pp. 561–567, 1982.

[25] C. R. McHenry, J. J. Piotrowski, D. Peterinic, and M. A. Malangoni, "Determinants of mortality for necrotising soft tissue infections," *Annals of Surgery*, vol. 221, no. 5, pp. 558–565, 1995.

[26] L. Steinstraesser, M. Sand, and H.-U. Steinau, "Giant VAC in a patient with extensive necrotizing fasciitis," *International Journal of Lower Extremity Wounds*, vol. 8, no. 1, pp. 28–30, 2009.

[27] Z. D. Mulla, "Streptococcal myositis," *British Journal of Plastic Surgery*, vol. 56, no. 4, article 424, 2003.

[28] Y. Jiménez, J. V. Bagán, J. Murillo, and R. Poveda, "Odontogenic infections. Complications. Systemic manifestations," *Medicina Oral, Patologia Oral y Cirugia Bucal*, vol. 9, pp. 143–143, 2004.

[29] S. Yadav, A. Verma, and A. Sachdeva, "Facial necrotizing fasciitis from an odontogenic infection," *Oral Surgery, Oral Medicine, Oral Pathology and Oral Radiology*, vol. 113, no. 2, pp. e1–e4, 2012.

35

Incidental Radiographic Discovery of a Screw in a Primary Molar

Farhin Katge, Sajjad Mithiborwala, and Thejokrishna Pammi

Department of Pedodontics & Preventive Dentistry, Terna Dental College, Sector 22, Plot No. 12, Nerul (W), Navi Mumbai 400706, Maharashtra, India

Correspondence should be addressed to Farhin Katge; pedotdc@gmail.com

Academic Editors: I. Anic, R. S. Brown, and W. L. Chai

Dentists often find foreign bodies in the primary dentition of children who habitually place objects in their mouths. The objects are frequently embedded in exposures that result from carious or traumatic lesions or from endodontic procedures that have been left open for drainage. Such bodies are often detected on routine radiographs and, less frequently, during clinical examination. We report a case of a 6-year-old boy who had inadvertently embedded a screw in his mandibular right first primary molar and had forgotten about it until it became symptomatic. The screw was impacted in the exposed pulp chamber due to a large carious lesion in the affected molar. This case report considers the possible medical and dental consequences of placing foreign bodies in the mouth.

1. Introduction

Many children are in the habit of exploring various objects in the oral cavity that can cause hard or soft tissue injuries. This practice may result in inadvertent insertion of foreign bodies within the pulp chamber or root canal [1]. Foreign objects are often discovered in the primary dentition during radiological examination. Radiographic examination assists in the determination of the number, type, composition, and position of the foreign object(s). Till date only two such cases of a screw impacted in a primary molar have been reported [2, 3].

2. Case Report

A 6 year old boy reported to the Department of Pedodontics, Terna Dental College, Navi Mumbai, India, complaining of pain in lower right back region of jaw, since 3–5 days. Intraoral clinical examination revealed deep occlusal caries and intraoral draining sinus in relation to #84. Vestibular tenderness and mobility were absent. An intraoral periapical radiograph of the tooth revealed presence of a linear radiopaque object (metallic screw) 6.5 × 4 mm in dimension, which was embedded in the pulp chamber of #84 (Figures 1 and 2). A clinical history revealed that the patient habitually

placed metal objects in his mouth; on one occasion, the screw had become lodged in the cavitated tooth. Several attempts by the child to retrieve it had proven futile. The child had not reported this incident to his parents for fear of punishment and had soon forgotten about it. A diagnosis of chronic dentoalveolar abscess with 84 was made. The treatment plan involved removal of foreign body from the pulp chamber of #84 followed by pulpectomy and stainless steel crown cementation.

Clinical procedure was embarked with hand excavation of the large carious lesion. Following excavation of the carious lesion the site was flushed with isotonic saline which then revealed the metallic screw. With the help of piezoelectric ultrasonics (Dentsply Tulsa Dental Specialties, USA) [4] at low intensity the screw was very slowly disengaged from the pulpal chamber taking care that the thin buccal and lingual walls did not fracture (Figure 3).

After the retrieval of the screw, the tooth was clinically evaluated for the signs of perforation of the pulpal floor. Careful biomechanical preparation of the root canals was done to avoid lateral root perforation. Concomitant copious irrigation with endodontic irrigants was done to debride the root canals. Following obturation with Vitapex (Neo Dental International, Inc., USA) the access cavity was restored with

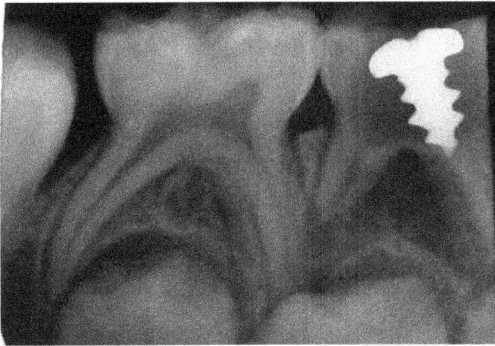

FIGURE 1: IOPA showing metallic screw in the pulp chamber of #84 with intact pulpal floor.

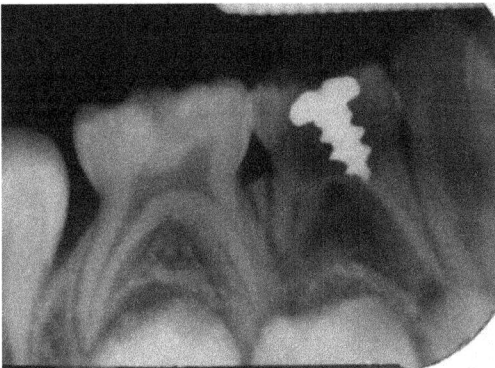

FIGURE 2: IOPA showing intact furcal area with no evidence of interradicular bone loss.

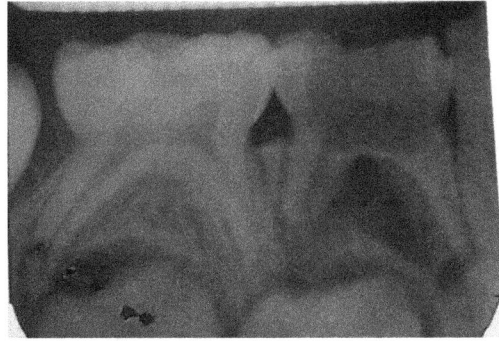

FIGURE 3: IOPA after retrieval of the metallic screw.

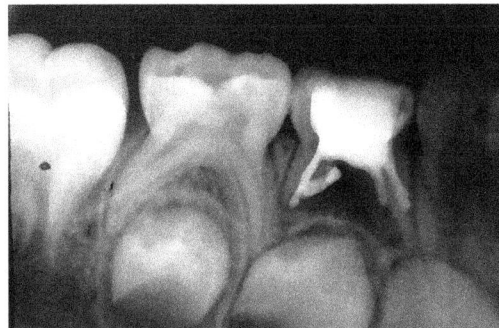

FIGURE 4: Obturation of the #84.

Ketac Molar (3M ESPE, USA) (Figure 4). The crown was then cemented with stainless steel crown (3M ESPE, USA) with luting cement.

The patient was kept under systemic antibiotic therapy, which was started one day prior to the clinical procedure (Amoxicillin 250 mg; Metronidazole 200 mg; and Tab Ibugesic kid 20 mg TID for 5 days). A tetanus toxoid vaccine (tetanus vaccine (adsorbed) Ip., Biological E. Limited, Hyderabad, India) was administered after the obturation of the tooth. One month recall examination showed complete healing of the intraoral sinus.

3. Discussion

Self-oral exploration, play while eating, imitation of peers or older siblings performing a similar behaviour, and attempts to relieve chronic irritation coupled with fear of dentistry are factors that may prompt children to place foreign objects in the mouth. A review of the literature reveals numerous reports describing the various foreign objects that have been inserted in the exposed pulp chambers or root canals. Most such case reports have dealt with anterior teeth. Objects such as wooden tooth picks, straws, pins, needles, a pencil tip, plastic objects, toothbrush bristles, crayons, beads, paper clip, and stapler pins [5–9] have been placed into the root canals of maxillary anteriors in an attempt to remove food plugs [10–12].

Within the oral cavity, foreign bodies may be embedded in the soft or hard tissue. Objects impacted within the periodontium are a potential source of infection and may lead to edema, hemorrhage, and abscess formation. In addition, foreign bodies in primary teeth can lead to the perforation of the pulp chamber floor space and possible trauma to the developing permanent dentition, depending on developmental stage. Trauma to the tooth in the initial stages of odontogenesis can destroy the permanent tooth bud completely or may result in disorganization of the tooth germ, forming a complex odontoma.

A force of lesser magnitude may result in a geminated and/or a hypoplastic successor tooth. Furthermore, the presence of a foreign body may impede the eruption of the underlying permanent tooth, resulting in ectopic or failed eruption. Such failure of the underlying tooth to erupt due to an overlying mechanical obstruction at the time of root formation may alter the angulation of its root, leading to dilaceration. A foreign object lodged in the tooth for a lengthy period of time is a potential source of infection and can lead to cyst formation. Therefore, the eruption of the permanent tooth should be closely and regularly monitored so that any anomaly can be detected at an incipient stage and treatment rendered accordingly.

The management of a foreign body impaction in a tooth depends on the location, accessibility, stage of tooth formation, restorability of the tooth, the patient's age, and level of cooperation. However, very few such cases have been reported in posterior teeth. Prabhakar et al. reported embedment of a screw in a permanent mandibular first molar; while Nadkarni et al. described retrieval of a needle fragment from the palatal root canal of a permanent maxillary first molar [13, 14]. A meticulous review of the literature reveals that our case report is unique as the tooth in question is a primary lower right first molar, and no similar report till date has been published.

A conventional practice employed during emergency root canal treatment involves leaving the pulp chamber open where pus continues to discharge through the canal and cannot be dried within a reasonable period of time. Weine recommends that the patient remains in office with a draining tooth for an hour or even more and finally ending the appointment by sealing the access cavity. With the access cavity closed, no new strains of microorganisms are introduced, and food debris and foreign body lodgement within the tooth can be avoided [15].

A radiograph can be of diagnostic significance especially if the foreign body is radiopaque. Mcauliffe et al. summarized various radiographic methods to be followed to localize a radiopaque foreign object as parallax views, vertex occlusal view, triangulation techniques, and stereo radiography and tomography. Parallax technique involves 2 radiographs taken at different horizontal angles with the same vertical direction. Due to parallax the objects appear to travel in the same direction as tube shifts, and the object closer to tube appears to move in opposite direction (the so-called Same Lingual Opposite Buccal—SLOB). Vertex occlusal view is no longer favored because of relatively high radiation exposure to the lens of the eye and because the primary beam is aimed towards the abdomen. Triangulation is by the use of two views right angle to one another. Interpretation is difficult because of the superimposition of the other incisor teeth over the root. Stereographic views and tomography were not considered due to minimal availability of these facilities in dental operatory. Specialized radiographic techniques such as radiovisiography and 3D CAT scans can play a role in localization of these foreign objects inside the root canal [16].

4. Conclusion

This case report would like to highlight the need of dental surgeons to establish good rapport with children, so that the history of foreign body impaction is not overlooked. Also evident is the need for an early radiological examination in cases of suspected "mouthing" of a foreign body. Moreover, teeth with traumatically or cariously exposed pulp should be coronally sealed whenever possible to avoid such complications. Moreover, a dire need exists to counsel parents in adopting basic home safety measures for children and vigilantly avoiding their having access to foreign objects within easy reach. In the present case, conservative method has been employed and extraction of the tooth prevented, since the patient had reported timely.

References

[1] I. B. Lamster and J. T. Barenie, "Foreign objects in the root canal. Review of the literature and report of two cases," *Oral Surgery Oral Medicine and Oral Pathology*, vol. 44, no. 3, pp. 483–486, 1977.

[2] L. Pomarico, L. G. Primo, and I. P. R. De Souza, "Images in paediatrics: unusual foreign body detected on routine dental radiograph," *Archives of Disease in Childhood*, vol. 90, no. 8, p. 825, 2005.

[3] U. Sharma and P. K. S. Virk, "Incidental discovery of a screw in a deciduous molar," *Oral Radiology*, vol. 27, no. 1, pp. 57–59, 2011.

[4] C. J. Ruddle, "Broken instrument removal. The endodontic challenge," *Dentistry Today*, vol. 21, no. 7, pp. 70–76, 2002.

[5] H. Nernst, "Foreign body in a root canal," *Quintessence International*, vol. 3, no. 8, pp. 33–34, 1972.

[6] W. E. Harris, "Foreign bodies in root canals: report of two cases," *The Journal of the American Dental Association*, vol. 85, no. 4, pp. 906–911, 1972.

[7] J. B. Hall, "Endodontics-performed," *Journal of Dentistry for Children*, vol. 36, pp. 213–215, 1969.

[8] W. E. Gelfman, L. J. Cheris, and A. C. Williams, "Self-attempted endodontics—a case report," *ASDC Journal of Dentistry for Children*, vol. 36, no. 4, pp. 283–284, 1969.

[9] J.-C. Shay, "Foreign body in a tooth," *Oral Surgery, Oral Medicine, Oral Pathology*, vol. 59, no. 4, p. 431, 1985.

[10] V. V. Subbareddy and D. S. Mehta, "Beads," *Oral Surgery Oral Medicine and Oral Pathology*, vol. 69, no. 6, pp. 769–770, 1990.

[11] E. Cataldo, "Unusual foreign objects in pulp canals," *Oral Surgery, Oral Medicine, Oral Pathology*, vol. 42, no. 6, p. 851, 1976.

[12] A. Rao and P. Sudha, "A case of stapler pin in the root canal—extending beyond the apex," *Indian Journal of Dental Research*, vol. 10, no. 3, pp. 104–107, 1999.

[13] U. M. Nadkarni, A. Munshi, S. G. Damle, and R. R. Kalaskar, "Retrieval of a foreign object from the palatal root canal of a permanent maxillary first molar: a case report," *Quintessence International*, vol. 33, no. 8, pp. 609–612, 2002.

[14] A. R. Prabhakar, N. Basappa, and O. S. Raju, "Foreign body in a mandibular permanent molar—a case report," *Journal of the Indian Society of Pedodontics and Preventive Dentistry*, vol. 16, no. 4, pp. 120–121, 1998.

[15] R. Aduri, R. E. Reddy, and K. Kiran, "Foreign objects in teeth: retrieval and management," *Journal of Indian Society of Pedodontics and Preventive Dentistry*, vol. 27, no. 3, pp. 179–183, 2009.

[16] N. Mcauliffe, N. A. Drage, and B. Hunter, "Staple diet: a foreign body in a tooth," *International Journal of Paediatric Dentistry*, vol. 15, no. 6, pp. 468–471, 2005.

36

Gingival Enlargement Induced by Felodipine Resolves with a Conventional Periodontal Treatment and Drug Modification

Nabil Khzam,[1] David Bailey,[1] Helen S. Yie,[2] and Mahmoud M. Bakr[3]

[1]DB Dental, Corner Tydeman & Pensioner Guard Roads, Perth, WA 6159, Australia
[2]Irwin Dental Centre, Irwin Barracks, Perth, WA 6010, Australia
[3]General Dental Practice, School of Dentistry and Oral Health, Griffith University, Gold Coast, QLD 4222, Australia

Correspondence should be addressed to Mahmoud M. Bakr; m.bakr@griffith.edu.au

Academic Editor: Ronald S. Brown

We present a case of a 47-year-old male who suffered from GE around his lower anterior teeth as soon as he started treatment with Felodipine 400 mg. We show that oral hygiene measures, antibiotics, and conventional periodontal treatment (scaling and root planing SRP) were all not sufficient to resolve the drug induced GE, which will persist and/or recur provided that systemic effect of the offending medication is still present. The condition immediately resolved after switching to a different medication. The mechanism of GE is complex and not fully understood yet. It is mainly due to overexpression of a number of growth factors due to high concentrations of calcium ions (Ca^{2+}). This affects fibroblasts proliferation and DNA synthesis and leads to a heavy chronic inflammatory cell infiltrate. Our case was managed according to the suggested protocols in previous case studies. The unique features in our case were the immediate onset of the adverse effect after starting the medication and the absence of any underlying medical condition apart from high blood pressure. Improving the oral hygiene together with SRP and cessation of the medication resolves drug induced GE.

1. Introduction

Different medications can cause a number of adverse reactions in the oral cavity including but not limited to oral ulceration, xerostomia, lichenoid reactions, oral pigmentations, burning mouth syndrome, tooth discoloration, and gingival hyperplasia [1]. Gingival enlargement (GE), also known as gingival overgrowth or hyperplasia, has a multifactorial aetiology including inflammation, neoplastic conditions, systemic disorders, and medications [2]. Drugs associated with GE can be grouped into anticonvulsant drugs (phenytoin) [3–5], potent immunosuppressants (cyclosporin) [6–8], and specific antihypertensive drugs (calcium channel blockers) [9–16].

The aetiology for GE is not fully understood. However, there has been a different correlation to different inflammatory and noninflammatory pathways. Individual's reaction or sensitivity towards a metabolic pathway could be a contributing factor as well [17]. Other nutritional and/or environmental factors may also play a role [18]. Untreated hyperplastic gingival tissue may lead to aesthetic, functional, and periodontal drawbacks and difficulties that affect the patient's well-being and may lead to an increased treatment cost on the long run [19].

Different studies aimed to investigate the possible factors contributing to drug induced GE. A study performed on patients receiving Phenytoin showed that the expression of some growth factors including Transforming Growth Factor (TGF-β1) and Platelet Derived Growth Factor (PDGF-BB) was significantly higher in GE areas when compared to nonenlarged gingival sites in the same patient and control patients not receiving Phenytoin [20]. Combinations of different drugs were also investigated and it was reported that these combinations increase the incidence and severity of GE [21]. A notorious combination is Cyclosporin and Nifedipine as the later could counteract the former's side effects of nephrotoxicity and hypertension [22]. It was proven that the above-mentioned combination increases the prevalence and intensity of GE when compared to using Cyclosporin with Amlodipine or Cyclosporin alone [23]. Furthermore,

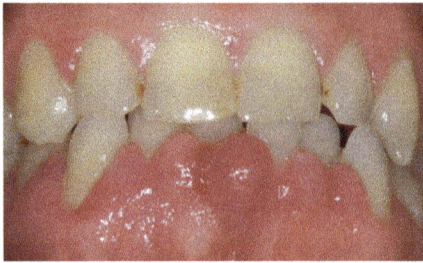

FIGURE 1: A photo showing the initial presentation of the GE associated with all lower anterior teeth.

prevalence of Amlodipine induced GE is as low as 1.3% [24].

2. Case Presentation

A 47-year-old male initially presented to a General Dentist for a regular dental check-up, where his enlarged gingiva was noted. On examination, there was gingival hyperplasia and pocketing of 5 mm (Figure 1). The patient was in pain and reported that the swelling started few days after a new antihypertensive medication (Felodipine) was prescribed. This was the first time ever the patient has had this kind of reaction to any medication as well as being the first time the patient experiences any gingival swellings. There was no pain associated with the swelling initially, but due to minimal trauma the pain started; small amount of bleeding was associated with the trauma.

A review of the patient's medical history revealed nothing significant other than high blood pressure (160/95) and family history of hypertension (father). A review of patient's medications showed that two months before presenting to the General Dentist, the patient was placed on Telmisartan 80 mg (Micardis) 28 tablets 1 tab daily and Felodipine (Plendil) 10 mg 30 tablets take 1 tab daily. A review of oral hygiene measures revealed the use of manual toothbrush twice daily but no flossing. Patient's oral hygiene was poor. Patient is a regular attender to dental appointment once a year for check-ups and cleans.

The General Dentist performed a deep scale and clean, removed some of the gingival tissue that is constantly being traumatized due to the swelling and prescribed Metronidazole 400 mg tid for a week, Panadeine Forte (Paracetamol 500 mg + Codeine Phosphate 30 mg), Ibuprofen 400 mg, and Savacol mouthwash (2 mg/mL Chlorhexidine Gluconate). There was no improvement in the gingival swelling despite the above treatment. However, the pain decreased.

The patient was referred to a specialist periodontist. A full comprehensive examination was done and revealed a periodontal diagnosis of mild to moderate generalized Chronic Periodontitis modified by poor oral hygiene and plaque induced GE affecting lower anterior teeth. The proposed treatment plan was patient education, oral hygiene instructions, SRP, surgical removal of the GE, the removed tissue to be submitted for a biopsy, reevaluation of periodontal tissue conditions in 3 months after completion of

the treatment and supportive periodontal treatment. Upper and lower Jaw debridement under local anaesthesia and an excisional biopsy including all labial GE around the lower anterior teeth were performed by the specialist periodontist. Communications to the patient's general practitioner regards the potential side effects of the antihypertensive medication and the possible correlations with the GE. The patient's general practitioner changed the antihypertensive medications to Coversyl (Perindopril) 30 tablets 10 mg 1 tab daily and Felodipine (Plendil) 10 mg 30 tablets take 1 tab daily.

Biopsy results showed the diagnosis was Fibrous Epulis with osseous metaplasia (Figure 2). In the first review appointment, the labial GE was still present. However, the degree of inflammation decreased (Figure 3). The overall oral hygiene of the patient was reasonable. Patient was scheduled for a second review in three months. Concerns were raised that Felodipine might be the cause of GE. Another communication to the patient's general practitioner resulted in changing his medication to Telmisartan 80 mg (Micardis) 28 tablets 1 tab daily and Moxonidine 400 mg (Physiotens) 30 tablets 1 tab daily.

The specialist periodontist contacted the patient, who reported disappearance of the GE immediately after cessation of Felodipine. In the second review appointment, there was a significant reduction in GE (Figure 4). A panoramic X-ray (OPG) was taken to be used as a base line to monitor the bone levels after regression of GE. The OPG showed mild to moderate horizontal bone around the lower anterior teeth (Figure 5). The importance of attending regular recall appointments in order to maintain the periodontal health of all teeth and specifically the lower anterior teeth was highly stressed.

3. Discussion

The response of gingival fibroblasts to calcium channel blockers has been investigated and mainly attributed to several mechanisms including high intracellular free Ca^{2+} concentration which results in cellular responses that affects growth factors, cell cycle regulators, cell proliferation, DNA, and collagen synthesis as well as intracellular cell talk [25]. Several therapeutic treatments were investigated in order to deplete the intracellular storage of Ca^{2+} including Tenidap and showed a degree of success on human cultured gingival fibroblasts [25].

Felodipine is an extended-release (ER) formula used to avoid the need for multiple daily doses and minimize side effects. When comparing the adverse effects Felodipine against those of other calcium channel blockers such as Nifedipine, a greater number of patients suffer from ankle oedema, nausea, and headache after receiving treatment with the former medication for mild to moderate hypertension [26]. This difference may be due to the different pharmacokinetic profiles of these two dihydropyridines; that is, with Felodipine ER the acute vasodilatory side effects are thought to be related to a rapid onset of action, high peak plasma concentrations, and large peak-trough concentration ratios. Such kinetic properties cause reflex sympathetic activation leading to the previously mentioned side effects [27]. We

(a)

(b)   (c)

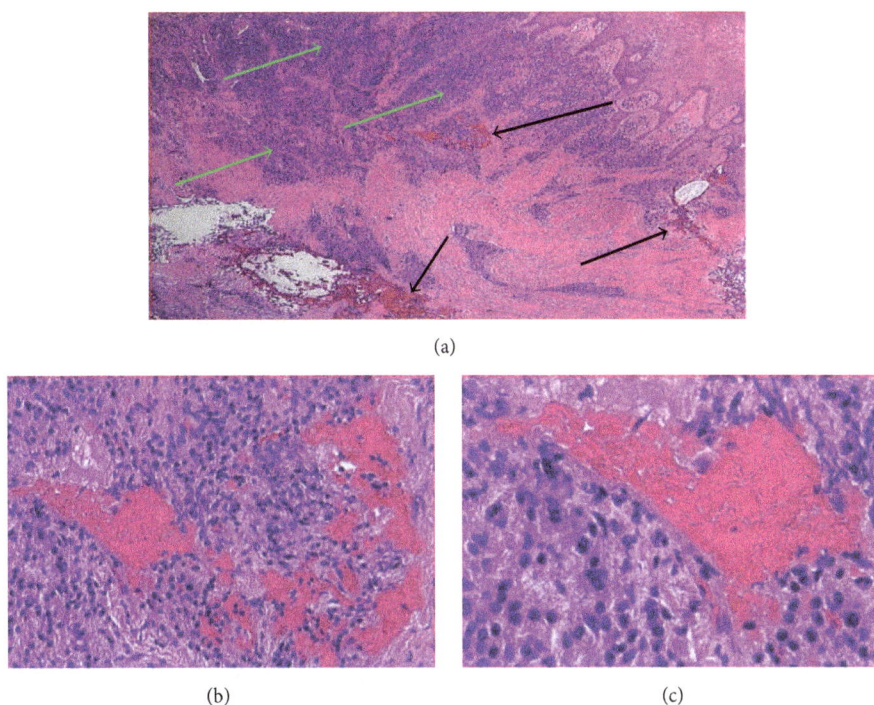

FIGURE 2: A photo showing the histopathological picture of the GE. (a) Showing heavy inflammatory cell infiltrate (green arrows) and osseous metaplasia (black arrows), H&E x2. (b) Showing a higher magnification of some areas of osseous metaplasia, H&E x20. (c) Showing an area of osseous metaplasia surrounded by chronic inflammatory cells, H&E x40.

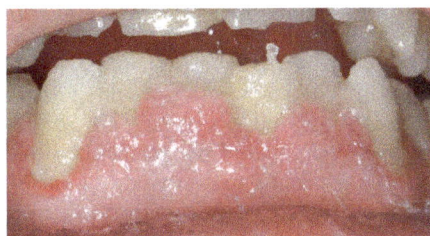

FIGURE 3: A photo showing the persistence of GE after the initial periodontal treatment. The inflammation decreased slightly. Oral hygiene improved after the initial treatment.

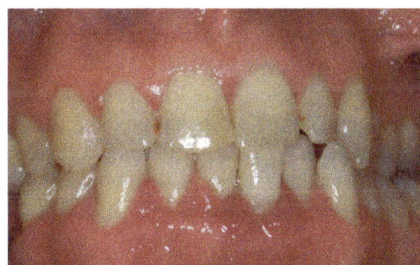

FIGURE 4: Showing disappearance of the GE and improvement of the overall periodontal condition after cessation of Felodipine together with strict oral hygiene measures.

believe that the GE could be attributed to the same above-mentioned pharmacological properties and mechanism.

Our histological findings were identical to another case report related to GE induced by Nifedipine. In both cases there was a heavy infiltration with chronic inflammatory cells and fibroblast proliferation [28, 29] which indicates a common mechanism is shared between both types of anti-hypertensive drugs regardless of their class and/or longevity of action. In addition to the above, there were osseous metaplasia and separate islands of bone seen in the deeper layers of gingival tissues. This can be explained by the presence of an underlying periodontal problem that adds to the adverse effects of the medication. Therefore, there is a high possibility that the lesion might reoccur if the plaque induced causative factor is not removed through conventional periodontal treatment.

In a previous case report of GE induced by Felodipine, it was shown that stopping the medication led to complete resolution of the gingival condition without any clinical intervention such as SRP or home care and oral hygiene measures [2]. It should be noted that in the above-mentioned case report the patient had an uncontrolled type II diabetes mellitus. In our case report, the patient was medically fit (apart from hypertension) and had no underlying medical problems that could have contributed to the GE other than the antihypertensive medication. In both cases no surgical interventions were needed to eliminate the GE permanently.

GE induced by calcium channel blockers does not require treatment with antibiotics as it is not a result of bacterial infection. This is in contrast with cases related to Cyclosporine-A where adjunctive treatment with Roxithromycin together

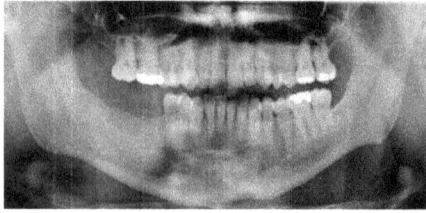

FIGURE 5: An orthopantograph (OPG) showing mild to moderate bone loss around lower anterior teeth, which compromises the long term prognosis of these teeth and mandates strict oral hygiene measures and careful and regular monitoring.

with SRP decreased levels of Transforming Growth Factor (TGF-β1) in gingival crevicular fluid, which improved the state of gingival tissue in immunocompromised patients [30]. We believe that the underlying suppressed immune system of patients on Cyclosporine-A justifies the need for supportive antibiotic therapy to enhance treatment outcomes.

With regard to the long term response to treatment in cases of GE, a recent study monitored patients with calcium channel blockers induced GE for 11 years and showed that 47.2% of patients suffered from recurrence of the GE during supportive periodontal therapy. In addition to that the long term tooth loss was higher in patients receiving calcium channel blockers [31]. Finally, replacement or withdrawal of the calcium channel blockers resulted in improvement of the GE; however, the condition did not heal completely, which indicates that there is an element of permanent damage that occurs after the use of these medications. The question of whether the oral hygiene status affects the long term prognosis is still debatable. Therefore, continuous follow-up is essential for our case in order to shed some light on the factors that influence a successful treatment outcome.

The key factors in our case management were drug substitution together with plaque control. This is in agreement with another case related to Amlodipine in a geriatric patient and the same treatment protocol was followed successfully [32]. Our biopsy results showed increased inflammatory cells infiltrate which is a very common well-documented feature of GE. Some authors even believe that the term gingival hyperplasia is not accurate as the GE does not result from an overproduction of cells. Instead it is a consequence of increased extracellular fluid due to chronic inflammatory cell infiltrate especially B-lymphocytes [33].

Recently, a universal hypothesis related to the mechanism of all drug categories that induce GE was suggested. Decreased cation influx of folic acid active transport within gingival fibroblasts leads to decreased cellular folate uptake, which in turn leads to changes in matrix metalloproteinases metabolism and the failure to activate collagenase. Decreased availability of activated collagenase results in decreased degradation of accumulated connective tissue which leads to GE [34]. Despite the fact that a universal theory for pathogenesis of drug induced GE could be accepted, the presentation of cases shows great variations. A classic case usually involves a high dose of the medication that has been used for at least 3–6 months. In our case the GE started

immediately after using Felodipine. In another case, GE was evident even with a small dose (5 mg) of Amlodipine [35].

Cessation of the offending drug and its replacement with a different one are a crucial step in management of drug induced GE. Even switching to another medication of the same therapeutic class can lead to a remarkable improvement [36]. Similarly switching Cyclosporin A to Tacrolimus in organ transplant patients resulted in control of GE [37]. In our case, switching the medication from Felodipine to Moxonidine (imidazoline$_1$ agonist) resulted in an immediate regression of the GE. Moxonidine exerts its blood pressure-lowering effect through stimulation of imidazoline type 1 (I$_1$) receptors in the cardiovascular regulatory centres of the medulla oblongata [38]. Up to the authors' knowledge, cases of GE associated with Moxonidine have not been reported. However, dry mouth (xerostomia) is a known side effect of this medication [39]. Therefore, this should be taken into consideration while planning for our patient's ongoing periodontal care. Regular follow-up appointments and maintaining periodontal health are important for the long term successful management of drug induced GE cases [40].

Furthermore, Moxonidine has an inhibitory effect on the sympathetic nervous system. Therefore, it produces an antihypertensive effect that is equivalent or superior to other classes of antihypertensive medications (including Felodipine) that act centrally on the nervous. In addition to the above, Moxonidine showed to have a better tolerance profile with less incidence of the most common side effects [41]. Of particular interest to our case, Moxonidine was reported to have an anti-inflammatory effect that is secondary to the decrease in the sympathetic system activity [42]. This potential anti-inflammatory effect would have a positive effect in counteracting any preexisting GE conditions and would explain the absence of documented cases of GE in conjunction with Moxonidine treatment.

Our case is unique as there was an immediate response to the change in medication within days. This is in contrast to other GE cases where regression of GE takes longer periods up to six months [19, 33]. The osseous metaplasia in the histopathological picture in our case was not previously documented. It is attributed to the presence of an existing periodontal condition that affects bone turnover. The bony islands are associated with the inflammatory GE condition and are expected to disappear after regression of GE and control of the periodontal condition. We endeavour to follow-up on this case and report any cases of recurrence of GE.

Conflict of Interests

The authors declare that there is no conflict of interests regarding the publication of this paper.

References

[1] M. Abdollahi and M. Radfar, "A review of drug induced oral reactions," *Journal of Contemporary Dental Practice*, vol. 4, no. 1, pp. 10–31, 2003.

[2] A. A. Fay, K. Satheesh, and R. Gapski, "Felodipine-influenced gingival enlargement in an uncontrolled type 2 diabetic patient," *Journal of Periodontology*, vol. 76, no. 7, pp. 1217–1222, 2005.

[3] T. M. Hassell and G. H. Gilbert, "Phenytoin sensitivity of fibroblasts as the basis for susceptibility to gingival enlargement," *The American Journal of Pathology*, vol. 112, no. 2, pp. 218–223, 1983.

[4] I. Casetta, E. Granieri, M. Desiderá et al., "Phenytoin-induced gingival overgrowth: a community-based cross-sectional study in Ferrara, Italy," *Neuroepidemiology*, vol. 16, no. 6, pp. 296–303, 1997.

[5] M. Brunsvold, J. Tomasovic, and D. Ruemping, "The measured effect of phenytoin withdrawal on gingival hyperplasia in children," *ASDC Journal of Dentistry for Children*, vol. 52, no. 6, pp. 417–421, 1985.

[6] E. M. Rateitschak-Pluss, A. Hefti, R. Lortscher, and G. Thiel, "Initial observation that cyclosporin-A induces gingival enlargement in man," *Journal of Clinical Periodontology*, vol. 10, no. 3, pp. 237–246, 1983.

[7] S. Pisanty, E. Rahamim, D. Ben-Ezra, and S. Shoshan, "Prolonged systemic administration of cyclosporin A affects gingival epithelium," *Journal of Periodontology*, vol. 61, no. 2, pp. 138–141, 1990.

[8] C. G. Daly, "Resolution of cyclosporin A (CsA)-induced gingival enlargement following reduction in CsA dosage," *Journal of Clinical Periodontology*, vol. 19, no. 2, pp. 143–145, 1992.

[9] S. Barak, I. S. Engelberg, and J. Hiss, "Gingival hyperplasia caused by nifedipine—histopathologic findings," *Journal of Periodontology*, vol. 58, no. 9, pp. 639–642, 1987.

[10] G. E. Romanos, C. Schroter-Kermani, N. Hinz, D. Herrmann, J. R. Strub, and J. P. Bernimoulin, "Extracellular matrix analysis of nifedipine-induced gingival overgrowth: immunohistochemical distribution of different collagen types as well as the glycoprotein flbronectin," *Journal of Periodontal Research*, vol. 28, no. 1, pp. 10–16, 1993.

[11] J. Miranda, L. Brunet, P. Roset, L. Berini, M. Farré, and C. Mendieta, "Prevalence and risk of gingival enlargement in patients treated with nifedipine," *Journal of Periodontology*, vol. 72, no. 5, pp. 605–611, 2001.

[12] H. E. Pernu, K. Oikarinen, J. Hietanen, and M. Knuuttila, "Verapamil-induced gingival overgrowth: a clinical, histologic, and biochemic approach," *Journal of Oral Pathology and Medicine*, vol. 18, no. 7, pp. 422–425, 1989.

[13] C. S. Miller and D. D. Damm, "Incidence of verapamil-induced gingival hyperplasia in a dental population," *Journal of Periodontology*, vol. 63, no. 5, pp. 453–456, 1992.

[14] A. V. Mehta, B. Chidambaram, and A. C. O'Riordan, "Verapamil-induced gingival hyperplasia in children," *American Heart Journal*, vol. 124, no. 2, pp. 535–536, 1992.

[15] S. Giustiniani, F. R. della Cuna, and M. Marieni, "Hyperplastic gingivitis during diltiazem therapy," *International Journal of Cardiology*, vol. 15, no. 2, pp. 247–249, 1987.

[16] L. Fattore, M. Stablein, G. Bredfeldt, T. Semla, M. Moran, and J. M. Doherty-Greenberg, "Gingival hyperplasia: a side effect of nifedipine and diltiazem," *Special Care in Dentistry*, vol. 11, no. 3, pp. 107–109, 1991.

[17] S. Tavassoli, N. Yamalik, F. Çağlayan, G. Çağlayan, and K. Eratalay, "The clinical effects of nifedipine on periodontal status," *Journal of Periodontology*, vol. 69, no. 2, pp. 108–112, 1998.

[18] L. M. Prisant and W. Herman, "Calcium channel blocker induced gingival overgrowth," *Journal of Clinical Hypertension*, vol. 4, no. 4, pp. 310–311, 2002.

[19] M. Sucu, M. Yuce, and V. Davutoglu, "Amlodipine-induced massive gingival hypertrophy," *Canadian Family Physician*, vol. 57, no. 4, pp. 436–437, 2011.

[20] L. Kuru, S. Yilmaz, B. Kuru, K. N. Köse, and Ü. Noyan, "Expression of growth factors in the gingival crevice fluid of patients with phenytoin-induced gingival enlargement," *Archives of Oral Biology*, vol. 49, no. 11, pp. 945–950, 2004.

[21] M. Varnfield and S. J. Botha, "Drug-induced gingival hyperplasia—a review," *SADJ*, vol. 55, no. 11, pp. 632–641, 2000.

[22] J. M. Thomason, R. A. Seymour, J. S. Ellis et al., "Iatrogenic gingival overgrowth in cardiac transplantation," *Journal of Periodontology*, vol. 66, no. 8, pp. 742–746, 1995.

[23] R. M. López-Pintor, G. Hernández, L. de Arriba, J. M. Morales, C. Jiménez, and A. de Andrés, "Amlodipine and nifedipine used with cyclosporine induce different effects on gingival enlargement," *Transplantation Proceedings*, vol. 41, no. 6, pp. 2351–2353, 2009.

[24] M. Ono, S. Tanaka, R. Takeuchi et al., "Prevalence of amlodipine-induced gingival overgrowth," *International Journal of Oral-Medical Sciences*, vol. 9, no. 2, pp. 96–100, 2010.

[25] H. Matsumoto, R. Takeuchi, M. Ono, Y. Akimoto, N. Kobayashi, and A. Fujii, "Drug-induced gingival overgrowth and its tentative pharmacotherapy," *Japanese Dental Science Review*, vol. 46, no. 1, pp. 11–16, 2010.

[26] J. P. Van Der Krogt, R. Brand, and E. C. Dawson, "Amlodipine versus extended-release felodipine in general practice: a randomized, parallel-group study in patients with mild-to-moderate hypertension," *Current Therapeutic Research—Clinical and Experimental*, vol. 57, no. 3, pp. 145–158, 1996.

[27] F. H. H. Leenen and D. L. Holliwell, "Antihypertensive effect of felodipine associated with persistent sympathetic activation and minimal regression of left ventricular hypertrophy," *The American Journal of Cardiology*, vol. 69, no. 6, pp. 639–645, 1992.

[28] E. E. van der Wall, D. B. Tuinzing, and J. Hes, "Gingival hyperplasia induced by nifedipine, an arterial vasodilating drug," *Oral Surgery, Oral Medicine, Oral Pathology*, vol. 60, no. 1, pp. 38–40, 1985.

[29] E. B. Nery, R. G. Edson, K. K. Lee, V. K. Pruthi, and J. Watson, "Prevalence of nifedipine-induced gingival hyperplasia," *Journal of Periodontology*, vol. 66, no. 7, pp. 572–578, 1995.

[30] Y. Gong, J. Lu, X. Ding, and Y. Yu, "Effect of adjunctive roxithromycin therapy on interleukin-1β, transforming growth factor-β1 and vascular endothelial growth factor in gingival crevicular fluid of cyclosporine A-treated patients with gingival overgrowth," *Journal of Periodontal Research*, vol. 49, no. 4, pp. 448–457, 2014.

[31] Ø. Fardal and H. Lygre, "Management of periodontal disease in patients using calcium channel blockers—gingival overgrowth, prescribed medications, treatment responses and added treatment costs," *Journal of Clinical Periodontology*, vol. 42, no. 7, pp. 640–646, 2015.

[32] R. Agnihotri, G. S. Bhat, and K. M. Bhat, "Amlodipine-induced gingival overgrowth: considerations in a geriatric patient," *Geriatrics and Gerontology International*, vol. 11, no. 3, pp. 365–368, 2011.

[33] V. Bhatia, A. Mittal, A. K. Parida, R. Talwar, and U. Kaul, "Amlodipine induced gingival hyperplasia: a rare entity," *International Journal of Cardiology*, vol. 122, no. 3, pp. e23–e24, 2007.

[34] R. S. Brown and P. R. Arany, "Mechanism of drug-induced gingival overgrowth revisited: a unifying hypothesis," *Oral Diseases*, vol. 21, no. 1, pp. e51–e61, 2015.

[35] S. Joshi and S. Bansal, "A rare case report of amlodipine-induced gingival enlargement and review of its pathogenesis," *Case Reports in Dentistry*, vol. 2013, Article ID 138248, 3 pages, 2013.

[36] P. Westbrook, E. M. Bednarczyk, M. Carlson, H. Sheehan, and N. F. Bissada, "Regression of nifedipine-induced gingival hyperplasia following switch to a same class calcium channel blocker, isradipine," *Journal of Periodontology*, vol. 68, no. 7, pp. 645–650, 1997.

[37] G. Hernández Vallejo, L. Arriba, M. C. Frías et al., "Conversion from Cyclosporin A to Tacrolimus as a non-surgical alternative to reduce gingival enlargement: a preliminary case series," *Journal of Periodontology*, vol. 74, no. 12, pp. 1816–1823, 2003.

[38] J. Waters, J. Ashford, B. Jäger, S. Wonnacott, and C. N. Verboom, "Use of moxonidine as initial therapy and in combination in the treatment of essential hypertension—results of the TOPIC (Trial Of Physiotens In Combination) Study," *Journal of Clinical and Basic Cardiology*, vol. 2, no. 2, pp. 219–224, 1999.

[39] P. Chrisp and D. Faulds, "Moxonidine: a review of its pharmacology, and therapeutic use in essential hypertension," *Drugs*, vol. 44, no. 6, pp. 993–1012, 1992.

[40] T. Ilgenli, G. Atilla, and H. Baylas, "Effectiveness of periodontal therapy in patients with drug-induced gingival overgrowth. Long-term results," *Journal of Periodontology*, vol. 70, no. 9, pp. 967–972, 1999.

[41] M. Schachter, "Moxonidine: a review of safety and tolerability after seven years of clinical experience," *Journal of Hypertension Supplement*, vol. 17, no. 3, pp. S37–S39, 1999.

[42] M. K. Pöyhönen-Alho, K. Manhem, P. Katzman et al., "Central sympatholytic therapy has anti-inflammatory properties in hypertensive postmenopausal women," *Journal of Hypertension*, vol. 26, no. 12, pp. 2445–2449, 2008.

37

Aesthetic Surgical Approach for Bone Dehiscence Treatment by Means of Single Implant and Interdental Tissue Regeneration

Giorgio Lombardo,[1] **Jacopo Pighi,**[1] **Giovanni Corrocher,**[1] **Anna Mascellaro,**[1] **Jeffrey Lehrberg,**[2] **Mauro Marincola,**[3] **and Pier Francesco Nocini**[1]

[1]*Clinic of Dentistry and Maxillofacial Surgery, University of Verona, Piazzale Ludovico Antonio Scuro 10, 37100 Verona, Italy*
[2]*Department of Biomaterials, Implant Dentistry Centre, 501 Arborway, Jamaica Plain, Boston, MA 02130, USA*
[3]*Universidad de Cartagena, Avenida del Consulado, Calle No. 30, No. 48-152, Cartagena, Bolívar, Colombia*

Correspondence should be addressed to Giorgio Lombardo; giorgio.lombardo@univr.it

Academic Editor: Adrian Kasaj

The replacement of single anterior teeth by means of endosseous implants implies the achievement of success in restoring both aesthetic and function. However, the presence of wide endoperiodontal lesions can lead to horizontal hard and soft tissues defects after tooth extraction, making it impossible to correctly place an implant in the compromised alveolar socket. Vertical augmentation procedures have been proposed to solve these clinical situations, but the amount of new regenerated bone is still not predictable. Furthermore, bone augmentation can be complicated by the presence of adjacent teeth, especially if they bring with them periodontal defects. Therefore, it is used to restore periodontal health of adjacent teeth before making any augmentation procedures and to wait a certain healing period before placing an implant in vertically augmented sites, otherwise risking to obtain a nonsatisfactory aesthetic result. All of these procedures, however, lead to an expansion of treatment time which should affect patient compliance. For this reason, this case report suggests a surgical technique to perform vertical bone augmentation at a single gap left by a central upper incisor while placing an implant and simultaneously to regenerate the periodontal attachment of an adjacent lateral incisor, without compromising the aesthetic result.

1. Introduction

Implant therapy was first introduced for the rehabilitation of completely edentulous jaws and has become today a viable option for the rehabilitation of partial and single edentulism [1]. In the anterior maxilla, a successful implant procedure requires not only well-anchored implants, but also natural looking result. The only way to gain this result is to correctly place implants in all the three dimensions of bone (i.e., apicocoronal, faciolingual, and mesiodistal) [2]. Unfortunately, this cannot always be achieved with dental implants due to the presence of alveolar defects. Several clinical and histologic studies have shown the dynamic resorptive process that unfolds after tooth extraction [3]. When the alveolar site presents deficiencies, many techniques can be used for its development. Vertical ridge augmentation has shown to be effective with several techniques, such as onlay autografts or particulate autogenous and xenogeneic bone covered by nonresorbable membranes [4–6]. Paramount to the success of vertical ridge augmentation are five crucial factors: biocompatibility, cell occlusion, space-provision, tissue integration, and ease of use [7].

Most of the published studies report on the outcomes of augmentation procedures in completely edentulous areas. The surgical management of edentulous ridges involves a simpler management of soft tissues in order to obtain a primary wound closure and reduce the risk of bacterial contamination. Alternatively, the presence of teeth in close proximity to the atrophic alveolar ridge can affect the procedure, in particular when teeth present periodontal

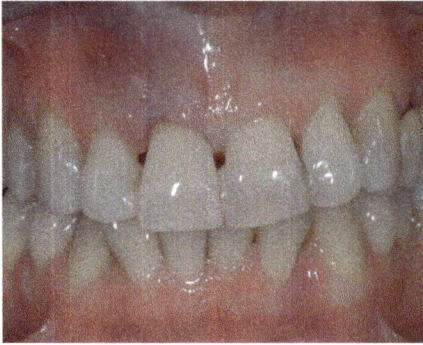

FIGURE 1: Front side view of patient upon presentation.

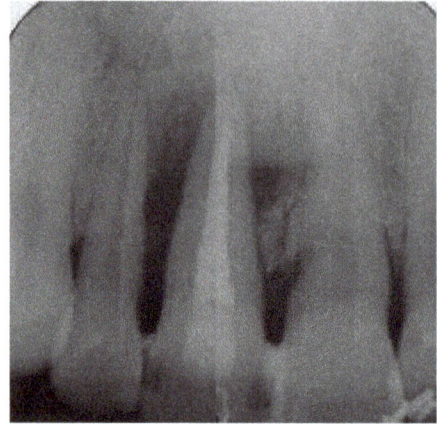

FIGURE 2: Intraoral periapical radiograph showing bone loss around the right central incisor and involving the mesial alveolar wall of the right lateral incisor.

morbidity [8]. The presence of horizontal defects on implant adjacent teeth limits the possibility of interproximal soft tissue overgrowth between teeth and implants, leading to the need to regenerate the lost periodontal attachment. While ridge augmentation has proven to be effective and predictable, supra-alveolar periodontal regeneration has not yet been demonstrated. Therefore, in clinical practice, periodontal regeneration should precede alveolar augmentation and implant placement. Furthermore, although vertical bone regeneration should occur, it is impossible to predict the amount of resorption of the grafted material, thus leading to the risk of finding part of the implant surface exposed after a certain period of time, if bone augmentation and implant placement are performed simultaneously.

Few reports can be found concerning the feasibility of regenerating a lost periodontal attachment around a tooth, while at the same time performing a vertical ridge augmentation to allow for the delayed placement of an implant [9].

The case report presented here illustrates a technique to regenerate the lost periodontal attachment, improve bone volumes, and allow the simultaneous placement of an implant in the adjacent edentulous alveolar ridge in order to achieve a good aesthetic result in a short rehabilitation time.

2. Case Presentation

A 43-year-old woman was referred to us presenting a hopeless upper left central incisor, affected by a large endoperiodontal lesion involving the buccal wall of the alveolar crest and the mesial aspect of the neighboring lateral incisor (Figures 1 and 2). The patient accepted the proposal of extracting the tooth and to replace it with an implant. The extraction was performed with minimal trauma and the extraction socket was filled with absorbable hemostatic gelatin sponge (Spongostan™ Dental, Ethicon, Edinburgh, UK) (Figures 3 and 4). The root of the extracted tooth was cut out and the remaining crown was used as provisional pontic element until the implant would have been placed (Figures 5 and 6).

After six weeks of healing soft tissues were well conditioned by the provisional pontic (Figures 7(a) and 7(b)) but a large bone defect was radiographically noticed (Figure 8). A full thickness flap was raised at the edentulous ridge and was continued on the palatal side with a partial thickness flap

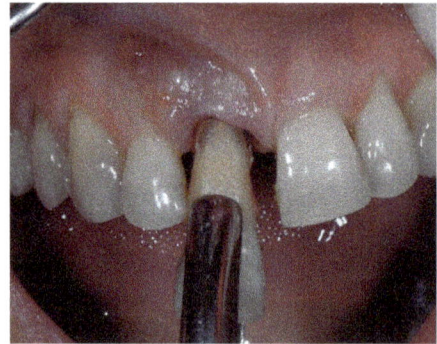

FIGURE 3: Plaque and calculus can be observed on the root surface at the time of extraction, performed with minimal trauma.

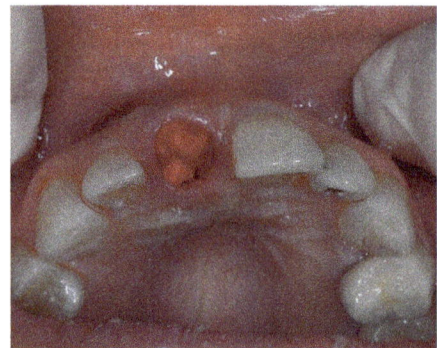

FIGURE 4: Occlusal view of the fresh alveolar socket after extraction and application of Spongostan™.

till the last molar (Figure 9), from where a free connective tissue graft was harvested (Figure 10). The alveolar defect was degranulated and the root surfaces of the adjacent elements were decontaminated using ultrasonic tips and then polished with low abrasive burs (Intensiv Perio Set®, Intensiv SA, Montagnola, Switzerland). After that a 5.0 × 8.0 mm, plateau

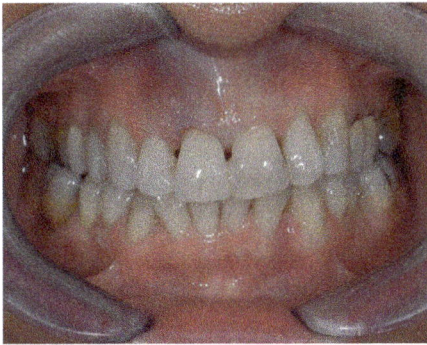

FIGURE 5: The crown of the extracted tooth was splinted to the adjacent elements and used as provisional pontic.

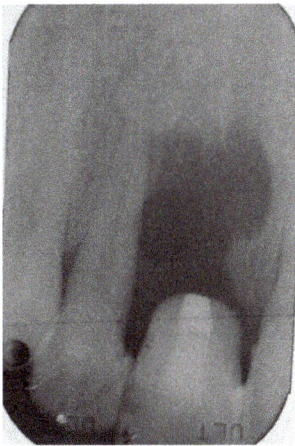

FIGURE 6: Postoperative X-ray after tooth extraction.

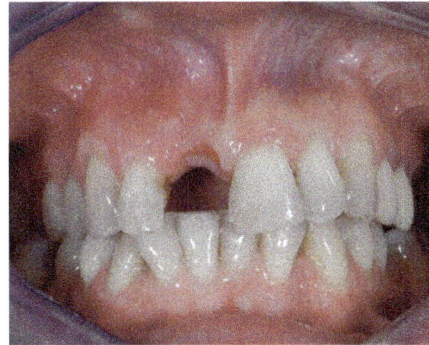

(a)

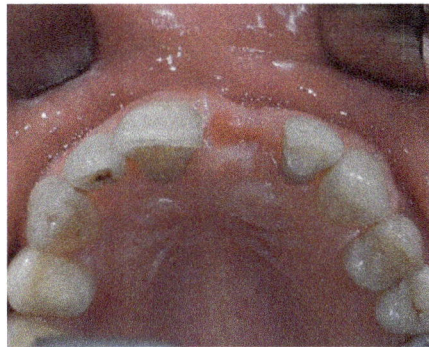

(b)

FIGURE 7: Frontal (a) and occlusal (b) views after six weeks of healing.

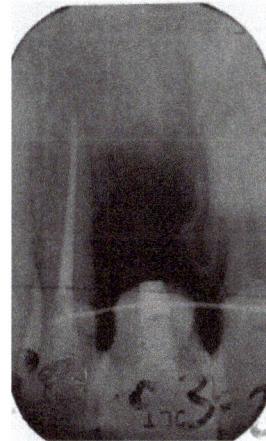

FIGURE 8: The radiograph taken before implant insertion shows a complete loss of the buccal and palatal bone.

design, locking-taper implant (Bicon LLC, Boston, MA) was placed under the buccal margin of the bone dehiscence (Figure 11). To maintain a proper bone and mucosal tunnel, a stealth abutment was modified on its top and then connected to the implant (Figures 12(a) and 12(b)), and in the meantime the connective graft was fixed to the buccal flap.

Following implant placement, the connective tissue graft was fixed to the buccal flap, and the compromised root surface of the lateral incisor was treated with a regenerative approach, using enamel matrix derivatives (Emdogain®, Straumann, Basel, Switzerland) (Figures 13(a) and 13(b)). A bovine xenograft material (Bio-Oss Collagen®, Geistlich Pharma, AG, Wolhusen, Switzerland) was grafted around facial and buccal aspects till the top of the implants abutment (Figure 14). The connective tissue graft was used as a membrane, over which the buccal flap was advanced and sutured to obtain a primary wound closure without tension (Figures 15(a) and 15(b)). After taking a postoperative radiograph (Figure 16), the provisional pontic was placed again and the patient was suggested to take oral antibiotics (Augmentin®, GlaxoSmithKline, UK) and to rinse the mouth twice a day using 0.2% chlorhexidine mouthrinse. Postoperative controls, during which professional oral hygiene was always performed, were made at one and two weeks and then once a month for four months. After four months, the implant and the grafting material appeared well integrated (Figures 17 and 18), so a small circular incision was made to allow for the removal of the customized abutment (Figures 19(a) and 19(b)), and a provisional integrated abutment crown was connected (Figures 20 and 21). To respect the new regenerated hard interproximal tissues, we chose an abutment with a long post (Figure 22). Six months after the

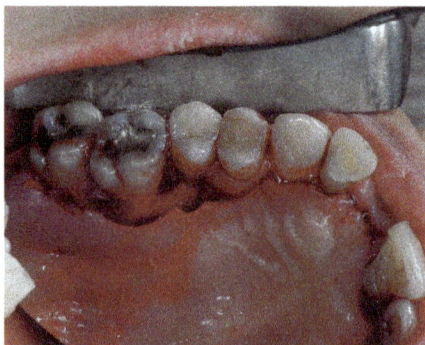

FIGURE 9: Occlusal view of the surgical incision at implant insertion time. A full thickness flap at the single gap continued with a partial thickness flap to harvest a connective tissue graft.

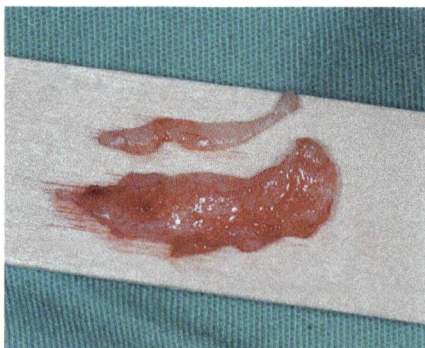

FIGURE 11: Surgical placement of the Bicon implant. The implant lies 1 mm below the margin of the buccal bone dehiscence.

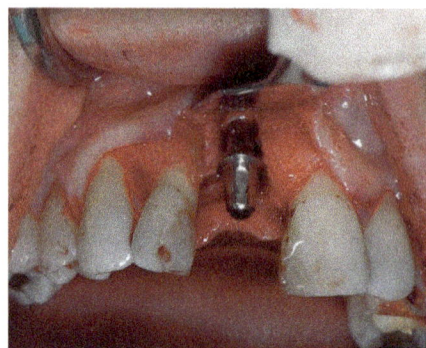

FIGURE 10: Aspect of the harvested connective tissue graft.

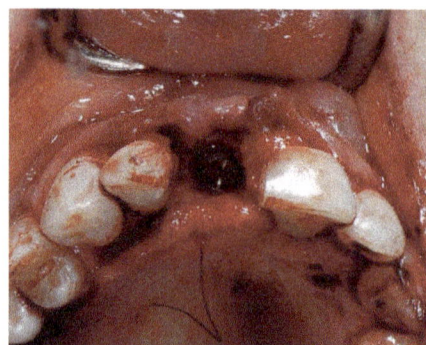

(a)

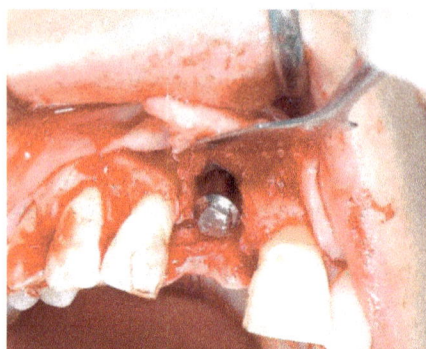

(b)

FIGURE 12: A stealth abutment was tested (a) and then modified on its top (b) to primarily close the wound maintaining a proper bone and mucosal tunnel.

contralateral incisors were endodontically treated and then reduced to abutment along with the right lateral incisor (Figure 23). Lateral/anterior protrusion of the definitive restorations was achieved using canine guidance: in this way, mutually protected occlusion prevented contact between incisors during all mandibular eccentric movements, and incisors came into contact with their antagonists only during maximum intercuspation. To orient the seating of the final abutment, a jig was fabricated and utilized to aid in correct positioning. A direct impression was then taken using a polyether impression material (Impregum Penta, 3MESPE, St. Paul, MN). A stone cast using type IV extra-hard dental stone was then prepared, from which the definitive abutment could be individually modified. Finally, four zirconia crowns were fabricated. The implant crown was cemented on the abutment using extraoral cement (RelyX Unicem, 3M ESPE, St. Paul, MN) (Figure 24). The abutment and crown were then tapped through the long axis of the post into the implant well using a 250 g mallet (Figures 25(a) and 25(b)). The other crowns were cemented on the natural abutments using a zinc phosphate definitive cement (Harvard Cement®, Harvard Dental International, Hoppegarten, Germany) (Figures 26–28).

3. Results

The patient returned to our observation after five years of prosthetic loading. The clinical follow-up examination revealed a satisfying aesthetic result, with adequate contours of peri-implant soft tissues and an almost complete filling of interproximal spaces (Figure 29). The periapical radiograph obtained showed the implant completely integrated in native bone, while new bone was visible around the implant abutment until the margins of the ceramic crowns (Figure 30).

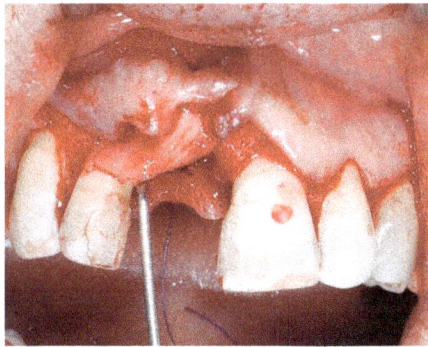

(a)

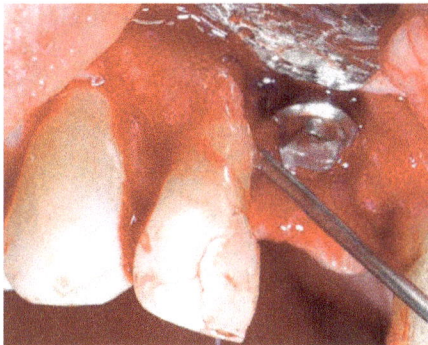

(b)

FIGURE 13: After fixation of the connective tissue graft to the buccal flap (a), Emdogain® was applied on the lateral incisor root surface to regenerate the lost periodontal attachment (b).

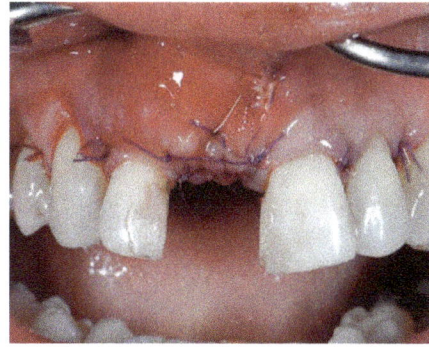

(a)

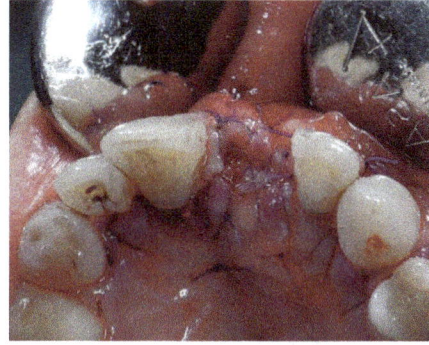

(b)

FIGURE 15: Frontal (a) and occlusal (b) view at the end of the surgical intervention.

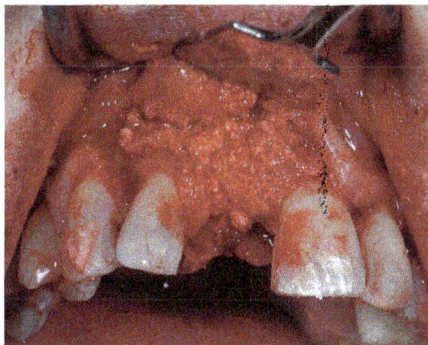

FIGURE 14: Bio-Oss® was applied to cover the defect around the implant.

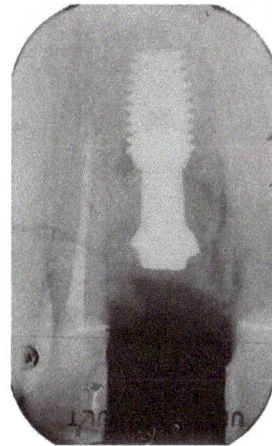

FIGURE 16: Postoperative X-ray shows fulfilling of the defect, with the implant lying in native bone below the grafted material.

The peri-implant tissues surrounding the implant were found to be in healthy conditions, free from any sign of inflammation and not bleeding after probing. Furthermore, the right lateral incisor presented probing depths below 5 mm, without bleeding after probing.

The patient concluded that she was fully satisfied with both the aesthetic and functional results of the procedure.

4. Discussion

In the present case report, the regeneration of a horizontal periodontal defect was achieved while simultaneously placing an implant and performing a vertical ridge augmentation. Success of periodontal regeneration usually depends on the initial probing depth in relation to the amount of the intrabony/vertical component [10]. In general, effectiveness

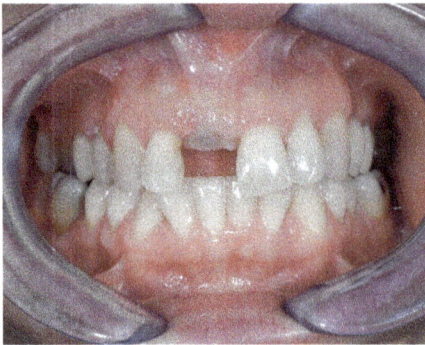

FIGURE 17: Frontal view following provisional pontic removal, after four months of healing.

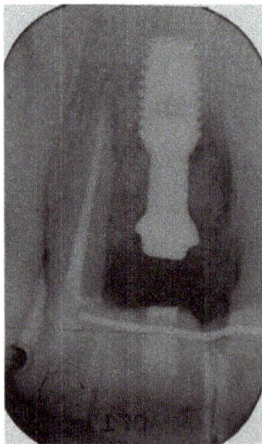

FIGURE 18: Radiograph at four months of healing showing good integration of the implant and the grafted material.

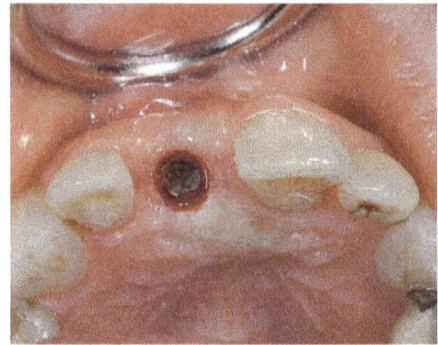

(a)

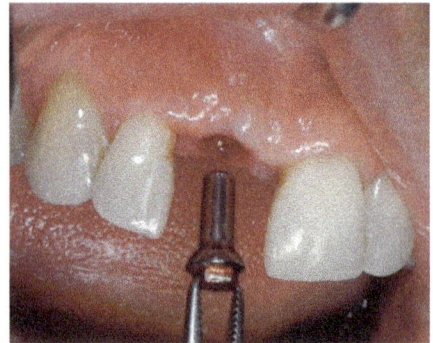

(b)

FIGURE 19: After performing a circular incision (a), the provisional stealth abutment was removed (b).

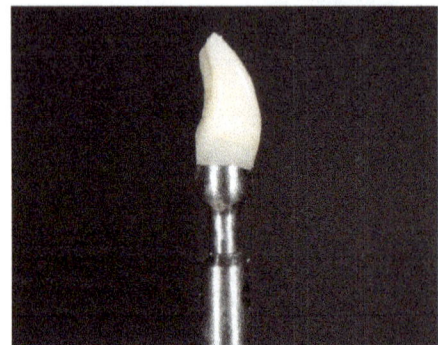

FIGURE 20: The provisional integrated abutment crown before fixation.

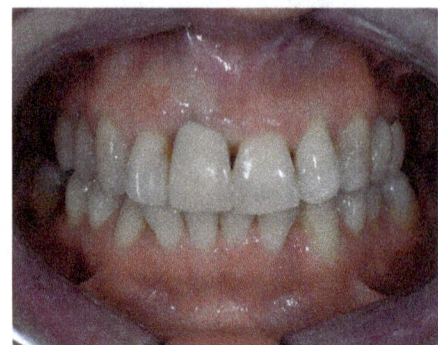

FIGURE 21: Frontal view after application of the provisional integrated abutment crown.

of enamel matrix derivatives in inducing periodontal regeneration of intrabony defects was proven to be almost equal if compared to guided tissue regeneration [11]. On the other hand, outcomes of regenerative therapy of periodontal supra-alveolar defects are known to be unpredictable, and there is little evidence to support such a procedure [4–6, 12]. In a recent animal trial, enamel matrix derivatives were combined with a scaffold material to obtain successful supracrestal bone regeneration around implants [13]. Also, with respect to vertical ridge augmentation, it is not possible to predict the amount of vertical bone gain; therefore, for both the procedures, we sought the use of a barrier able to provide stable space for tissue regeneration against the pressure made by the uppermost soft tissues and to avoid the migration of epithelial cells. Under this point of view, however, both nonresorbable and resorbable barriers have resulted in the same performance [14]. Despite this, a disadvantage of using nonresorbable barriers is that they need a second intervention for their removal. Membranes, however—particularly nonresorbable membranes—are susceptible to exposure during the healing-phase, leading to only a partial regeneration. Assuming that the placement of an implant occurred followed by membrane exposure, then the aesthetic

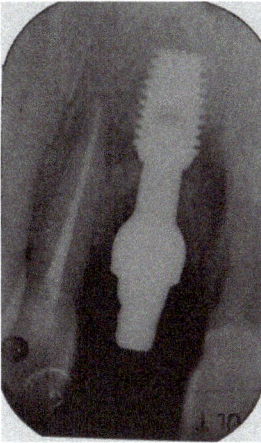

FIGURE 22: Radiograph showing the long abutment post, chosen to respect the bone and mucosal tunnel.

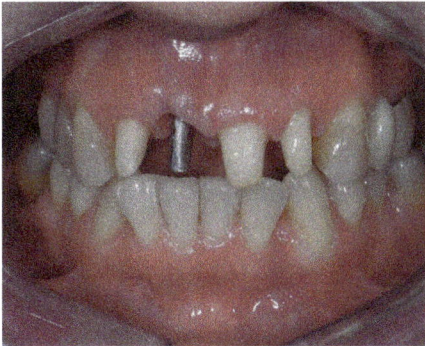

FIGURE 23: Frontal view before prostheses delivery. The implant abutment was tested before extraoral cementation of the crown.

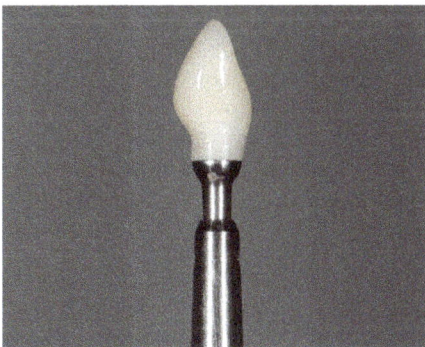

FIGURE 24: Aspect of the implant crown after extraoral cementation.

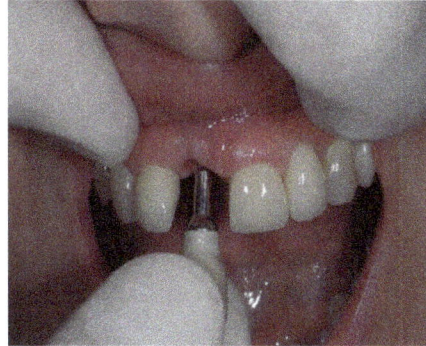

(a)

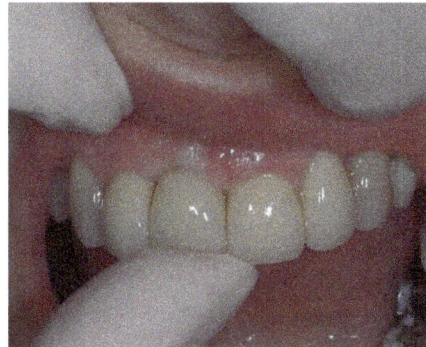

(b)

FIGURE 25: The abutment and crown were inserted through the long axis of the implant well (a) and then manually pressed (b) before tapping with mallet.

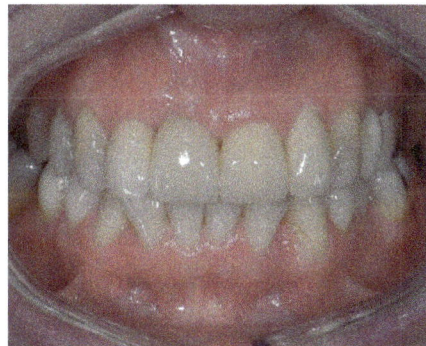

FIGURE 26: Frontal view after prostheses delivery.

appearance of soft tissues might be negatively affected, thus compromising the overall success of implant therapy in the anterior maxilla.

Tooth loss in aesthetic areas has a profoundly negative impact on the patient's social life, and attempts to reduce rehabilitation times were of primary concern; for this reason,

a simultaneous approach for periodontal regeneration, alveolar regeneration, and implant insertion was attempted.

Therefore, to reduce rehabilitation time, we forgo the use of membrane and we used a subepithelial free connective tissue graft to protect the underlying grafting material and to prop up peri-implant soft tissues. The use of free or pedicle soft tissue grafts to preserve gingival color and tissue characteristics is supported by the literature [15–17]. Moreover, connective tissue grafts have proven their capability of performing an effective barrier function [18–20].

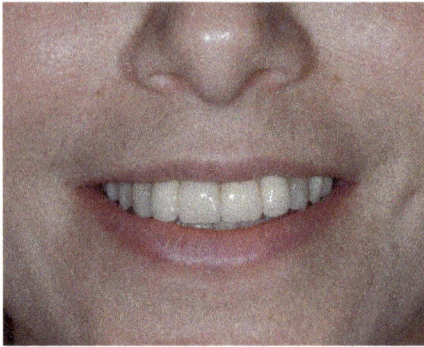

FIGURE 27: The patient's natural looking smile at the end of the therapy.

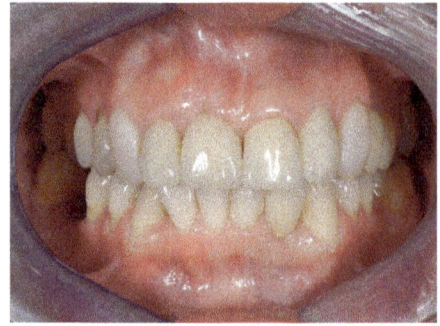

FIGURE 29: Frontal view showing the aesthetic result at the five-year follow-up examination.

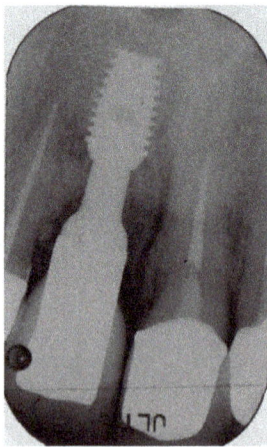

FIGURE 28: Control X-ray at the end of therapy.

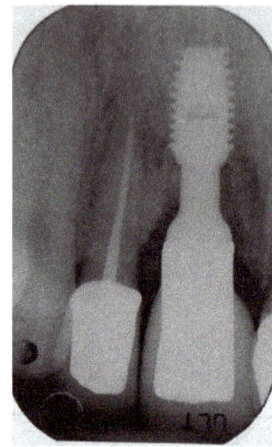

FIGURE 30: The radiograph performed after five years shows full integration of the implant and good stability of interproximal soft tissues, along with almost full filling of the lateral incisor's periodontal defect.

Vertical ridge augmentation was also performed due to the presence of the customized abutment connected to the implant at the time of its insertion, which maintained the space for grafting material preventing any possible collapse due to compression. As a result of the subcrestal placement and vertical ridge augmentation, the abutment post had to cross a long transmucosal tunnel to connect to the implant. Implant subcrestal placement should lead to further bone resorption in presence of microgaps located at the implant-abutment connection. However, the literature has shown that some locking-taper implant-abutment connections, like the one used in this study, are resistant to bacterial leakage [21, 22], and some studies have demonstrated minimal bone resorption around similar implants placed subcrestally [23, 24].

While the sloping shoulder design of the implant used provides space for interproximal bone regeneration, only histological analysis could distinguish the presence of new bone or simply a filled defect. Nevertheless, the absence of inflammation, along with radiological findings, indicates that the material is well integrated and does not induce a deleterious immunological response. Furthermore, the implant was placed in native bone immediately under the buccal ridge of the alveolar defect, in order to prevent

complications if graft resorption occurred. This means that the regenerated hard tissue served to give support to peri-implant soft tissues, to ensure their stability, and to improve the periodontal attachment of the lateral incisor. Finally, for the case shown here, a time period of five years has shown to be sufficient to permit the stability of peri-implant tissues using this aforementioned approach.

To the best of our knowledge, this is the first report concerning the simultaneous application of periodontal and alveolar regeneration at the implant surgery stage. Based on the positive aesthetic and functional results obtained with the subcrestal placement of a locking-taper connection implant in the anterior maxilla, we look forward to further investigate the efficacy of this treatment as a therapeutic approach.

Disclosure

Jeffrey Lehrberg, Ph.D. (JL), received research support from Bicon LLC (Boston, MA) and consults Bicon LLC on matters pertaining to scientific research. Jeffrey Lehrberg is not involved with any aspect of Bicon LLC sales, marketing, or equivalent business practices; furthermore, Jeffrey Lehrberg understands his obligation to share scientific results and materials with the scientific community, when appropriate and/or applicable. No manager, employee, or other agents associated with Bicon LLC have had any role in the current study's design, data collection methods, analysis, decision to publish, or preparation. At the time of the submission of the report, none of the other authors report any conflict of interests that might raise questions about sources of bias.

Conflict of Interests

Jeffrey Lehrberg is funded in part by Bicon LLC. The funder had no role in study design, data collection and analysis, decision to publish, or preparation of the paper. The authors declare that there is no conflict of interests regarding the publication of this paper.

References

[1] M. Esposito, M. G. Grusovin, M. Willings, P. Coulthard, and H. V. Worthington, "The effectiveness of immediate, early, and conventional loading of dental implants: a cochrane systematic review of randomized controlled clinical trials," *International Journal of Oral and Maxillofacial Implants*, vol. 22, no. 6, pp. 893–904, 2007.

[2] F. L. Higginbottom and T. G. Wilson Jr., "Three-dimensional templates for placement of root-form dental implants: a technical note," *International Journal of Oral and Maxillofacial Implants*, vol. 11, no. 6, pp. 787–793, 1996.

[3] M. G. Araújo, F. Sukekava, J. L. Wennström, and J. Lindhe, "Ridge alterations following implant placement in fresh extraction sockets: an experimental study in the dog," *Journal of Clinical Periodontology*, vol. 32, no. 6, pp. 645–652, 2005.

[4] Z. Artzi, D. Dayan, Y. Alpern, and C. E. Nemcovsky, "Vertical ridge augmentation using xenogenic material supported by a configured titanium mesh: clinicohistopathologic and histochemical study," *The International Journal of Oral & Maxillofacial Implants*, vol. 18, no. 3, pp. 440–446, 2003.

[5] L. Canullo, P. Trisi, and M. Simion, "Vertical ridge augmentation around implants using e-PTFE titanium-reinforced membrane and deproteinized bovine bone mineral (bio-oss): a case report," *International Journal of Periodontics and Restorative Dentistry*, vol. 26, no. 4, pp. 355–361, 2006.

[6] J. D. Kassolis and G. M. Bowers, "Supracrestal bone regeneration: a pilot study," *International Journal of Periodontics and Restorative Dentistry*, vol. 19, no. 2, pp. 131–139, 1999.

[7] T. V. Scantlebury, "1982–1992: a decade of technology development for guided tissue regeneration," *Journal of Periodontology*, vol. 64, no. 11, pp. 1129–1137, 1993.

[8] N. U. Zitzmann, P. Schärer, and C. P. Marinello, "Factors influencing the success of GBR. Smoking, timing of implant placement, implant location, bone quality and provisional restoration," *Journal of Clinical Periodontology*, vol. 26, no. 10, pp. 673–682, 1999.

[9] P. Windisch, D. Szendrói-Kiss, A. Horváth, Z. Suba, I. Gera, and A. Sculean, "Reconstructive periodontal therapy with simultaneous ridge augmentation. A clinical and histological case series report," *Clinical Oral Investigations*, vol. 12, no. 3, pp. 257–264, 2008.

[10] M. S. Tonetti, G. P. Prato, and P. Cortellini, "Factors affecting the healing response of intrabony defects following guided tissue regeneration and access flap surgery," *Journal of Clinical Periodontology*, vol. 23, no. 6, pp. 548–556, 1996.

[11] M. G. Grusovin and M. Esposito, "The efficacy of enamel matrix derivative (Emdogain) for the treatment of deep infrabony periodontal defects: a placebo-controlled randomised clinical trial," *European Journal of Oral Implantology*, vol. 2, no. 1, pp. 43–54, 2009.

[12] S. S. Stahl and S. Froum, "Human suprabony healing responses following root demineralization and coronal flap anchorage. Histologic responses in 7 sites," *Journal of Clinical Periodontology*, vol. 18, no. 9, pp. 685–689, 1991.

[13] B. Wen, Z. Li, R. Nie et al., "Influence of biphasic calcium phosphate surfaces coated with Enamel Matrix Derivative on vertical bone growth in an extra-oral rabbit model," *Clinical Oral Implants Research*, 2015.

[14] M. Merli, M. Moscatelli, G. Mariotti, R. Rotundo, F. Bernardelli, and M. Nieri, "Bone level variation after vertical ridge augmentation: resorbable barriers versus titanium-reinforced barriers. A 6-year double-blind randomized clinical trial," *The International Journal of Oral & Maxillofacial Implants*, vol. 29, no. 4, pp. 905–913, 2014.

[15] S. Yoshino, J. Y. K. Kan, K. Rungcharassaeng, P. Roe, and J. L. Lozada, "Effects of connective tissue grafting on the facial gingival level following single immediate implant placement and provisionalization in the esthetic zone: a 1-year randomized controlled prospective study," *The International Journal of Oral & Maxillofacial Implants*, vol. 29, no. 2, pp. 432–440, 2014.

[16] P. Adriaenssens, M. Hermans, A. Ingber, V. Prestipino, P. Daelemans, and C. Malevez, "Palatal sliding strip flap: soft tissue management to restore maxillary anterior esthetics at stage 2 surgery: a clinical report," *The International Journal of Oral & Maxillofacial Implants*, vol. 14, no. 1, pp. 30–36, 1999.

[17] C. E. Nemcovsky and O. Moses, "Rotated palatal flap. A surgical approach to increase keratinized tissue width in maxillary implant uncovering: technique and clinical evaluation," *International Journal of Periodontics and Restorative Dentistry*, vol. 22, no. 6, pp. 607–612, 2002.

[18] M. Santagata, L. Guariniello, R. V. E. Prisco, G. Tartaro, and S. D'Amato, "Use of subepithelial connective tissue graft as a biological barrier: a human clinical and histologic case report," *The Journal of Oral Implantology*, vol. 40, no. 4, pp. 465–468, 2014.

[19] U. Covani, S. Marconcini, G. Galassini, R. Cornelini, S. Santini, and A. Barone, "Connective tissue graft used as a biologic barrier to cover an immediate implant," *Journal of Periodontology*, vol. 78, no. 8, pp. 1644–1649, 2007.

[20] S. G. Jyothi, M. G. Triveni, D. S. Mehta, and K. Nandakumar, "Evaluation of single-tooth replacement by an immediate implant covered with connective tissue graft as a biologic barrier," *Journal of Indian Society of Periodontology*, vol. 17, no. 3, pp. 354–360, 2013.

[21] G. Sannino and A. Barlattani, "Mechanical evaluation of an implant-abutment self-locking taper connection: finite element analysis and experimental tests," *The International Journal of Oral & Maxillofacial Implants*, vol. 28, no. 1, pp. e17–e26, 2013.

[22] S. Pappalardo, I. Milazzo, G. Nicoletti et al., "Dental implants with locking taper connection versus screwed connection: microbiologic and scanning electron microscope study," *The International Journal of Immunopathology & Pharmacology*, vol. 20, no. 1, pp. 13–17, 2007.

[23] G. Lombardo, G. Corrocher, J. Pighi et al., "The impact of subcrestal placement on short locking-taper implants placed in posterior maxilla and mandible: a retrospective evaluation on hard and soft tissues stability after 2 years of loading," *Minerva Stomatologica*, vol. 63, no. 11-12, pp. 391–402, 2014.

[24] M. Fetner, A. Fetner, T. Koutouzis et al., "The effects of subcrestal implant placement on crestal bone levels and bone-to-abutment contact: a microcomputed tomographic and histologic study in dogs," *The International Journal of Oral & Maxillofacial Implants*, vol. 30, no. 5, pp. 1068–1075, 2015.

38

Fabrication of Customized Sectional Impression Trays in Management of Patients with Limited Mouth Opening

Vamsi Krishna CH, K. Mahendranadh Reddy, Nidhi Gupta, Y. Mahadev Shastry, N. Chandra Sekhar, Venkat Aditya, and G. V. K. Mohan Reddy

Department of Prosthodontics, Sri Sai College of Dental Surgery, Kothrepally, Vikarabad 501101, India

Correspondence should be addressed to Vamsi Krishna CH; chvk_guntur@yahoo.co.in

Academic Editors: I. El-Hakim and C. Ledesma-Montes

Impression making is not only important but is also the most significant step in the fabrication of any fixed or removable prosthesis. Proper impression making may be hindered by certain pathologic conditions. Reduced mouth opening is one of the common mechanical obstructions for proper orientation of the impression tray in the patient's mouth. In patients with trismus induced by submucous fibrosis, the procedure may be even more difficult to carry out because of reduced tissue resiliency and obliteration of vestibular spaces. Use of sectional trays offers one of the alternatives to overcome the problem of restricted mouth opening. Fabrication of customized impression trays according to the patient dentition improves the accuracy of impression making. The present case reports describe the fabrication of sectional custom trays designed for dentulous patients with chronic tobacco-induced submucous fibrosis.

1. Introduction

Reduced mouth opening poses a challenge and is often a daunting task for the operator to perform any intraoral procedures. Reportedly, this problem has been associated commonly with orofacial cancer surgeries, scleroderma, traumatic injuries, temporomandibular joint disorders, oral submucous fibrosis, and so forth. One of the most commonly observed pathologies associated with limited mouth opening is oral submucous fibrosis. Rajendran, in 1994 [1], reported and named this condition as "atrophia idiopathica (tropica) mucosae oris" involving oral mucosa, palate, and pillars of the fauces. Later, it was termed as oral sub mucous fibrosis. It is called by various synonyms like "diffuse oral sub mucous fibrosis," "idiopathic scleroderma of the mouth," "idiopathic palatal fibrosis," "sclerosing stomatitis," and "juxta-epithelial fibrosis" [2]. The characteristic finding observed in these patients is pale mucosa with loss of elasticity and resiliency. Formation of fibrous bands in sub mucous connective tissue was reported to be the root cause behind gradual reduction in mouth opening. Prosthetic intervention for these patients entails an accurate impression of the patient's mouth. Difficulties in impression making encountered due to reduced access to the oral cavity can be overcome by the use of sectional trays. Various types of sectional trays held together by different mechanisms have been designed and described in the literature. Present case reports describe simple and economic methods of fabrication of two-piece custom sectional trays for patients with oral sub mucous fibrosis.

2. Case Reports

45-year-old male patient and 31-year-old female patient, who were suffering from chronic oral sub mucous fibrosis, were reported to the department of prosthodontics (Sri Sai college of dental surgery, India) with a chief complaint of a missing teeth. On oral examination, maximum mouth opening was reported to be 2 cm and 2.4 cm, respectively, between incisal edges of maxillary and mandibular anteriors (Figure 1).

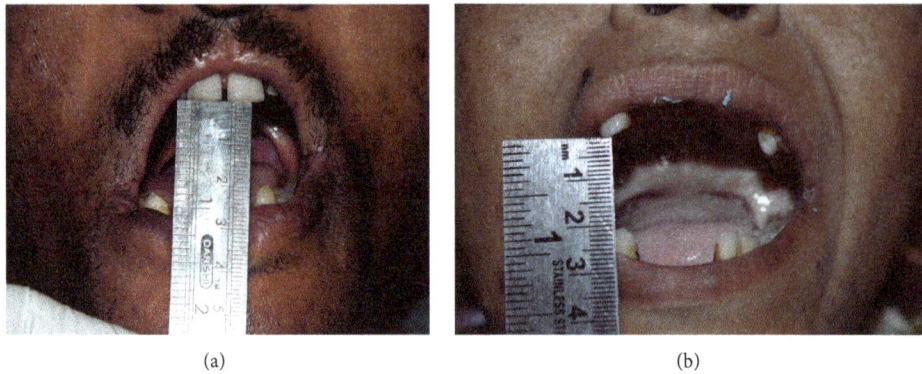

(a)   (b)

FIGURE 1: Maximum mouth openings.

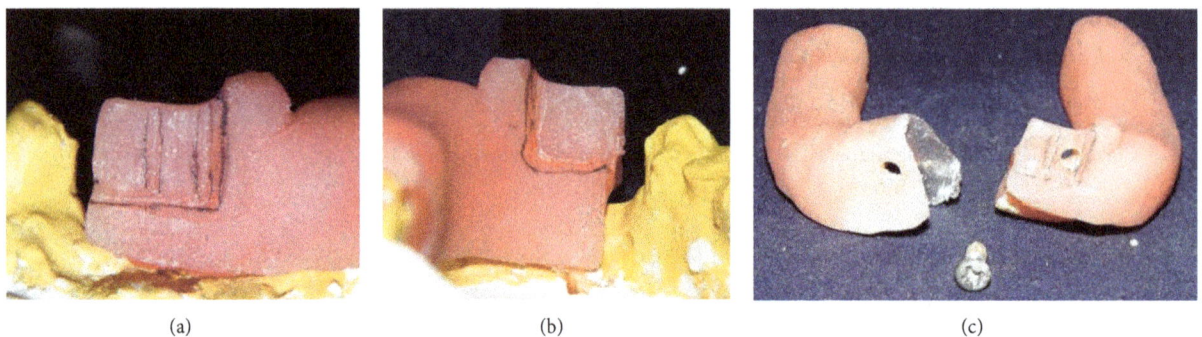

(a)   (b)   (c)

FIGURE 2: Fabrication technique for the sectional tray—Design 1.

Prognosis and probable prosthetic treatment options were explained to the patients, and informed consents were obtained.

Because of restricted size of oral orifice and severe intraoral fibrous bands, preliminary impressions were made with polyvinyl siloxane putty material. Flexible impression tray technique described by Whitsitt and Battle [3] was used to make preliminary impressions. The material was manipulated, rolled, and adapted on to the hard and soft tissues. Catalyst proportion was altered to reduce setting time to 1 min. Once the material had been set, the impression was folded and removed from the patient's mouth. The flexible impressions were stabilized using plaster and models obtained using pumice plaster method. Two-piece custom trays were designed and fabricated on the models.

2.1. Fabrication of Custom Trays

Design 1. The custom tray was designed making sure that the sections of the tray could be joined firmly and oriented accurately both in patient's mouth and after removal of the tray from the mouth. A 2 mm thick wax spacer was adapted with four occlusal stops. Autopolymerizing resin was mixed and adapted using finger adaptation dough method on one side on the cast crossing midline. After the material polymerized, tray section was removed, trimmed, and designed using an acrylic trimmer as shown in Figure 2. The orientation

grooves helped in three-dimensional stabilization of the tray. After designing the lock system for the first tray segment, a tin foil was adapted over that, and the second tray section was fabricated. After fabrication of the second segment, both the sections were approximated and secured using a screw. The screw helped in securing the tray segments together in a predetermined relationship (Figure 2).

Design 2. Fabrication of maxillary sectional tray was demonstrated here. After proper relief and block out, wax spacer was adapted on to the model. The first section of the tray was fabricated by adapting self-activated resin and incorporating female compartment of the press button on the center of the tray. Orientation lock was designed on the handle using acrylic trimmer as shown in Figure 3. After adapting tin foil separating medium, male part of the button was attached to female part, and the second segment tray was fabricated. During fabrication of the second segment, acrylic material was extended on to the orientation lock on the first segment near the handle of the tray. The female part of the button was retrieved along with the second section of the tray (Figure 3).

2.2. Impression Making.
After completion of the special tray fabrication, the first segment was used to make the first section of the impression. Wax spacer was removed, and the tray was loaded with polyvinyl siloxane, and sectional impression was made. Sectional impression was removed,

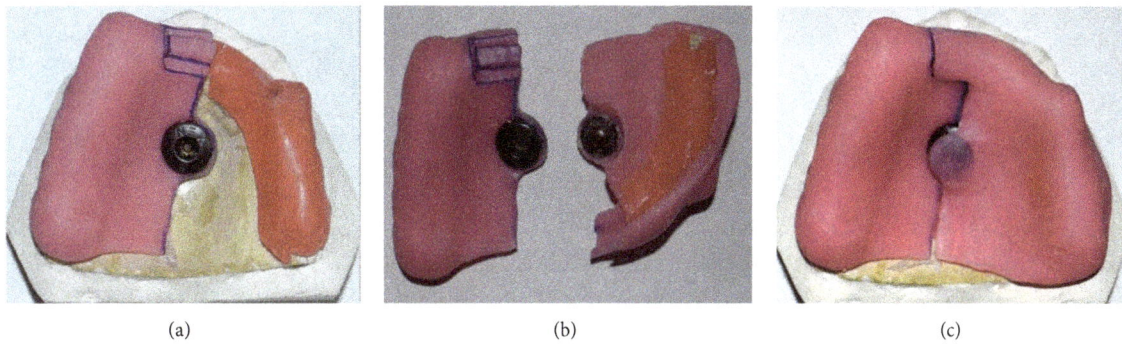

(a)   (b)   (c)

FIGURE 3: Fabrication technique for the sectional tray—Design 2.

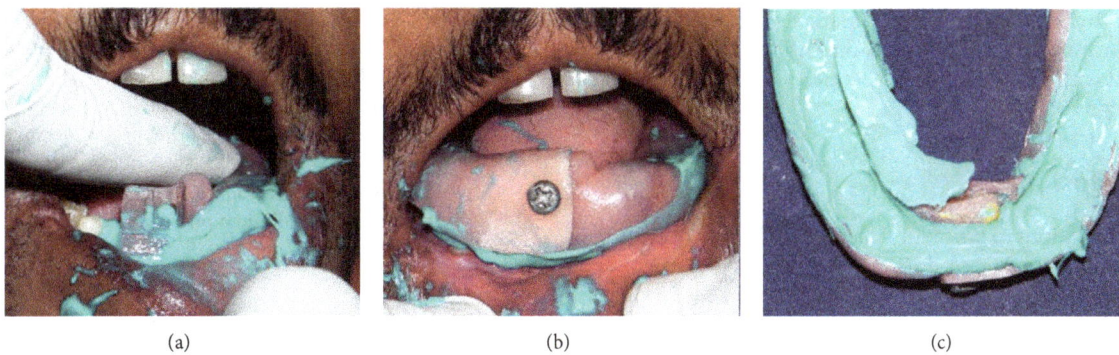

(a)   (b)   (c)

FIGURE 4: Impression making using the sectional tray Design 1.

and the excess material flown on to the lock region and the screw hole was removed. The impression was placed back in the patient's mouth. The second part of the tray was loaded with the same impression material and oriented onto the first segment.

In the first case report, after proper orientation of the tray, a screw was used to secure the segments together before the material set. The screw helped in securing the orientation of the sections of the tray properly within the patient's mouth. After the material had beenset, the screw was removed, and the sections were removed separately. Both the sections were approximated and secured using the screw after removal from the mouth (Figure 4).

In the second case report, the sections of the tray were oriented making sure that the male part of the button was seated properly onto the female part. After the material had been set, both the sections were separated and removed from mouth. Both the sections of the tray were joined together with the help of the locking button (Figure 5).

3. Discussion

Impression making in patients that planned for fixed or removable partial denture with restricted mouth opening is a challenging task as it requires more accuracy and precision. The present case reports described simplified locking designs of the tray segments which could be used for both dentulous and edentulous patients for fabrication of custom trays.

In case report I, the patient was planned to receive a fixed partial denture replacing missing mandibular incisors. Patient in case report II was planned to receive a flexible removable partial denture to replace multiple missing teeth. Recording abutment finish line along with the remaining teeth is important for fabricating fixed partial denture. Similarly for fabrication of removable partial denture, the teeth along with functional depth of the sulcus have to be recorded. Practical difficulties of reduced mouth opening were overcome by designing sectional custom tray which provided an alternative for making an accurate impression.

Simple and economic sectional tray design was fallowed in the present case reports. Male and female segments of the tray were oriented by the locking mechanism which was designed using acrylic trimmer. Use of screws and press buttons helped in securing tray segments more accurately together with precession. Many techniques were described in the literature for impression making in dentulous and edentulous patients with limited mouth opening. Various mechanisms like hinges [4], locking levers [5], plastic blocks [6, 7], orthodontic expansion screws [8], magnet systems [9], parallel pins [10], and so forth were used so far for fabricating sectional trays. In the present case reports, incorporation of complicated locking devices was avoided by designing a locking mechanism within the tray handle to secure the tray segments three dimensionally. Manual locks designed with trimmer on the surface of acrylic lack accuracy and precession. Incorporation of screw and press button into the

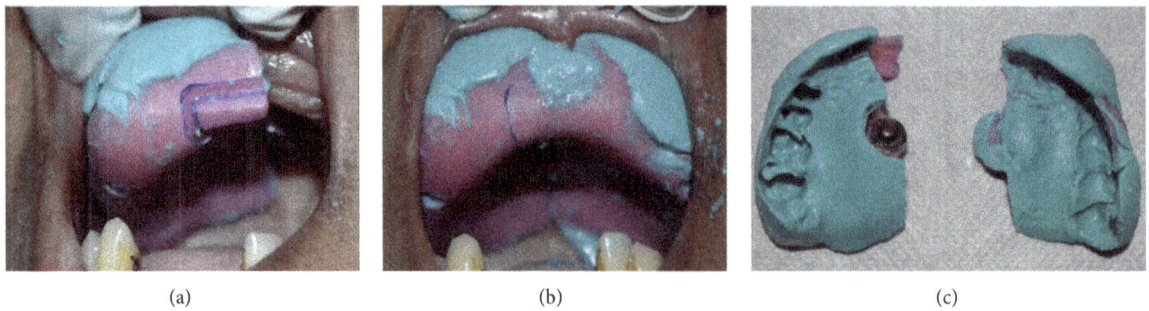

(a)   (b)   (c)

FIGURE 5: Impression making using the sectional tray Design 2.

design provides the precession in securing the trays together firmly. Accurate fit of fixed and removable prostheses was reported with the impressions obtained from both sectional tray designs.

4. Conclusions

Simple alterations in procedural techniques help to overcome clinical difficulties faced during prosthetic management of patients with oral sub mucous fibrosis. Present case reports facilitated the operator to obtain accurate impressions for patients with limited mouth opening. These simple and logical sectional tray designs are easy to fabricate, consume less time, and require inexpensive locking mechanisms.

Conflict of Interests

The authors declare that they have no conflict of interests.

References

[1] R. Rajendran, "Oral submucous fibrosis: etiology, pathogenesis, and future research," *Bulletin of the World Health Organization*, vol. 72, no. 6, pp. 985–996, 1994.

[2] J. J. Pindborg and S. M. Sirsat, "Oral submucous fibrosis," *Oral Surgery, Oral Medicine, Oral Pathology*, vol. 22, no. 6, pp. 764–779, 1966.

[3] J. A. Whitsitt and L. W. Battle, "Technique for making flexible impression trays for the microstomic patient," *The Journal of Prosthetic Dentistry*, vol. 52, no. 4, pp. 608–609, 1984.

[4] B. Conroy and M. Reitzik, "Prosthetic restoration in microstomia," *The Journal of Prosthetic Dentistry*, vol. 26, no. 3, pp. 324–327, 1971.

[5] P. S. Baker, R. L. Brandt, and G. Boyajian, "Impression procedure for patients with severely limited mouth opening," *Journal of Prosthetic Dentistry*, vol. 84, no. 2, pp. 241–244, 2000.

[6] R. J. Luebke, "Sectional impression tray for patients with constricted oral opening," *The Journal of Prosthetic Dentistry*, vol. 52, no. 1, pp. 135–137, 1984.

[7] Y. Suzuki, M. Abe, T. Hosoi, and K. S. Kurtz, "Sectional collapsed denture for a partially edentulous patient with microstomia: a clinical report," *Journal of Prosthetic Dentistry*, vol. 84, no. 3, pp. 256–259, 2000.

[8] A. Mirfazaelian, "Use of orthodontic expansion screw in fabricating section custom trays," *Journal of Prosthetic Dentistry*, vol. 83, no. 3, pp. 474–475, 2000.

[9] S. S. Colvenkar, "Sectional impression tray and sectional denture for a microstomia patient," *Journal of Prosthodontics*, vol. 19, no. 2, pp. 161–165, 2010.

[10] S. Kumar, A. Arora, and R. Yadav, "Prosthetic rehabilitation of edentulous patient with limited oral access: a clinical report," *Contemporary Clinical Dentistry*, vol. 3, no. 3, pp. 349–351, 2012.

39

Oral Myiasis Affecting Gingiva in a Child Patient

Fareedi Mukram Ali,[1] Kishor Patil,[2] Sanjay Kar,[3]
Atulkumar A. Patil,[4] and Shabeer Ahamed[5]

[1]Department of Oral and Maxillofacial Surgery, SMBT Dental College and Hospital, Sangamner, Maharashtra 422608, India
[2]Department of Oral Pathology and Microbiology, SMBT Dental College and Hospital, Sangamner, Maharashtra 422608, India
[3]Department of Oral and Maxillofacial Surgery, Mansarovar Dental College, Hospital & Research Centre,
 Bhopal, Madhya Pradesh 462001, India
[4]Department of Dentistry, Dr. Vaishampayan Memorial Government Medical College, Solapur, Maharashtra, India
[5]Department of Periodontics, Malabar Dental College, Edapal, Kerala 679578, India

Correspondence should be addressed to Kishor Patil; drpatilkishor1@gmail.com

Academic Editor: Yousef S. Khader

Certain dipteran flies larvae causing invasion of the tissues and organs of the humans or other vertebrates are called as myiasis, which feed on hosts dead or living tissues. It is well documented in the skin and hot climate regions; underdeveloped countries are affected more commonly. Oral cavity is affected rarely and it can be secondary to serious medical conditions. Poor oral hygiene, alcoholism, senility, or suppurating lesions can be associated with the oral myiasis. Inflammatory and allergic reactions are the commonest clinical manifestations of the disease. In the present case, gingiva of maxillary anterior region was affected by larval infection in a 13-year-old mentally retarded patient.

1. Introduction

The term myiasis is derived from the Greek word "myia," which is used for fly and it means invasion of organs or tissues of vertebrate animals or humans by dipteral larvae. The term myiasis was coined in 1940 by *F. W. Hope. Zumpt* defined myiasis as the dipterous larva invading the human or other vertebrate animals and feeding on host's dead or living tissue, liquid body substances, and ingested food for certain period of time [1–3].

It is restricted to summer months in temperate zones and all year round in the tropics, as the flies which are responsible for myiasis prefer a warm and humid environment. Myiasis is less common in humans than in the vertebrate animals [4].

The ear, nose, eyes, lungs, skin, anus, and vagina are the most common sites affected in myiasis [1, 5]. The oral tissues are not permanently exposed to the external environment and thus the oral cavity rarely provides a favorable environment for the growth of the larvae [6, 7].

The predisposing factors like poor oral hygiene, presence of periodontal pockets, open bite in the anterior part, mouth breathing during sleep, ulcerative lesions, and carcinoma can be present in the patients of oral myiasis. Most of the patients are mentally retarded, senile, immunocompromised, alcoholics, and living in poor conditions [8, 9]. In the Hindu mythology, similar condition was considered in old times as the "God's" punishment to sinners [1].

The present paper describes a rare case of gingival myiasis in a 13-year-old mentally retarded patient.

2. Case Report

A 13-year-old male patient presented to the hospital with a complaint of swelling and discomfort in maxillary anterior region since 10–12 days. On medical examination, the patient was found to be mentally retarded. The patient was from low socioeconomic background and residing in a rural area. On extra oral examination, the upper lip was swollen causing

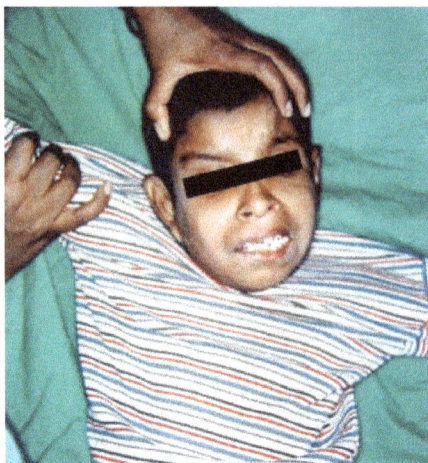

FIGURE 1: Extraoral appearance of the patient at the time of presentation.

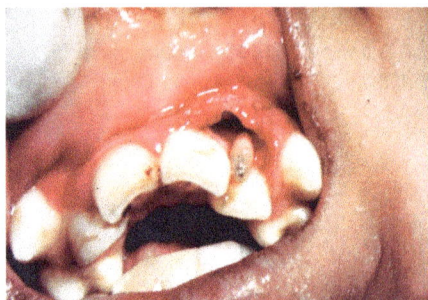

FIGURE 2: Intraoral photograph showing maggots (larvae) coming out from the maxillary anterior region after application of the turpentine oil.

slight protrusion on the left side (Figure 1). Systemic examination of the patient was normal with normal body temperature and the regional lymph nodes were not palpable. Intraoral examination revealed an ulcerated area in the maxillary left labial vestibular region at 21 and 22. It was of 1.8 × 1.0 cm in size and a number of maggots were seen in the ulcerated area. The surrounding area of the ulcer was erythematous and swollen (Figure 2). On instrumentation, the teeth in the involved area had no mobility and his oral hygiene was poor. Based on the clinical findings, the case was provisionally diagnosed as oral myiasis. His hematological analysis was within normal limits.

2.1. Treatment. The most common protocol followed for the myiasis was given for this patient. It consists of flushing affected area with turpentine oil, followed by administration of local anesthesia and removal of maggots by simple tweezers. Around 11–13 maggots were removed from the affected site (Figure 3). Ivermectin 6 mg OD for 3 days, along with metronidazole 400 mg for 5 days and analgesic, and ibuprofen with paracetamol were given to the patient. The area was then washed with saline and irrigation was done with Betadine. The procedure was repeated for 3 consecutive days until

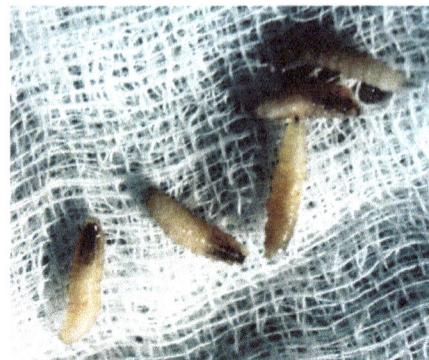

FIGURE 3: Maggots retrieved from the lesion.

all the maggots were removed and the area was completely cleaned. On the fourth day, the site was examined for any remaining larvae and control of the infection. Then, it was sutured with 3–0 silk. Personal hygiene instructions were given to the parents of the patient.

The maggots were preserved in 10% formalin and sent to a parasitology department of medical college for identification, where they were identified as larvae of *Musca domestica* (common housefly). The larvae of the housefly were of cylindrical shape but tapering towards the head, were typical creamy white in color, and had 13 segments, of which 12 were apparent, as the first 2 were partly fused. The head was containing one pair of dark hooks.

2.2. Outcome and Follow-Up. After 1 month, the lesional site was found to be healed properly. On the follow-up of the patient, after 6 months, he was absolutely alright and no parasitic infestation was found in oral cavity.

3. Discussion

The oral myiasis, parasitic infestation of the human, is a rare condition, which mainly occurs in the rural areas. The flies of the order Diptera (maggots) are the main parasites affecting humans [1, 6]. The most common causative agent of myiasis is dipteran clade Calyptratae. It consists of four families: Calliphoridae, Sarcophagidae, Oestridae, and Muscoidea [10].

In the present case, the causative agent was identified to be of common housefly. Similar type of case reports of common housefly affecting maxillary anterior region intraorally was also reported by Bhagawati et al. [11] and Pereira et al. [1].

The life cycle of a fly consists of 4 stages: egg stage, larval stage, the pupa, and finally the adult fly. Direct inoculation into wounds and ingestion of infected materials like meat are the two ways causing infestation of the maggots in the humans. For the larval development of these flies, the intermediate host is required and the flies can lay more than 500 eggs at a time directly over the diseased tissue [3, 6, 12]. After the gravid female flies lay eggs in the tissues, the larvae hatch in about 8–10 hours, after which they invade into the surrounding tissues and cause inflammation and discomfort to the patient [1, 6, 13].

The action of proteolytic enzymes released by the surrounding bacteria causes decomposition of the tissue and helps in the feeding of the maggots [3, 14]. Larval growth causes progressive destruction and cavitation and finally forms a fibrous capsule to which they firmly adhere and cause more difficulty in dissection during surgical procedures [6, 15]. The burrowing of the larvae causes the separation of the mucoperiosteum from the bone and mild to acute pain. Thus, a patent opening is maintained with induration of the marginal tissues and raising a dome shaped "warble." Infestation is mostly seen subcutaneously and may produce a furunculated or boil-like lesion, also called as berne [6, 15].

Larvae position themselves with their heads down to expose their posterior spiracles to the air, which makes their respiration possible. Approximately 8–10 days are required for the larvae to develop into prepupal stage after their penetration into the tissues and then they leave the host. The backward segmental hooks are useful for the anchoring of the larvae to the surrounding tissue. The larvae are photophobic; hence, they tend to hide deep into the tissues for a suitable niche to develop into pupa [1, 6].

Oral myiasis usually has male predilection because of outdoor activities and habit of neglecting oral hygiene. It is commonly seen in adults, but cases in children have also been reported. In case of oral myiasis, the most common site involved is the anterior segments of the maxillary and mandibular jaws and the palate [4, 6].

In the present case, gingiva of the maxillary anterior site was affected. Reddy et al. [8], Bhagawati et al. [11], Moshref et al. [13], Mohammadzadeh et al. [16], and Govindaraju et al. [17] also reported a case of oral myiasis affecting gingiva of the maxillary anterior region.

Clinical picture of the pulsating larvae is sufficient for the diagnosis of the oral myiasis and for the species identification it should be sent to the specialized laboratories. Mechanical removal of larvae is the most commonly used treatment [3, 6]. Local application of substances like mineral oil, ether, oil of turpentine, chloroform, mercuric chloride, ethyl chloride, creosote, phenol, saline, calomel, gentian violet, white head varnish, olive oil, and iodoform can be used for ensuring the complete removal of all larvae [6, 18, 19]. Treatment of the surrounding bacterial infection with broad-spectrum antibiotics and nutritional support of the patient with multivitamin tablets are also important. Commonly used antibiotics include ampicillin, amoxicillin, or metronidazole. Topical use of nitrofurazone and ivermectin has also been useful [3, 20, 21].

In our case, turpentine oil was applied followed by local anaesthesia and removal of the maggots by tweezer followed by antibiotic course of ivermectin, which was similar to the treatment suggested by Reddy et al. [8], Sankari and Ramakrishnan [14], Kumar and Srikumar [5], Pereira et al. [1], and Bhagawati et al. [11].

4. Conclusion

Oral myiasis is an uncommon condition. Parasitic infestations can be reduced by raising the quality of life and improving the personal hygiene measurements. Mental and physically disabled patients need special care to maintain oral hygiene. As dentists, it is our duty to raise awareness that a special needs patient should be exposed to proper dental intervention on regular basis as early as possible to promote cooperation and to prevent the occurrence of the disease.

Conflict of Interests

The authors declare that there is no conflict of interests regarding the publication of this paper.

References

[1] T. Pereira, A. P. Tamgadge, M. S. Chande, S. Bhalerao, and S. Tamgadge, "Oral myiasis," *Contemporary Clinical Dentistry*, vol. 1, no. 4, pp. 275–276, 2010.

[2] S. Sheikh, S. Pallagatti, I. Singla, A. Kalucha, A. Aggarwal, and H. Kaur, "Oral myiasis—a review," *Journal of Clinical and Experimental Dentistry*, vol. 3, no. 5, pp. e465–e468, 2011.

[3] R. Srivastava, P. Devi, V. B. Thimmarasa, and S. Jayadev, "Flies blown disease—oral myiasis," *Indian Journal of Dental Research*, vol. 22, no. 4, p. 615, 2011.

[4] E. B. Droma, A. Wilamowski, H. Schnur, N. Yarom, E. Scheuer, and E. Schwartz, "Oral myiasis: a case report and literature review," *Oral Surgery, Oral Medicine, Oral Pathology, Oral Radiology, and Endodontics*, vol. 103, no. 1, pp. 92–96, 2007.

[5] P. Kumar and G. P. V. Srikumar, "Oral myiasis in a maxillofacial trauma patient," *Contemporary Clinical Dentistry*, vol. 3, no. 2, pp. 202–204, 2012.

[6] L. K. Surej Kumar, S. Manuel, T. V. John, and M. P. Sivan, "Extensive gingival myiasis—diagnosis, treatment, and prevention," *Journal of Oral and Maxillofacial Pathology*, vol. 15, no. 3, pp. 340–343, 2011.

[7] A. A. G. Khan and K. M. Shah, "Primary oral myiasis: a clinical presentation in cerebral palsy," *International Journal of Case Reports and Images*, vol. 4, no. 2, pp. 95–98, 2013.

[8] M. H. R. Reddy, N. Das, and M. R. Vivekananda, "Oral myiasis in children," *Contemporary Clinical Dentistry*, vol. 3, no. 5, pp. S19–S22, 2012.

[9] T. Rossi-Schneider, K. Cherubini, L. S. Yurgel, F. Salum, and M. A. Figueiredo, "Oral myiasis: a case report," *Journal of Oral Science*, vol. 49, no. 1, pp. 85–88, 2007.

[10] M. Jang, S.-M. Ryu, S.-C. Kwon et al., "A case of oral myiasis caused by *Lucilia sericata* (Diptera: Calliphoridae) in Korea," *Korean Journal of Parasitology*, vol. 51, no. 1, pp. 119–123, 2013.

[11] B. T. Bhagawati, M. Gupta, and S. Singh, "Oral myiasis: a rare entity," *European Journal of General Dentistry*, vol. 2, no. 3, pp. 312–314, 2013.

[12] R. Ramli and R. A. Rahman, "Oral myiasis: case report," *Malaysian Journal of Medical Sciences*, vol. 9, no. 2, pp. 47–50, 2002.

[13] M. Moshref, G. Ansari, and A. Lotfi, "Oral gingival myiasis: a case report," *International Journal of Tropical Medicine*, vol. 3, no. 4, pp. 97–100, 2008.

[14] L. S. Sankari and K. Ramakrishnan, "Oral myiasis caused by *Chrysomya bezziana*," *Journal of Oral and Maxillofacial Pathology*, vol. 14, no. 1, pp. 16–18, 2010.

[15] R. R. Felices and K. U. E. Ogbureke, "Oral myiasis: report of case and review of management," *Journal of Oral and Maxillofacial Surgery*, vol. 54, no. 2, pp. 219–220, 1996.

[16] T. Mohammadzadeh, R. Hadadzadeh, F. Esfandiari, and S. M. Sadjjadi, "A case of gingival myiasis caused by wohlfahrtia magnifica," *Iranian Journal of Arthropod-Borne Diseases*, vol. 2, no. 1, pp. 53–56, 2008.

[17] R. Govindaraju, V. M. Rajshekar, M. P. David, and S. Shivraj, "'Wriggling rotters' in the oral cavity: a rare case report," *Journal of Indian Academy of Oral Medicine and Radiology*, vol. 26, no. 4, pp. 442–445, 2014.

[18] C.-J. Wu, T.-S. Chang, and S.-T. Chu, "Nasal myiasis in a bedridden patient and literature review," *Journal of Medical Sciences*, vol. 32, no. 1, pp. 39–41, 2012.

[19] M. A. Sikder, L. Pradhan, F. Ferdousi, and M. K. Parvin, "Oral myiasis: a case report," *Bangladesh Journal of Medical Science*, vol. 10, no. 3, pp. 206–208, 2011.

[20] S. M. Lima Júnior, L. Asprino, Â. P. Prado, R. W. F. Moreira, and M. de Moraes, "Oral myiasis caused by *Cochliomyia hominivorax* treated nonsurgically with nitrofurazone: report of 2 cases," *Oral Surgery, Oral Medicine, Oral Pathology, Oral Radiology and Endodontology*, vol. 109, no. 3, pp. e70–e73, 2010.

[21] E. H. Shinohara, M. Z. Martini, H. G. Oliveira Neto, and A. Takahashi, "Oral myiasis treated with ivermectin: case report," *Brazilian Dental Journal*, vol. 15, no. 1, pp. 79–81, 2004.

40

Altered Apical Morphology (Reverse Architecture): Use of Indirect Ultrasonic Technique for Orthograde MTA Placement in Maxillary Premolars

Kapoor Sonali, Agrawal Vineet Suresh, Patel Abhishek, and Patel Jenish

Department of Conservative and Endodontics, M. P. Dental College and Hospital, Vadodara 390011, India

Correspondence should be addressed to Agrawal Vineet Suresh; vineetdent@yahoo.co.in

Academic Editor: Jiiang H. Jeng

Aim. To report the management and orthograde technique of MTA placement in case of reverse architecture maxillary premolars. *Summary.* Two cases of 17-year-old and 21-year-old female patients were referred to endodontic speciality for management of maxillary premolar having reverse architecture with wide immature open apex like a bell mouth. In both the cases, after control of intraradicular infection, it was decided to use MTA for apexification and obturation of canals. Orthograde placement of MTA is a challenging procedure in terms of length control and condensation especially in divergent irregular reverse architecture wide open apex. A novel technique with the help of finger plugger, sterilized paper point, and ultrasonic agitation for 3D compaction of MTA at apical reverse architecture was used. Thickening of the canal wall and complete apical closure were confirmed one year after the treatment.

1. Introduction

The treatment of pulpal injury after eruption of teeth, during the period, that is, 3 yrs, for completion of root development and closure of apex, provides significant challenge for endodontist [1, 2]. During this period, if pulpal exposure occurs due to trauma or caries, necrosis of pulp takes place, ceasing dentin formation and arresting root growth. Resultant immature root will have a wide open apex termed as blunderbuss canal [3].

Bell mouth-like open apex has reverse architecture, that is, larger apical diameter and smaller coronal diameter, leading to improper root canal debridement [4]. It leads to difficulty during filling of root canal due to lack of resistance from apical tissues and absence of natural constriction [4]. Wide apical foramen requires large volume of filling material to be condensed apically, which may extrude in periapical region due to lack of apical seat leading to foreign body reactions [5]. Also, the thin root canal walls will make the tooth more prone to fracture [4].

Apexification is defined as "a method of inducing a calcified barrier in a root with an open apex or the continued apical development of an incompletely formed root in teeth with necrotic pulp" [6]. The classical apexification process with calcium hydroxide is associated with some problems, such as long-term treatment and the risk of teeth fracture [7]. Presently, mineral trioxide aggregate (MTA) obturation technique has become a more favourable option in treating necrotized teeth with open apex owing to its good canal sealing property, biocompatibility, and ability to promote pulp and periapical tissue regeneration [8, 9]. Also, reduced treatment time, less chance of tooth fractures, and fewer dental appointments have added to its advantage [9]. However, orthograde placement of MTA is a challenging procedure in terms of length control in reverse architecture open apex cases which require a specialized sensitive placement technique.

Reverse architecture or wide open apex cases mostly reported in literature are in maxillary anterior teeth and rarely in maxillary premolars [7]. The purpose of this report is to present successful management of two rare cases of maxillary premolars with necrotic pulp and open apex with reverse architecture obturated with MTA. Also, the cases illustrate proper MTA placement technique in reverse architecture wide open apex teeth.

2. Case Reports

Case 1. A 17-year-old, medically free female patient was referred by some general dentist to the Department of Conservative Dentistry and Endodontics after performing emergency root canal opening in upper right first premolar. Patient suffered from severe pain and intraoral swelling in maxillary right first premolar. These symptoms occurred frequently during the last 5-6 years but have never been treated.

On clinical examination, there was root canal opening performed in 14 with some carious tooth structure still remaining. No mobility was present but 14 was tender on percussion. Radiographically, tooth appeared to have reverse architecture with wide immature open apex like a bell mouth with thinner root wall and periradicular radiolucency (Figure 1(a)). It was decided that MTA will be used for apexification and complete obturation of both root canals after thorough debridement.

After rubber dam isolation, access cavity was prepared and remaining caries was removed with Endo-Z Bur (Dentsply Maillefer) to enhance the visibility of root canal. An approximate working length was estimated on radiograph for both the buccal and the palatal canals (Figure 1(b)). Both the canals showed lack of resistance in periapical region indicating open apex in both the roots (buccal and palatal). The root canal walls were gently instrumented with stainless steel K-files and irrigated with 5 mL of 2.5% sodium hypochlorite (NaOCl). Canals were dried with paper points. A thick mixture of calcium hydroxide was placed in the canals for 2-week interval and temporary coronal seal was established with CAVIT (3M ESPE, St. Paul, MN, USA).

When patient returned, she was asymptomatic. Calcium hydroxide was removed from the canals using 5 mL of 2.5% NaOCl, and the canals were dried with paper points. A mixture of ProRoot MTA powder (ProRoot MTA, Dentsply Tulsa Dental Specialties, Johnson City, TN, USA) and distilled water was prepared as per manufacturer's instruction. Then, the MTA was placed by orthograde technique in both canals individually as described below.

At first, few mm of MTA was taken on applicator instrument and placed at canal orifice. Using an endodontic finger plugger and back end of sterilized paper point, premeasured to be within 0.5–1 mm of the working length, MTA was packed towards the apex. At this point, indirect ultrasonic agitation (Satelec Acteon, Mérignac, France) of MTA material via plugger was done to create sort of a wet sand flow effect and again it was condensed using back end of sterilized paper point ensuring 3D compaction of MTA at bell mouth-like open apex. Radiograph was taken to confirm correct location of the first pack of MTA apically. After confirmation of proper position, the rest of the canal was filled with MTA incrementally as well as condensing with plugger and paper point. A moist cotton pellet was placed above this condensed MTA for setting and access cavity was temporized with CAVIT (3M ESPE, St. Paul, MN, USA).

At the next appointment, after verifying set of MTA, the tooth was permanently restored with the dentin bonded composite resin (Filtek Z350 XT, 3M ESPE, St. Paul, MN, USA) (Figure 1(c)). The clinical follow-up at 1 year revealed adequate clinical function without clinical symptoms, such as percussion pain, palpation pain, or swelling. Follow-up radiograph at 6 months (Figure 1(d)) also revealed healing of periradicular region.

Case 2. A 21-year-old, medically free female patient was again referred by some general dentist to the Department of Conservative Dentistry and Endodontics after performing emergency root canal opening in upper left second premolar. Patient suffered from severe pain in maxillary left second premolar. Patient complained of similar pain 8-9 years back giving history of chewing something hard on the same side with pain subsiding on its own.

On clinical examination, there was root canal opening performed in 25 and no mobility was present. Radiographically, tooth appeared to have reverse architecture with wide immature open apex like a bell mouth with thinner root wall and periradicular radiolucency (Figure 2(a)). It was decided that MTA will be used for apexification and complete obturation of the root canal after thorough debridement.

Following the same protocol in Case 1, after rubber dam isolation, access cavity was prepared, working length radiograph was taken (only 1 canal was present in this case) (Figure 2(b)), minimal instrumentation with K-files was done, irrigation with 2.5% NaOCl was performed, and calcium hydroxide dressing was given for 2 weeks. After 2 weeks, calcium hydroxide was removed and MTA was placed in orthograde manner following similar technique described in Case 1. After setting of MTA, permanent restoration was done with composite restoration (Filtek Z350 XT, 3M ESPE, St. Paul, MN, USA) (Figure 2(c)).

Follow-up at 1 year revealed no clinical symptoms and radiograph (Figure 2(d)) shows complete healing of the periapical lesion with regenerated bone and periodontal ligament-like space.

3. Discussion

Successful healing of odontogenic tissues, from both a periodontal and endodontic aspect, has developed a quest for such material since last decade. Introduction of MTA has led to this solution as it can induce healing of periapical tissues, such as periodontal ligament, bone, and cementum. MTA has led to thicker and less porous dentin bridge formation and less pulp inflammation compared with calcium hydroxide [7, 10]. MTA induces recruitment and proliferation of undifferentiated cells to form a dentin bridge while reducing inflammation compared with calcium hydroxide [7]. Also, MTA when placed in direct contact with the human dental pulp cells (DPCs) differentiated them into odontoblast-like cells [11]. MTA has also been shown to permit cementoblast attachment and growth as well as the production of mineralized matrix gene and protein expression [12]. *In vitro* experiments have shown that MTA upregulated the expression of type I collagen and osteocalcin in osteoblasts

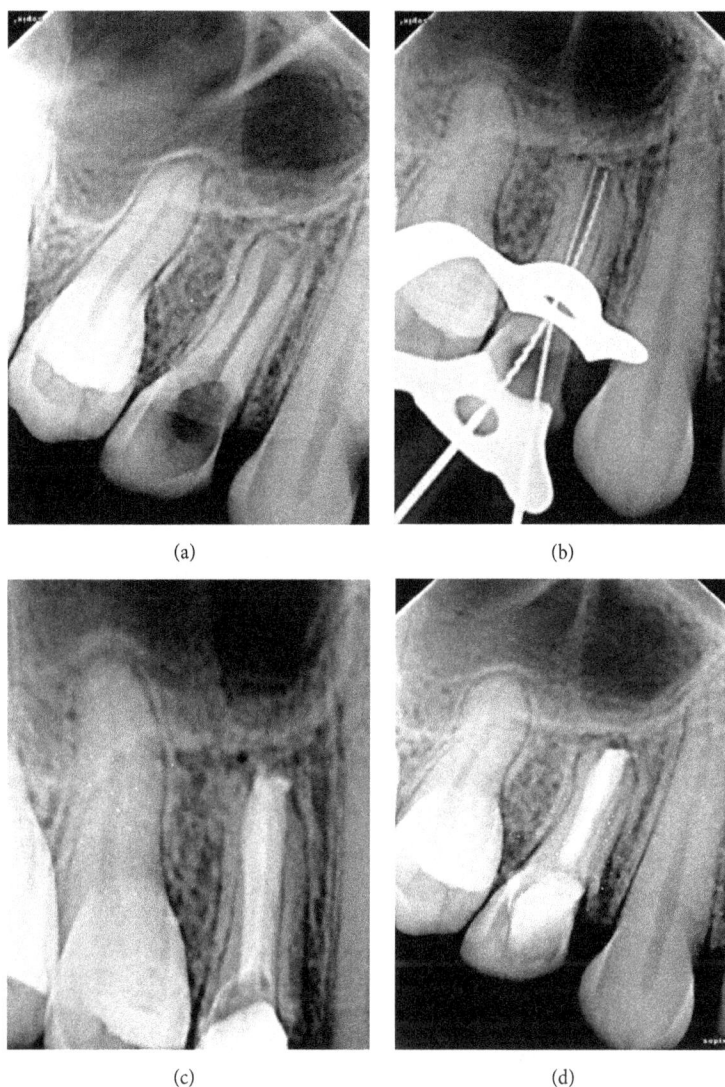

FIGURE 1: (a) Preoperative radiograph (Case 1). (b) Working length radiograph (Case 1). (c) MTA obturation (Case 1). (d) One-year follow-up radiograph (Case 1).

after 24 h [12]. Other research studies have shown that MTA stimulates the proliferation of cementoblasts, fibroblasts, and osteoblasts [10–12].

From a clinical point of view, in cases with immature apex with necrotic pulp and inflamed periapical lesion, there is always the presence of tissue fluid or exudation [5]. MTA has unique advantage that is able to set in the presence of moisture. When treating nonvital teeth, main issue is eliminating bacteria from the root canal system. In the above cases, in order to limit bacterial infection before obturation with MTA, irrigation with sodium hypochlorite was done and short-term intracanal calcium hydroxide medication was placed within the canal for two weeks. The rationale was, as instrumentation should be minimal due to thin dentinal walls, complete debridement depends on irrigation and intracanal medicament.

In immature teeth with reverse architecture, the absence of apical constriction complicates the proper placement of MTA within root canal confinements. In addition, the inherent irregularities and divergent nature of the tooth anatomy may affect its adaptation to the dentin walls, predisposing the material to marginal gaps at the dentin interface. In the above cases, access cavities were modified to have enhanced visibility and straight access to root. Orthograde method of MTA placement is more technique sensitive than retrograde method but Hachmeister et al. [13] found that sealing ability of MTA is superior when using orthogradely as apical plug. Aminoshariae et al. [14] reported that hand condensation resulted in better adaptation and fewer voids. Hence, in the above cases, hand condensation technique along with indirect ultrasonic agitation was used for MTA condensation to obtain proper seal and flow of MTA in area of

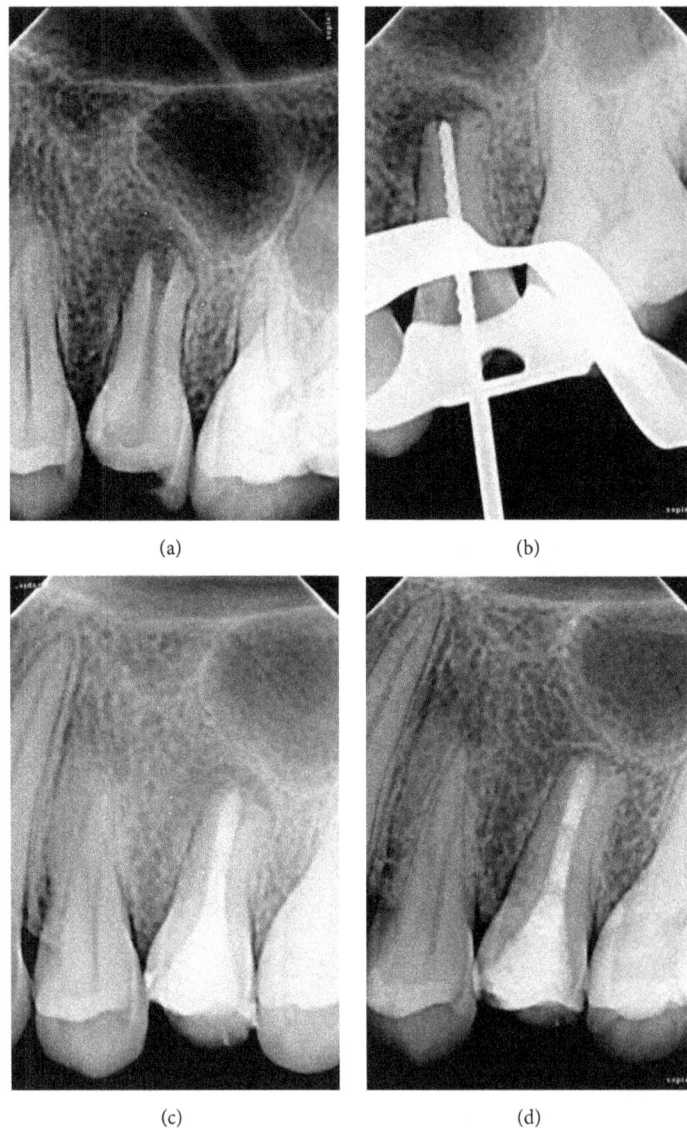

FIGURE 2: (a) Preoperative radiograph (Case 2). (b) Working length radiograph (Case 2). (c) MTA obturation (Case 2). (d) One-year follow-up radiograph (Case 2).

reverse architecture. Various instruments can be used for this precision of MTA placement such as paper points, ultrasonic agitation of the material (creating sort of a wet sand flow effect), and larger hand-files that have been flattened at the tip. Indirect ultrasonic activation means touching the ultrasonic tip with any instrument such as plugger and transforming the vibrating energy to MTA leading to its proper condensation in bell mouth-like area. A study by Yeung et al. [15], comparing the fill density of MTA by hand and ultrasonic compaction, showed that ultrasonication produced a denser MTA fill. A recent study by Parashos et al. [16] concluded that the use of ultrasonics with MTA was useful in improving flow and compaction of MTA, but excessive ultrasonication can adversely impact MTA properties. A suggested time of 2 seconds of ultrasonication per increment presented the best

compromise between microhardness values, dye penetration depths, and lack of radiographic voids [16].

MTA has a profound advantage when used as a canal obturation material because of its superior physicochemical and bioactive properties. A study by Hatibović-Kofman et al. [17], on fracture resistance and histological findings of immature teeth treated with mineral trioxide aggregate, showed that the teeth with root treatment with MTA showed the highest fracture resistance at 1 year. As in the above cases, there were thinner root dentin walls remaining, and hence to reinforce the tooth entire canal was obturated with MTA. It has an added advantage of speed of completion of therapy and periapical healing that follows.

Both clinical and radiological examination in follow-up showed healing of periapical lesion and hard tissue formation in apical area of affected teeth. Hence, MTA can be considered very effective in management of immature permanent teeth with open apices and reverse architecture if placed with proper condensation technique. We cannot confirmatively say that regeneration, revascularization, repair, or apexification has taken place in our cases due to the limitation of clinical cases as we cannot take the histological sections to know which type of tissue and cells has led to healing.

Competing Interests

The authors declare that they have no competing interests.

References

[1] S. N. Bhasker, *Orban's Oral Histology and Embryology*, Mosby-Year Book, St Louis, Miss, USA, 11th edition, 1991.

[2] S. Singh, S. Singh, S. Mugana, and G. S. Maurya, "Induced apical closure of nonvital immature root apices with MTA," *Journal of Orofacial Research*, vol. 4, no. 1, pp. 46–49, 2014.

[3] T. B. Kardos, "The mechanism of tooth eruption," *British Dental Journal*, vol. 181, no. 3, pp. 91–95, 1996.

[4] J.-B. Park and J.-H. Lee, "Use of mineral trioxide aggregate in the open apex of a maxillary first premolar," *Journal of Oral Science*, vol. 50, no. 3, pp. 355–358, 2008.

[5] S.-W. Chang, T.-S. Oh, W. Lee, G. S. Cheung, and H.-C. Kim, "Long-term observation of the mineral trioxide aggregate extrusion into the periapical lesion: a case series," *International Journal of Oral Science*, vol. 5, no. 1, pp. 54–57, 2013.

[6] G. N. Glickman, A. K. Mickel, L. G. Levin, A. F. Fouad, and W. T. Johnson, *Glossary of Endodontic Terms*, American Association of Endodontists, Chicago, Ill, USA, 7th edition, 2003.

[7] S. Chala, R. Abouqal, and S. Rida, "Apexification of immature teeth with calcium hydroxide or mineral trioxide aggregate: systematic review and meta-analysis," *Oral Surgery, Oral Medicine, Oral Pathology, Oral Radiology and Endodontology*, vol. 112, no. 4, pp. e36–e42, 2011.

[8] M. Torabinejad and N. Chivian, "Clinical applications of mineral trioxide aggregate," *Journal of Endodontics*, vol. 25, no. 3, pp. 197–205, 1999.

[9] S. Simon, F. Rilliard, A. Berdal, and P. Machtou, "The use of mineral trioxide aggregate in one-visit apexification treatment: a prospective study," *International Endodontic Journal*, vol. 40, no. 3, pp. 186–197, 2007.

[10] S. G. Floratos, I. N. Tsatsoulis, and E. G. Kontakiotis, "Apical barrier formation after incomplete Orthograde MTA apical plug placement in teeth with open apex—report of two cases," *Brazilian Dental Journal*, vol. 24, no. 2, pp. 163–166, 2013.

[11] S. S. Hakki, S. B. Bozkurt, E. E. Hakki, and S. Belli, "Effects of mineral trioxide aggregate on cell survival, gene expression associated with mineralized tissues, and biomineralization of cementoblasts," *Journal of Endodontics*, vol. 35, no. 4, pp. 513–519, 2009.

[12] V. D'Antò, M. P. Di Caprio, G. Ametrano, M. Simeone, S. Rengo, and G. Spagnuolo, "Effect of mineral trioxide aggregate on mesenchymal stem cells," *Journal of Endodontics*, vol. 36, no. 11, pp. 1839–1843, 2010.

[13] D. R. Hachmeister, W. G. Schindler, W. A. Walker III, and D. D. Thomas, "The sealing ability and retention characteristics of mineral trioxide aggregate in a model of apexification," *Journal of Endodontics*, vol. 28, no. 5, pp. 386–390, 2002.

[14] A. Aminoshariae, G. R. Hartwell, and P. C. Moon, "Placement of mineral trioxide aggregate using two different techniques," *Journal of Endodontics*, vol. 29, no. 10, pp. 679–682, 2003.

[15] P. Yeung, F. R. Liewehr, and P. C. Moon, "A quantitative comparison of the fill density of mta produced by two placement techniques," *Journal of Endodontics*, vol. 32, no. 5, pp. 456–459, 2006.

[16] P. Parashos, A. Phoon, and C. Sathorn, "Effect of ultrasonication on physical properties of mineral trioxide aggregate," *BioMed Research International*, vol. 2014, Article ID 191984, 4 pages, 2014.

[17] Š. Hatibović-Kofman, L. Raimundo, L. Zheng, L. Chong, M. Friedman, and J. O. Andreasen, "Fracture resistance and histological findings of immature teeth treated with mineral trioxide aggregate," *Dental Traumatology*, vol. 24, no. 3, pp. 272–276, 2008.

41

Unilateral Absence of Mental Foramen with Surgical Exploration in a Living Human Subject

Murat Ulu,[1] Elif Tarim Ertas,[2] Fatih Gunhan,[1] Meral Yircali Atici,[2] and Huseyin Akcay[1]

[1]*Department of Oral and Maxillofacial Surgery, Faculty of Dentistry, Izmir Katip Celebi University, 35640 Izmir, Turkey*
[2]*Department of Oral and Maxillofacial Radiology, Faculty of Dentistry, Izmir Katip Celebi University, 35640 Izmir, Turkey*

Correspondence should be addressed to Fatih Gunhan; fatihgunhan44@hotmail.com

Academic Editor: Asja Celebić

The mental foramen (MF) is an important anatomic landmark of the mandible, in which the somatic afferent sensory nerve of the mandibular nerve emerges as mental nerve and blood vessels. The identification and actual location of MF are important in order to avoid sensory dysfunction or paresthesia due to mental nerve injury. In the literature there are some rare reports on the anatomical variations of the MF such as its location or presence of accessory foramina. The present report describes the absence of mental foramina on the left side of the mandible, as detected by cone-beam computed tomography before impacted tooth removal and observed directly during surgery.

1. Introduction

The mental foramen (MF) nerves divide into several branches to provide sensorial innervation of the angle of the mouth with its angular branch: the skin of the lower lip, oral mucosa, and gingiva up to the second premolar with its medial and lateral inferior labial branches and the skin of the mental region with its mental branch [1]. MF is generally located in the area of premolar region as bilateral oval or round openings, although race and ethnicity may affect its location [2]. Radiographically, the MF can be seen as a round or oval radiolucent area on both the right and left sides of the mandible [3, 4].

The identification and actual location of MF are important in order to avoid sensory dysfunction or paresthesia during any surgical procedures in this area, as well as achieving effective anesthesia [3, 5, 6]. Since the conventional radiographs such as periapical and panoramic films provide two-dimensional images of the mandible [2, 7], the MF may not be observed in some cases due to the superimposition of anatomic landmarks [5, 8], the pattern of trabecular bone [4], and the thinning of the mandible [5]. In the literature, variations of the MF such as its location or presence of accessory foramina are reported in several articles but the absence of MF is extremely rare [5, 5].

We present here a case of unilateral absence of the mental foramen in a living patient detected on cone-beam computed tomography (CBCT) images and surgical exploration during lower impacted 2nd and 3rd molar extraction. According to our knowledge there is a very extremely rare case report in the literature which indicates absence of mental foramen with CBCT image and by surgical exploration.

2. Case Report

A 20-year-old male patient was referred to Izmir Katip Celebi University Faculty of Dentistry with a chief complaint of pain in left posterior mandible. A panoramic radiograph disclosed the presence of fully impacted mandibular 2nd and 3rd left molars with horizontally overlapped position (Figure 1). A radiolucent area around impacted molars and bone resorption distal side of 1st molar was observed. Extraction was decided for both of the impacted teeth. In order to evaluate the relation between the impacted 2nd molar and inferior alveolar nerve, CBCT (NewTom 5G®, QR, Verona, Italy) examination was performed before surgery. All axial, coronal, and 3D images were carefully explored. During CBCT examination an uncommon anatomic variation drew our attention. In the left mandible MF could not be seen

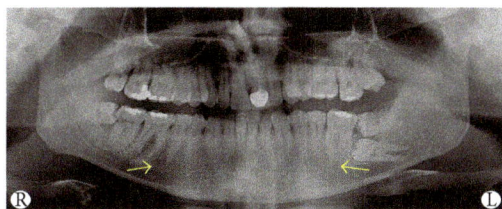

FIGURE 1: 20-year-old patient's panoramic radiograph in which the images of the right MF and the end of the left mandibular canal are pointed by the arrows.

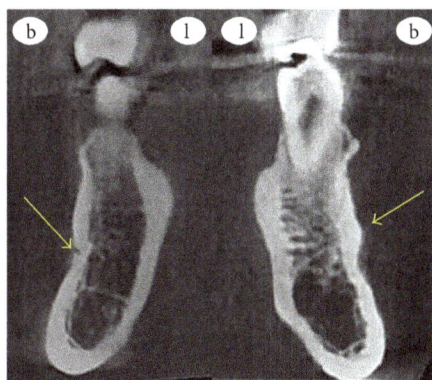

FIGURE 2: Coronal CBCT slice in which the openings of the right MF and the left protuberance at the MF area are pointed by the arrows.

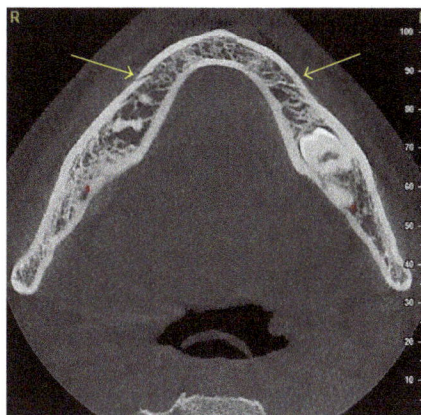

FIGURE 3: Transverse CBCT slice of the right MF is pointed by the arrow and the left MF area protuberance is pointed by the arrow.

and on the right side there was a slight foramen between the 1st and 2nd premolars. We assessed axial and coronal images (Figures 2 and 3) carefully and then made a 3D construction (Figure 4). On the left side MF was absent but the patient did not complain about sensory deficiency. Using the fine slices from the CBCT, we analysed the mandibular images with Mimics software (Materialise, Leuven, Belgium) and reconstructed the data into 3D images. By segmenting the mandibular canals, we revealed their courses within the mandible. Although right mandibular nerve exists into the MF at the 1st premolar region, the left canal could not be identified after the region of tooth 35 (Figure 5). We could not identify incisive canal on the left side.

Prior to surgical removal of the impacted teeth the patient was informed about paresthesia. Inferior alveolar nerve block anesthesia was achieved with 4 mL local anesthetic (Ultracaine D-S Fort, Sanofi Aventis, Istanbul, Turkey). Sulcular incision, which extended to the middle of the 1st premolar, was combined with two releasing incisions and then a mucoperiosteal envelope flap was reflected. At the 1/3 apical level of the 2nd premolar, bone prominence was seen; there was no foramen (Figure 6). After providing a clear exposure the 3rd molar was divided into small pieces with tungsten round and fissure bur and then extracted with a Bein elevator. After that 2nd molar was extracted with the same procedure. Finally, the granulation tissue was scraped from the cavity and the flap was repositioned in its original place and then sutured with 3-0 silk (Dogsan, Trabzon, Turkey). Antibiotic and nonsteroidal anti-inflammatory drugs were

prescribed after surgery. We did not notice nerve disturbance during suture removing seance.

3. Discussion

In recent years with the improvement of implant dentistry and its growing popularity, the possibility of surgical procedures near the MF has increased. Therefore, detailed anatomical knowledge of the region and MF's variations is crucial. MF is an important anatomical landmark of the mandible during surgical procedures in order to achieve effective mental nerve block anesthesia and to prevent mental nerve injuries of the lower jaw [9].

The location of MF shows changes in different races [2]. It is usually located apical to the second premolar or between apices of the premolars and first molars [9]. In the first years of life before tooth eruption, the MF exists closer to the alveolar margin; in time it is observed closer to the inferior border, and with aging related to tooth loss and bone resorption the MF is found closer to the alveolar border [7].

Usually the MFs are observed as bilateral oval or round opening on the lateral surface of the mandible, but some variations of MF have been reported in the literature. However, accessory foramina, retromolar foramen, and abnormal courses of the inferior alveolar neurovascular bundle were recorded as normal variations in the studies [6, 10]. The size of MF varies individually. Greenstein and Tarnow [5] assessed the size of MF by using morphometric skull and reported the following mean values: height (3.47 mm; range 2.5–5.5 mm), width (3.59 mm; range 2–5.5 mm), and diameter (3.5 and 5 mm wide). In our case, we measured the dimensions of the right MF using transversal CBCT slices and values are as follows: height 1.1 mm, width 1.2 mm. The left MF of the patient was absent.

There is a limited publication about the exact prevalence of MF agenesis in the literature. De Freitas et al. [11] examined 1,435 dry human mandibles and they could not detect MF only in three cases. The limitations of 2D radiographs may be the possible explanation for this lack of data, because conventional panoramic radiographs are not reliable for true

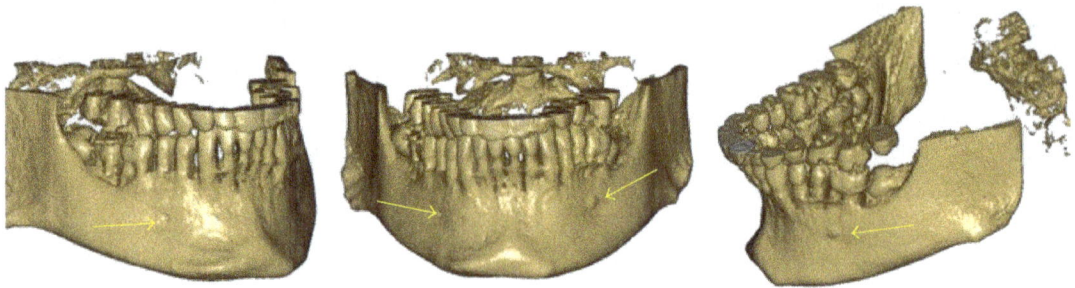

FIGURE 4: 3D reconstruction of the patient's right side, left side, and frontal appearance showing hypoplastic foramen and protuberance at the MF area.

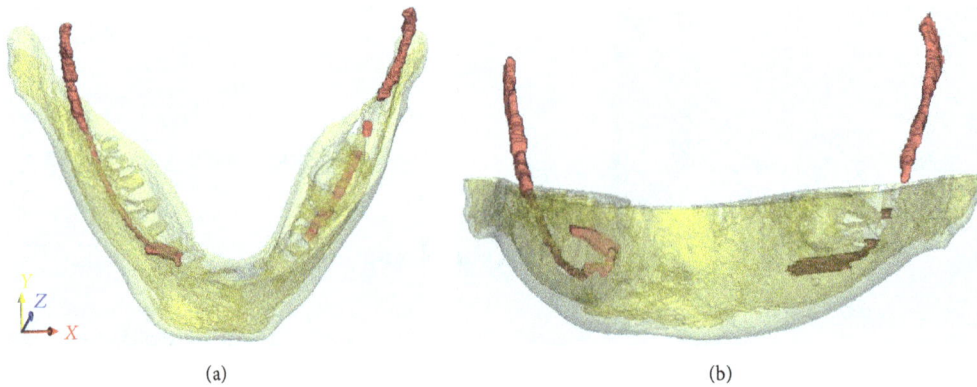

(a)   (b)

FIGURE 5: Segmentation of the mandibular canal by using CBCT images with Mimics software.

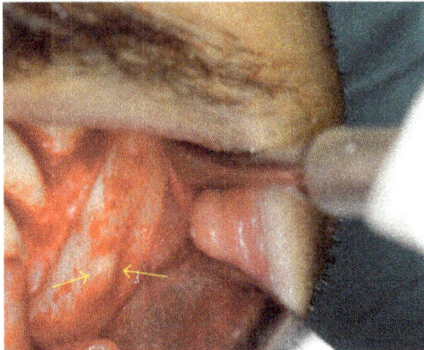

FIGURE 6: Clinical appearance of the protuberance at the mental foramen area on the left mandible.

diagnosis due to the superimposition of teeth, trabecular pattern of bone, thinning of mandible, or patient positioning and processing errors. This imaging method provided insufficient information to diagnose accurately the width and height of the bone and exact relationship with the adjacent structures especially before implant surgeries. CBCT is a more effective method that provides three-dimensional (3D) imaging and exact linear measurements for presurgical assessment, evaluation of the bone quality, and the possible anatomic variations [2]. In addition, acquisition of 3D reconstructions and use of lower radiation doses in comparison to medical CT are some of other advantages of the system [1, 6] which may play a key role in elucidating details of these normal variations [9].

There is a rare case report about absence of MF in the literature. In 2011, da Silva Ramos Fernandes et al. [1] detected unilateral absence of the MF and hypoplasia on the other side in a patient undergoing CBCT prior to orthodontic examination which was the first case in the literature of MF absence seen in CBCT images of a living patient. In 2013 Matsumoto et al. [9] reported bilateral absence of the MF, which was detected incidentally by CBCT performed prior to dental implant surgery. In most recent case reported by Lauhr et al. [2], they incidentally discovered bilateral absence of MF during CBCT examination before implant surgery. In the present case report, unilateral MF agenesis which was detected incidentally by CBCT prior to impacted teeth extraction is represented in the literature.

The reason for the absence of the MF is unclear [9]. The underlying cause seems most likely to be congenital agenesis because in all of the reported cases (including our case) no evidence of trauma existed and the mandibles were otherwise healthy with normal morphology [7]. da Silva Ramos Fernandes et al. [1] detected unilateral MF absence in female patient's mandible and then they examined her mother CBCT; there was unilateral hypoplasia of the MF; they concluded that variations of the MF may partly arise through genetic factors.

Our patient did not complain of any nerve or developmental disturbances around his mentum and lower lip. In the previously mentioned case reports none of the authors reported any innervation or vascularization disturbance [1, 9]. Therefore the authors concluded that the mental nerve and blood vessels serving the mental region might be very thin but surely present and may run with an alternative course, which could go undetected [1, 9].

Particular attention should be paid to such variations as indicated in the literature since knowledge about the morphology of the jaw and position of the mandibular foramen helps dental and oral and maxillofacial surgeons to carry out successful local anesthetic blocks and surgical procedures without postoperative complications.

Conflict of Interests

The authors have not received any funding or grant for this work from organizations or foundations. The authors declare that they have no conflict of interests.

References

[1] L. M. P. da Silva Ramos Fernandes, A. L. Á. Capelozza, and I. R. F. Rubira-Bullen, "Absence and hypoplasia of the mental foramen detected in CBCT images: a case report," *Surgical and Radiologic Anatomy*, vol. 33, no. 8, pp. 731–734, 2011.

[2] G. Lauhr, J. C. Coutant, E. Normand, M. Laurenjoye, and B. Ella, "Bilateral absence of mental foramen in a living human subject," *Surgical and Radiologic Anatomy*, vol. 37, pp. 403–405, 2015.

[3] W. Apinhasmit, D. Methathrathip, S. Chompoopong, and S. Sangvichien, "Mental foramen in Thais: an anatomical variation related to gender and side," *Surgical and Radiologic Anatomy*, vol. 28, no. 5, pp. 529–533, 2006.

[4] S. Haghanifar and M. Rokouei, "Radiographic evaluation of the mental foramen in a selected Iranian population," *Indian Journal of Dental Research*, vol. 20, no. 2, pp. 150–152, 2009.

[5] G. Greenstein and D. Tarnow, "The mental foramen and nerve: clinical and anatomical factors related to dental implant placement: a literature review," *Journal of Periodontology*, vol. 77, no. 12, pp. 1933–1943, 2006.

[6] M. Naitoh, Y. Hiraiwa, H. Aimiya, K. Gotoh, and E. Ariji, "Accessory mental foramen assessment using cone-beam computed tomography," *Oral Surgery, Oral Medicine, Oral Pathology, Oral Radiology and Endodontology*, vol. 107, no. 2, pp. 289–294, 2009.

[7] T. Hasan, M. Fauzi, and D. Hasan, "Bilateral absence of mental foramen—a rare variation postoperative," *International Journal of Anatomical Variations*, vol. 3, pp. 167–169, 2010.

[8] R. Jacobs, N. Mraiwa, D. Van Steenberghe, G. Sanderink, and M. Quirynen, "Appearance of the mandibular incisive canal on panoramic radiographs," *Surgical and Radiologic Anatomy*, vol. 26, no. 4, pp. 329–333, 2004.

[9] K. Matsumoto, M. Araki, and K. Honda, "Bilateral absence of the mental foramen detected by cone-beam computed tomography," *Oral Radiology*, vol. 29, no. 2, pp. 198–201, 2013.

[10] K. Katakami, A. Mishima, K. Shiozaki, S. Shimoda, Y. Hamada, and K. Kobayashi, "Characteristics of accessory mental foramina observed on limited cone-beam computed tomography images," *Journal of Endodontics*, vol. 34, no. 12, pp. 1441–1445, 2008.

[11] V. De Freitas, M. C. Madeira, J. L. Toledo Filho, and C. F. Chagas, "Absence of the mental foramen in dry human mandibles," *Acta Anatomica*, vol. 104, no. 3, pp. 353–355, 1979.

42

The Hybrid Aesthetic Functional (HAF) Appliance: A Less Visible Proposal for Functional Orthodontics

Christos Livas

Department of Orthodontics, University of Groningen, University Medical Center Groningen, Hanzeplein 1. Postbus 30.001, 9700 RB Groningen, The Netherlands

Correspondence should be addressed to Christos Livas; c.livas@umcg.nl

Academic Editors: G. Gómez-Moreno, M. A. de A. M. Machado, and U. Zilberman

In modern orthodontics, aesthetics appear to have a decisive influence on orthodontic appliance preferences and acceptability. This paper reports the early application of a newly emerged functional device with enhanced aesthetics in a Class II treatment. Patient perspectives and technical considerations are discussed along with recommendations for further design development. It can be assumed that the use of thermoplastic material-based appliances may meet both the therapeutic and aesthetic demands of young age groups.

1. Introduction

Contemporary orthodontic technology is undoubtedly driven by the growing interest of the public for aesthetically advanced treatment options. Reflecting this trend, alternative orthodontic systems, such as clear aligners and lingual appliances, have been perceived by patients as the most appealing in relation to different types of buccal fixed attachments [1, 2]. Acceptability and attractiveness of vacuum formed aligners were rated also high in children and adolescents and showed an increase by age evolution pattern, resembling the conclusions of adult studies [3]. Moreover, appliance nonvisibility has been attributed greater intellectual ability, a finding which, even in its extremity, may indicate the impact of orthodontic appliance design on social perceptions [2]. Clinicians are nowadays enabled to select from a wide variety of clear tray trademarks that guide gradual tooth movement by means of a series of custom-made removable devices to satisfy patient's aesthetic demands with respect to appliance appearance.

To our knowledge, up to this date, thermoplastic materials have not been engaged in the construction of functional orthopaedic devices. This article describes the design and clinical application of the prototype of the novel HAF appliance, a concept, which may bridge the gap between aesthetic preferences of young patients and hitherto dento-facial orthopaedics.

2. Appliance Design and Fabrication

As the title implies, HAF appliance is intended to integrate aesthetics in functional orthodontic therapy. It is of double plate design, consisting of thermoplastic and acrylic parts (Figure 1). The upper component is a vacuum formed plate, made of transparent hard-elastic polyethylene sheet with 2 mm-thickness, equipped with an acrylic advancement bar positioned in the anterior midpalatal region. Similarly, the lower plate is constructed by thermoplastic material of the same width that covers totally the six anterior teeth. An acrylic guidance surface is placed over the plastic coverage on the lingual surfaces of lower incisors and canines, aimed to fit the upper bar. Two-sided arms are extended from the acrylic resin body up to second molars adapted to the morphology of lingual vestibule. To obtain optimal shape matching of the opposing attachments, the working casts are mounted on a semiadjustable articulator to contact in an end-to-end relationship, previously clinically registered with a construction bite. Posterior teeth are intentionally exposed to facilitate eruption and leveling of a deep curve of Spee. White colored acrylic resin is used for the fabrication

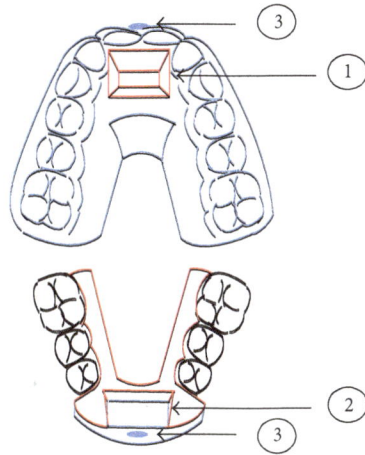

FIGURE 1: Schematic diagram of HAF appliance design. (1) Advancement bar. (2) Guiding surface. (3) Buttons (in blue ink: thermoplastic parts, in red ink: acrylic parts).

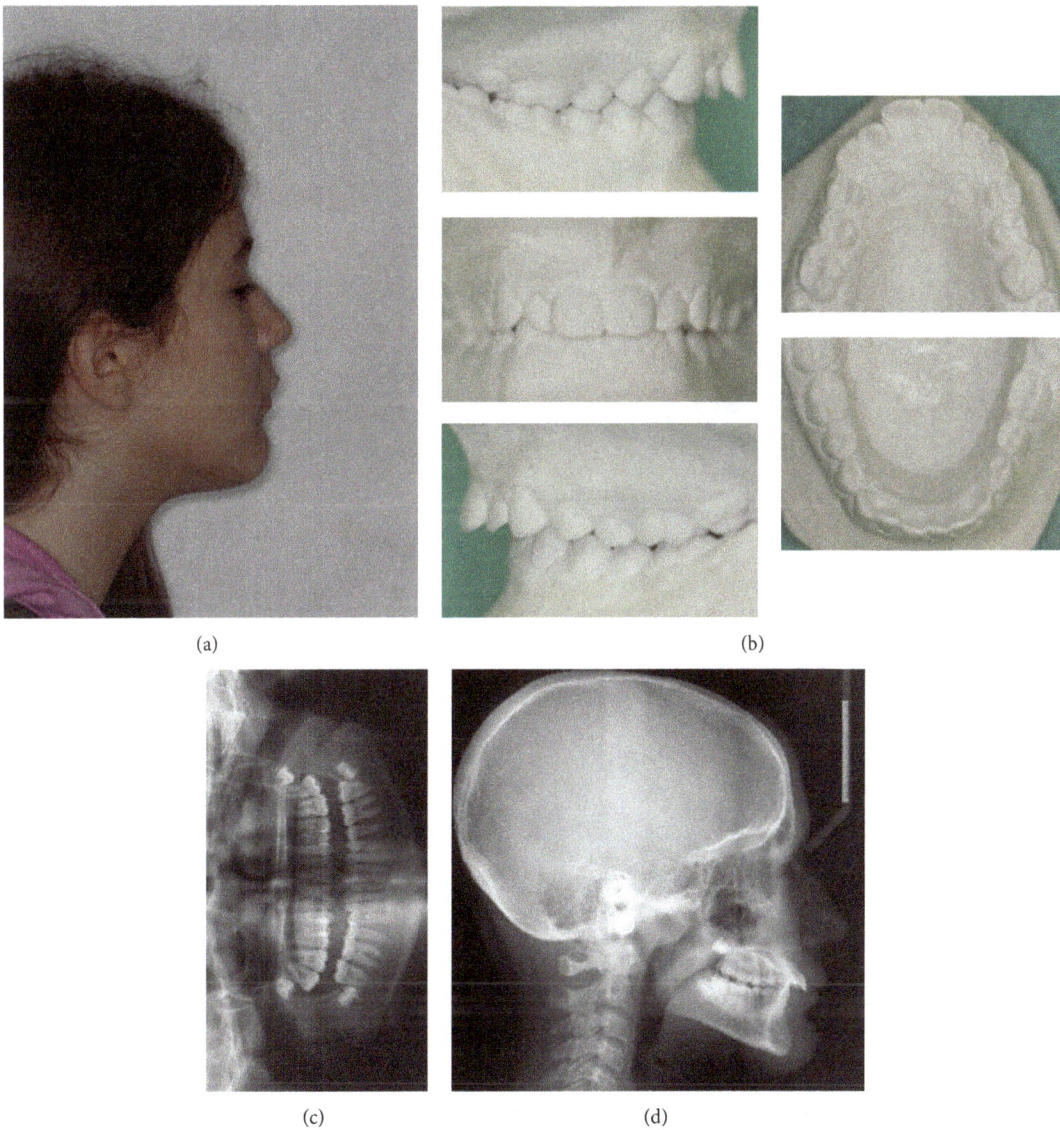

(a)   (b)

(c)   (d)

FIGURE 2: Pretreatment records: (a) extraoral profile photo, (b) dental casts, (c) panoramic radiograph, and (d) cephalometric radiograph.

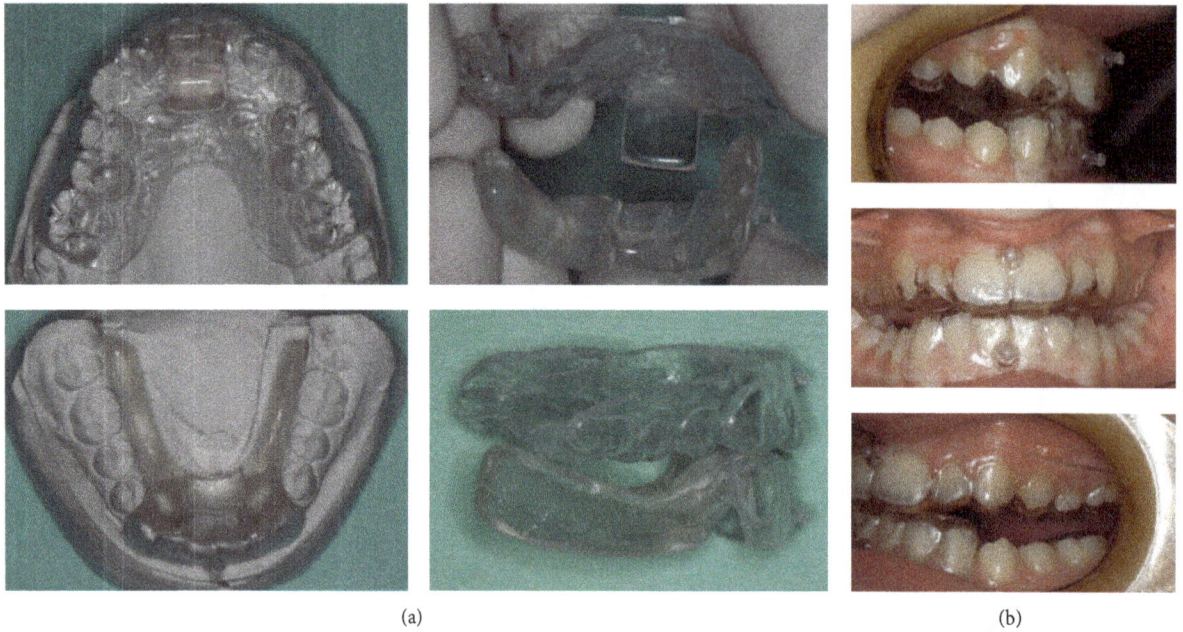

(a)   (b)

FIGURE 3: (a) Extraoral and (b) intraoral views of the HAF appliance used in this treatment.

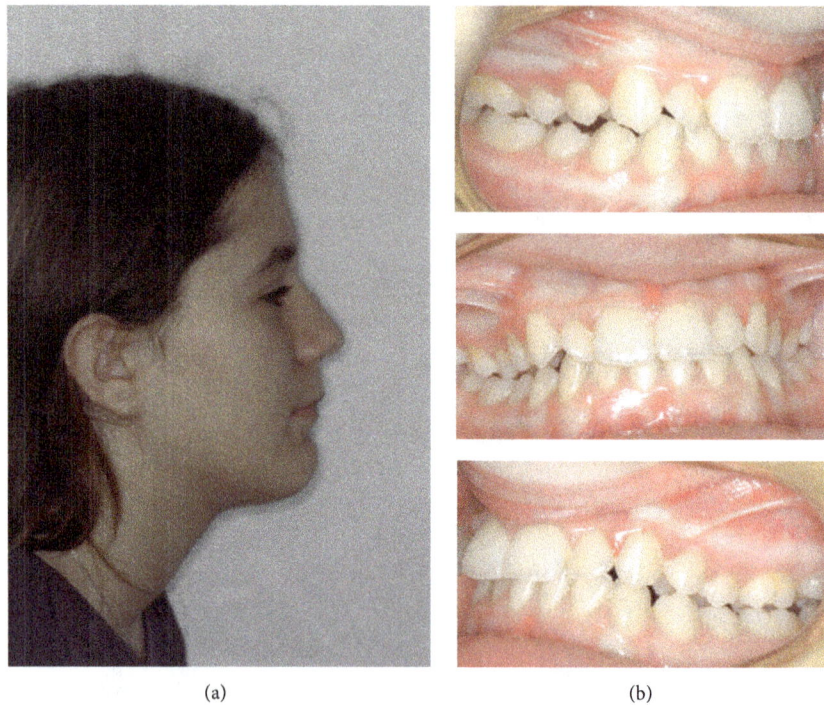

(a)   (b)

FIGURE 4: Intermediate records: (a) extraoral profile photo and (b) intraoral photos.

of acrylic parts to enhance esthetics. By means of a special plier, buttons are formed at the cervical third of upper and lower dental midlines to enable night-time wear of vertical elastics. Alternatively, light-cured composite resin combined with appropriate transparent matrices can be used for button construction.

3. Case

3.1. Diagnosis and Treatment Plan. An 11.6-year-old female was diagnosed with bilateral full cusp width Class II relationship, overjet of 11 mm, overbite of 5 mm, and mild crowded dental arches (Figure 2). Extraorally, the patient presented

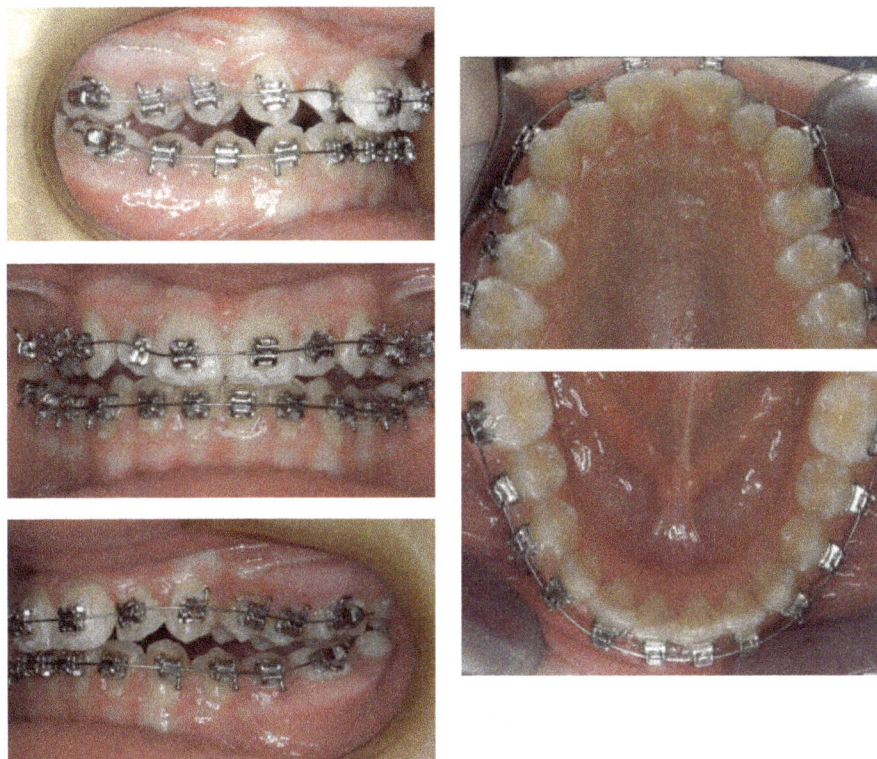

FIGURE 5: Intraoral photos with fixed appliances placed on both arches after a 10-month period in treatment.

a convex profile with slightly prominent chin. Radiographic examination revealed signs of external apical root resorption for maxillary incisors, probably due to past occlusal trauma during bruxism activity. The treatment plan included two phases, an initial functional appliance stage for sagittal correction through mandibular advancement, following by limited full fixed mechanics to establish favorable tooth alignment and intercuspation. Appointments were determined on 4-week intervals, as generally suggested for compliance-dependent appliances [4].

3.2. Treatment Progress and Results. Thorough instructions were given to the patient and her parents for appliance insertion, removal, and maintenance (Figure 3). The patient was tutored in front of a mirror to advance her mandible while closing the mouth in order to achieve matching of the acrylic surfaces. A minimum of 14 hours including bed time was prescribed for appliance wearing. Vertical intermaxillary elastic use was advised during sleeping to ensure mouth closure in the desired end-to-end relationship. Finally, the patient was asked to record herself the daily appliance wear, which was checked by the specialist at the beginning of each session.

Class I molar relationship was reached within eight months (Figure 4). Immediately after, Quick System (Forestadent, Pforzheim, Germany; http://www.forestadent.de/) self-ligating brackets (.022″ slots, Roth prescription) were bonded in the mandibular arch, while the upper plate served shortly as anterior bite plane. Eight weeks later, fixed appliances were also placed on maxillary teeth, from first molar to first molar (Figure 5). Light force application was practised throughout fixed appliance phase to prevent aggravation of root resorption [5]. Without persisting on detailed root positioning, appliances were debonded after seven months (Figure 6). Pretreatment overjet and overbite values were reduced to 4 and 2 mm, respectively. In total, the two-stage treatment lasted seventeen months. Canine-to-canine bonded flexible spiral wire lingual retainers were placed on both arches for permanent retention. Additionally, an upper Hawley type retainer with anterior bite plane was prescribed for night-time wear aiming to prevent deep bite relapse.

4. Discussion

This case report has demonstrated a successful 2-phase treatment of a Class II division 1 malocclusion including sequential use of a new "jumping the bite" device and fixed orthodontics. As indicated by the superimposition of the pre- and posttreatment cephalometric radiographs (Figure 7), the initial anteroposterior discrepancy has been corrected by treatment and growth associated effects, namely, forward and downward translation of the mandible in combination with reciprocal and opposite in direction maxillary and mandibular incisor tooth movement. Randomized clinical trials that investigated potential skeletal outcomes of various functional

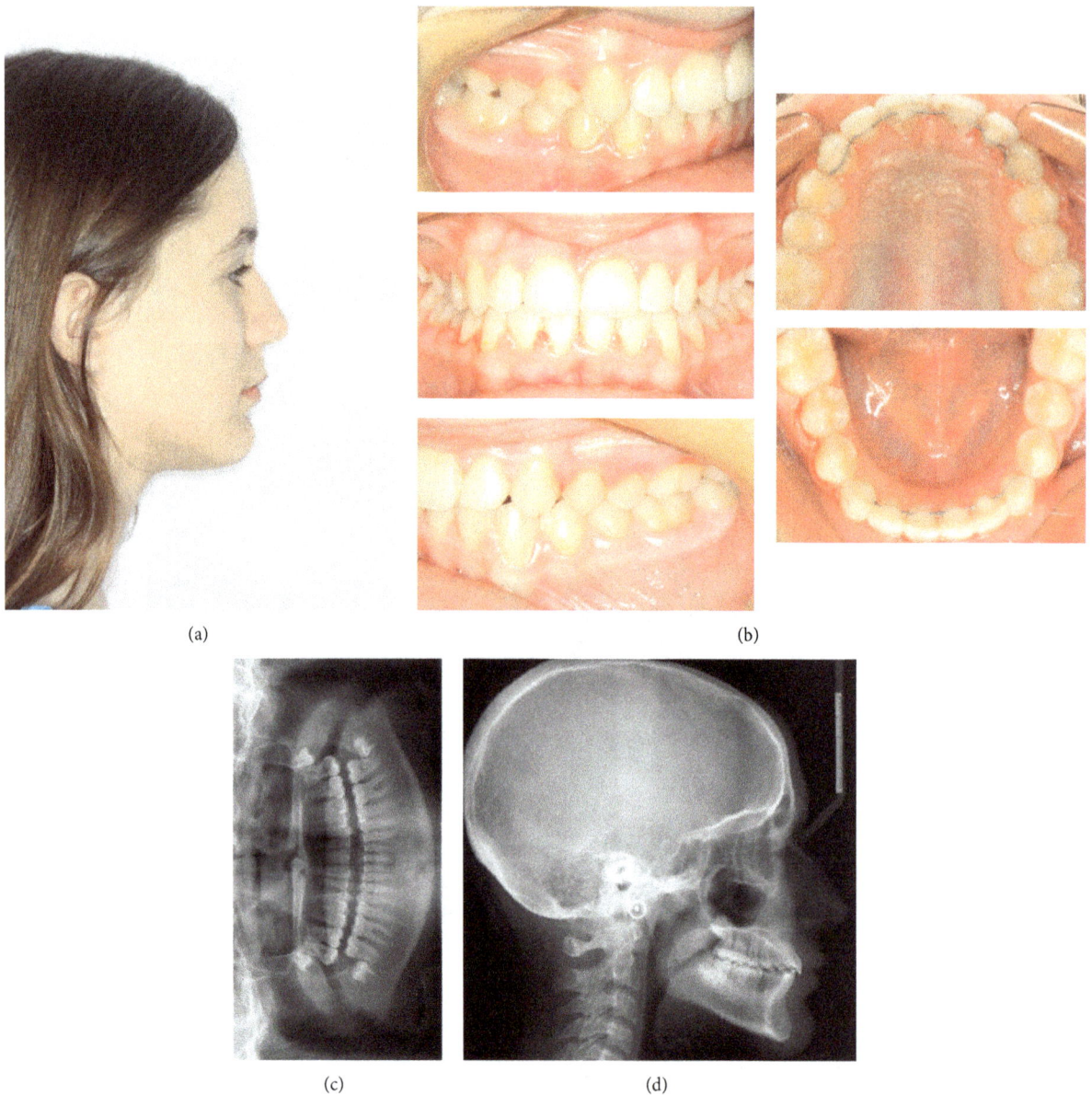

FIGURE 6: Posttreatment records: (a) extraoral profile photo, (b) dental casts, (c) panoramic radiograph, and (d) cephalometric radiograph.

appliances [6–8] demonstrated small but statistically significant differences in mandibular length and especially higher effectiveness of "jumping the bite" appliances such as Herbst and Twin-Block compared to Andresen activator and related passive devices [9].

We were motivated to devise an aesthetically attractive removable appliance with complete lack of metal parts, largely transparent appearance, diminished bulkiness to avoid patient discomfort, and relatively less demanding laboratory fabrication. Ziuchkovski et al. [1] concluded that appliance attractiveness is inversely affected by the amount of visibility of metal parts. Likewise, best accepted functional appliances have been found to be the ones with reduced acrylic coverage occupying little space intraorally. On the contrary, appliances of design and shape causing excessive

interocclusal opening with subsequent soft tissue tension and lip incompetence or constraining the tongue were the least approved [10].

Patient compliance manifested as sufficient wear time of the removable appliance is a major prerequisite for treatment success. Wear time prescription usually ranges from 13 to 16 hours per day and derives from empirical, nonevidence-based data owing to lack of objective measures and documentation. However, when it comes to real life, 8 out of 10 children may appear unwilling to extend plate use beyond night span [11]. Under such conditions, the actual wear time might decline to 9.5 hours daily and jeopardize a successful therapeutic outcome. According to the case records, the patient appeared to wear the appliance for approximately 12.5 each day, which practically proved to be sufficient to fulfill

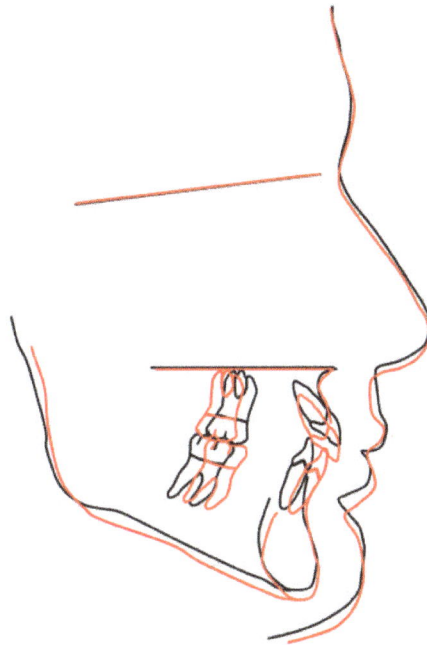

FIGURE 7: Superimposition of pre- and posttreatment cephalometric tracings.

treatment requirements. Interestingly, she found it difficult to keep the intermaxillary elastics in place while sleeping and eventually abandoned elastic use. From a technical perspective, this fact questions the number and location of buttons, or even the presence of this feature per se in prospective versions. Modifications such as extension of the plastic coverage of the lower plate in favour of retention, radical reduction of the acrylic resin, and revision of matching of anterior attachments may be as well considered.

Our initiative was to demonstrate one of our first attempts to produce a less visible and patient friendly functional device. Case reports inherently do not add rigorous scientific evidence. Thus, definite statements on the clinical performance of HAF appliance cannot be made. Overall, the development of a new appliance concept is a time-consuming process that necessitates meticulous observation and respective structural adjustment. Albeit the limited impact of our case presentation and early developmental stage of the device, HAF appliance treatment appeared to be beneficial and may deserve further research attention.

To conclude, using subsequently a novel functional device and fixed appliances, the sagittal skeletal discrepancy of a young female was corrected. Auxiliary development and clinical testing are required to augment the technical features and elucidate the treatment efficiency and effects of HAF appliance. On the whole, thermoplastic materials may be potentially utilized in the fabrication of functional orthodontic appliances.

Acknowledgment

The author wishes to thank MSgt. (DT) Panagiotis Mouratidis, laboratory technician, Department of Orthodontics, 251 Hellenic Air Force VA General Hospital, Athens, Greece, for technical support.

References

[1] J. P. Ziuchkovski, H. W. Fields, W. M. Johnston, and D. T. Lindsey, "Assessment of perceived orthodontic appliance attractiveness," *The American Journal of Orthodontics and Dentofacial Orthopedics*, vol. 133, supplement 4, pp. S68–S78, 2008.

[2] H. G. Jeremiah, D. Bister, and J. T. Newton, "Social perceptions of adults wearing orthodontic appliances: a cross-sectional study," *European Journal of Orthodontics*, vol. 33, no. 5, pp. 476–482, 2011.

[3] D. K. Walton, H. W. Fields, W. M. Johnston, S. F. Rosenstiel, A. R. Firestone, and J. C. Christensen, "Orthodontic appliance preferences of children and adolescents," *The American Journal of Orthodontics and Dentofacial Orthopedics*, vol. 138, no. 6, pp. 698.e1–698.e12, 2010.

[4] L. Jerrold and N. Naghavi, "Evidence-based considerations for determining appointment intervals," *Journal of Clinical Orthodontics*, vol. 45, no. 7, pp. 379–383, 2011.

[5] B. Weltman, K. W. L. Vig, H. W. Fields, S. Shanker, and E. E. Kaizar, "Root resorption associated with orthodontic tooth movement: a systematic review," *The American Journal of Orthodontics and Dentofacial Orthopedics*, vol. 137, no. 4, pp. 462–476, 2010.

[6] H. Pancherz, "The mechanism of Class II correction in Herbst appliance treatment. A cephalometric investigation," *The American Journal of Orthodontics*, vol. 82, no. 2, pp. 104–113, 1982.

[7] D. I. Lund and P. J. Sandler, "The effects of twin blocks: a prospective controlled study," *The American Journal of Orthodontics and Dentofacial Orthopedics*, vol. 113, no. 1, pp. 104–110, 1998.

[8] K. O'Brien, J. Wright, F. Conboy et al., "Effectiveness of early orthodontic treatment with the twin-block appliance: a multi-center, randomized, controlled trial—part 1: dental and skeletal effects," *The American Journal of Orthodontics and Dentofacial Orthopedics*, vol. 124, no. 3, pp. 234–243, 2003.

[9] M. C. Meikle, "Remodeling the dentofacial skeleton: the biological basis of orthodontics and dentofacial orthopedics," *Journal of Dental Research*, vol. 86, no. 1, pp. 12–24, 2007.

[10] H. G. Sergl and A. Zentner, "A comparative assessment of acceptance of different types of functional appliances," *European Journal of Orthodontics*, vol. 20, no. 5, pp. 517–524, 1998.

[11] T. C. Schott and G. Göz, "Young patients' attitudes toward removable appliance wear times, wear-time instructions and electronic wear-time measurements—results of a questionnaire study," *Journal of Orofacial Orthopedics*, vol. 71, no. 2, pp. 108–116, 2010.

43

A Novel Technique of Impression Procedure in a Hemimaxillectomy Patient with Microstomia

Suryakant C. Deogade

Department of Prosthodontics, Hitkarini Dental College & Hospital, Jabalpur, Madhya Pradesh 482005, India

Correspondence should be addressed to Suryakant C. Deogade, dr_deogade@yahoo.co.in

Academic Editors: T. Hata and L. Junquera

A restricted mouth opening in hemimaxillectomy patient can create a significant problem with the insertion and the removal of the obturator prosthesis. Even it poses a problem in impression making due to small oral opening. A modification of the standard impression procedure is often necessary to accomplish an acceptable impression in the fabrication of a successful prosthesis. Sectional trays are a good option for such patients. This paper describes a novel technique of impression procedure and a method of fabricating a sectional tray with the anterior and the posterior locking mechanism for a hemimaxillectomy patient with limited oral opening.

1. Introduction

Patients with extensive head and neck injuries due to trauma and/or extensive surgical procedures often exhibit a severely limited ability to open the mouth. For the dentist involved in prosthodontic treatment of such patients, restricted maximal opening commonly leads to compromised impressions and prostheses. In prosthodontic treatment, the loaded impression tray is the largest item requiring intraoral placement. During impression procedures, wide mouth opening is required for proper tray insertion and alignment. Because this is not possible in patients with restricted opening ability, a modification of the standard impression procedure is often necessary to accomplish this fundamental step in the fabrication of a successful prosthesis [1].

Microstomia is defined as an abnormally small oral orifice [2]. Other causes of microstomia are scleroderma, oral submucous fibrosis, sequelae of burns, genetic disorders, Plummer Vinson's syndrome, surgical resection of facial and oral neoplasms, and temporomandibular joint disorders [3–6]. Patients with microstomia due to pathology or extensive surgical procedures often exhibit severely limited ability to open the mouth. As the size of the oral opening decreases, the difficulty in the planned treatment procedures also increases.

The reduced mouth opening hinders conventional dental treatment; hence, alternative treatment procedures have to be chosen to overcome the clinical difficulties while managing such a patient. Several stock and custom tray designs have been described in the literature. Sectional impression trays have been fabricated using, orthodontic expansion screws [7], metal pins and acrylic resin block [8], lego blocks [9], dowel plug holes and a screw joint for rigid connection [10], locking levers [11], and interlocking tray segments [12]. Flexible impression tray with silicone putty has been also used in microstomia patient [13].

This paper presents a novel modification of previously described methods used in the fabrication of custom sectional tray with additional anterior and posterior locking mechanism by using press buttons and acrylic resin blocks. It also describes an alternative impression procedure for the prosthetic rehabilitation of a hemimaxillectomy patient with limited mouth opening.

2. Clinical Report

A 70-year-old man visited the Department of Prosthodontics, Hitkarini dental college and hospital, Jabalpur (India), for the fabrication of definitive obturator prosthesis. He

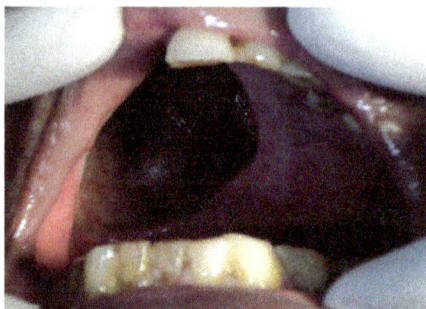

FIGURE 1: Intraoral view of defect.

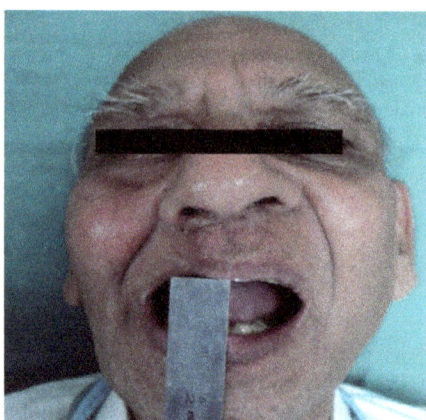

FIGURE 2: Restricted mouth opening.

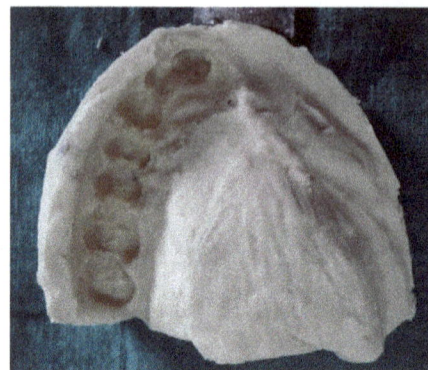

FIGURE 3: Primary impression.

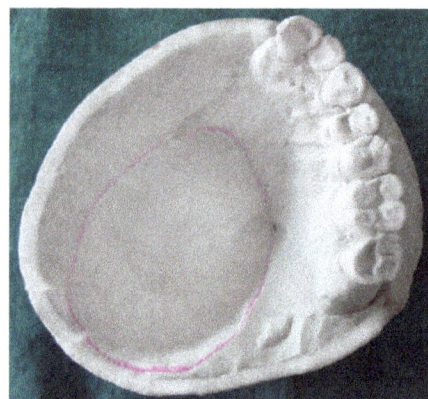

FIGURE 4: Primary cast.

underwent right hemimaxillectomy procedure to treat squamous cell carcinoma. The patient presented with an obvious and typical nasal twang, and he was experiencing difficulty in speech and deglutition.

Intraoral examination revealed a large but well-healed Armany's class I defect [14] on the right side of the maxilla along with loss of dentition on the same side (Figure 1). Patient had a severe restricted mouth opening of 18–20 mm due to postsurgical scar formation and radiation therapy (Figure 2). Hence, the decision was made to fabricate a custom sectional tray for definitive impression procedures.

3. Preliminary Impression

Because of limited mouth opening, the suitable perforated stock tray was selected whose flange on the defect side was shortened until it could be inserted in patient's mouth, and the impression was made with irreversible hydrocolloid (Dentalgin; Prime Dental Products, Mumbai, India) (Figure 3).

After retrieval of the tray, the cast was poured with type II gypsum material (Figure 4). After that, wax spacers (modeling wax; Deepti Dental Products, Ratnagiri, India) were adapted such that there were four tissue stops in each section to stabilize the tray when used in sections in maxillary arch.

4. Fabrication of Custom Sectional Tray

Acrylic resin blocks are used for the fabrication of the handle of the tray, whereas the press buttons (press button; Needle industries India Pvt. Ltd., Nilgiris, Tamilnadu) are used as the locks. Press buttons have a male and female parts (Figures 5(a), 5(b), and 5(c)). These buttons are commercially available. The handle and the press button functions as an anterior and posterior locks.

The sectional tray was designed into right and left section (Figures 6, 7, 8 and 9). These sections could be detached and then joined together in the correct original position with the help of snap fit buttons (Figures 10 and 11).

Autopolymerizing acrylic resin (DPI cold cure; Dental Products of India, Mumbai, India) was used for the fabrication of the tray. After removing the wax spacers, impressions of each half of the arches were carried out separately.

5. Definitive Impression

A medium and light viscosity poly (vinyl siloxane) elastomeric impression material (Reprosil; Dentsply DeTrey GmbH, Konstanz, Germany) is used to minimize errors due to manipulation distortion after setting. In order to make a definitive impression, and following step-by-step procedure is performed.

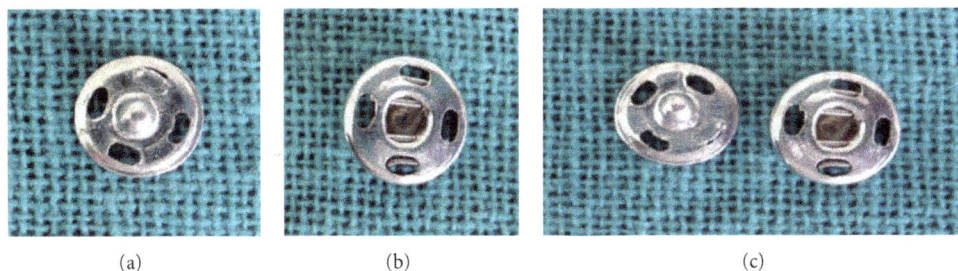

FIGURE 5: (a) Male button, (b) Female button, (c) Press button.

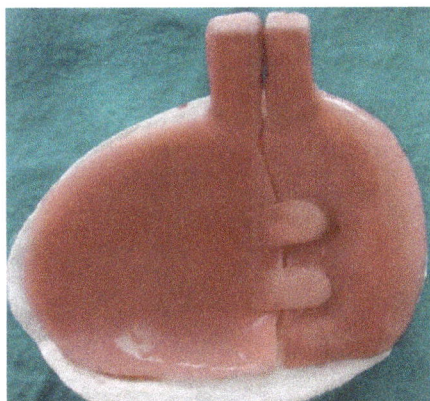

FIGURE 6: Custom sectional tray.

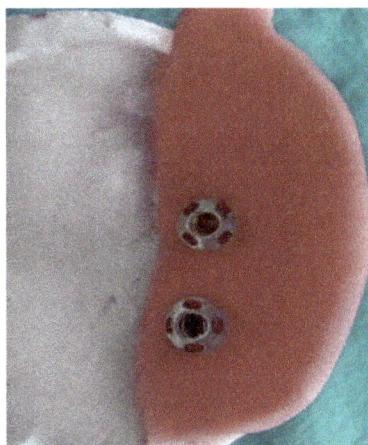

FIGURE 8: Female part.

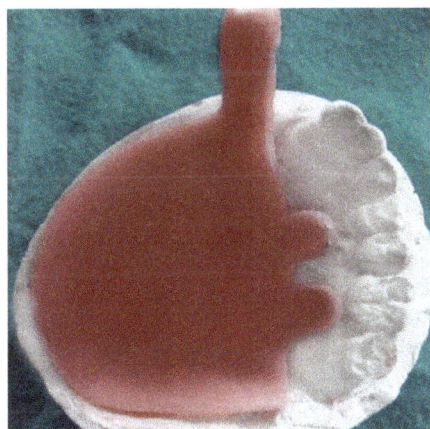

FIGURE 7: Male part.

(1) Make an impression with the first half of the tray. After removing it from the patient's mouth, trim the impression material so that it flush with the medial edge of the tray.

(2) For the parts of the impression tray or material that will contact the second half tray, lubricate them and reinsert the tray in the mouth.

(3) Load the second tray half with impression material and insert it in the mouth. Squeeze together the two tray parts at the handle. After ensuring precise fit,

snap fit buttons are pressed firmly and allow the material to set.

(4) Unpress the snap fit buttons and remove the parts individually (Figure 12).

(5) Reassemble the tray outside the mouth; sticky wax or modeling plastic may be placed across the external tray component joints to stabilize the tray assembly (Figure 13).

(6) Conventional prosthodontic protocols of boxing and pouring the impression were used with type III gypsum material (Kalstone; Kalabhai Karson, Mumbai, India) to create a definitive cast (Figure 14).

6. Discussion

The prosthodontist plays an important role in the rehabilitation of maxillofacial defects with limited mouth opening. A method of overcoming impression difficulties that uses a sectional custom impression tray that results in an accurate impression for such patients is described.

In the present case, mouth opening was about 18 mm which posed a significant problem while making impressions. The patient was treated for squamous cell carcinoma and was having the classical Armany's class I defect. As the resection bed was treated postoperatively with radiation therapy, it resulted in limited oral opening.

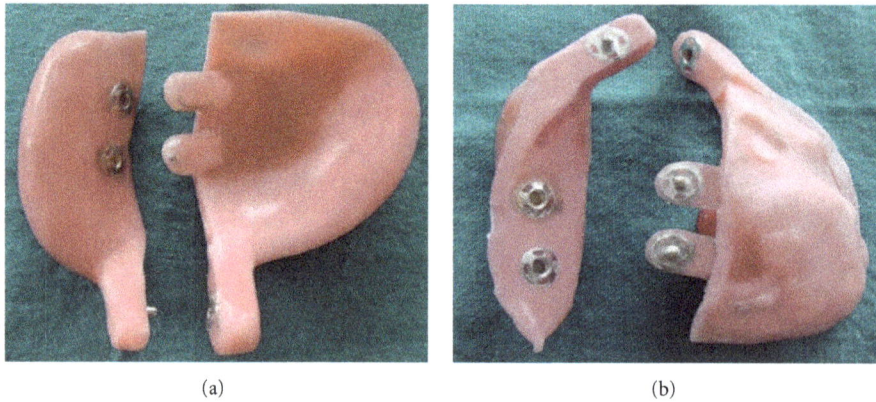

(a)

(b)

FIGURE 9: (a) and (b) Showing anterior and posterior locking mechanism.

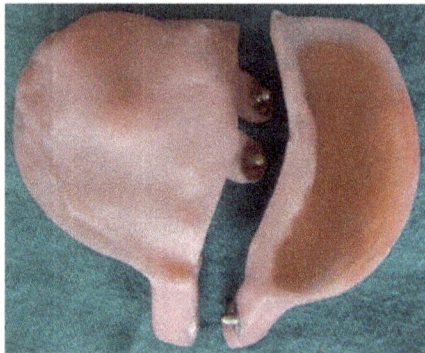

FIGURE 10: Dissembled sectional tray.

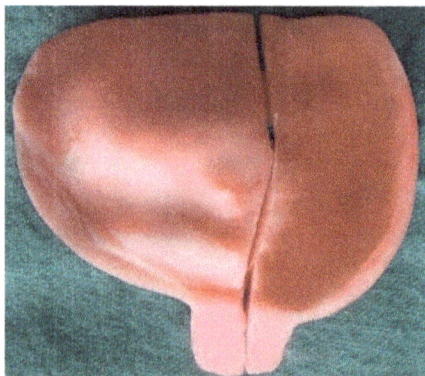

FIGURE 12: Dissembled impression.

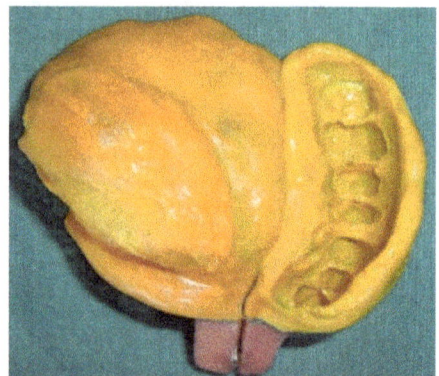

FIGURE 11: Assembled sectional tray.

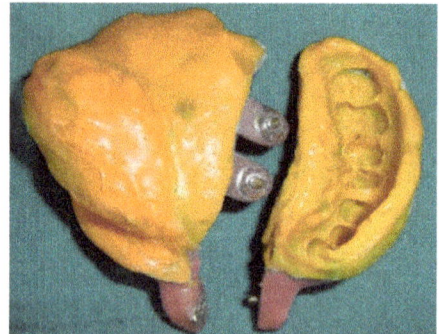

FIGURE 13: Assembled impression.

Limited mouth opening often complicates and compromises the treatment of patients. Sectional trays are an alternative treatments in such conditions [11]. One of the requirements of the sectional trays are the ease of reassembling and disassembling the tray in the mouth. This feature necessitated to incorporate an easy locking mechanism [10]. It is observed that in the absence of a posterior lock, the tray would separate in the posterior palatal seal region making the

impression difficult. This realized the need of using posterior lock in the maxillary sectional tray, as in the current design.

Hence, the decision was taken to fabricate the sectional tray with the help of readily available options like acrylic blocks and snap fit buttons. The trays could be detached and reattached again which made a very good option for the patient. Advantages of the technique include very economical simplified tray manipulation and decreased patient trauma, the ability to use a custom fabricated tray for optimal impression material thickness, and precise intraoral positioning and

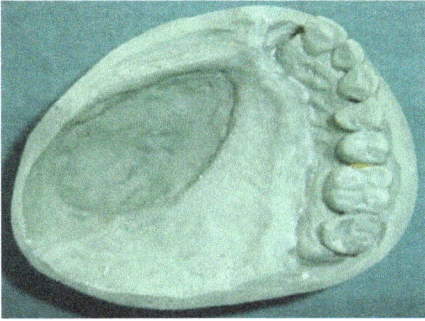

FIGURE 14: Master cast.

stability. Disadvantages are the additional time, materials, and labor required for precise fabrication of the sectional tray and secondary impression and the requirement for correct fitting of the components to produce an accurate cast.

7. Conclusion

Restricted mouth opening in hemimaxillectomy patients is a common scenario due to postsurgical scar formation and radiation therapy. Making good impressions is an important step in prosthodontic management of such patients. Keeping this in mind, we have to modify the routinely used trays and provide newly designed trays for ease and betterment. This paper describes very simple, quick, economical, and readily available methods of dealing with patients in whom placement of full size impression tray is hindered by microstomia.

Alignment and stability of a reassembled sectional tray is necessary, and it can be achieved by using an anterior and posterior lock. These features are present in the current design that helps to overcome difficulties while making impressions in such patients.

References

[1] P. S. Baker, R. L. Brandt, and G. Boyajian, "Impression procedure for patients with severely limited mouth opening," *Journal of Prosthetic Dentistry*, vol. 84, no. 2, pp. 241–244, 2000.

[2] "The glossary of prosthodontic terms," *Journal of Prosthetic Dentistry*, vol. 94, pp. 10–92, 2005.

[3] W. D. Martins, F. H. Westphalen, and V. P. Westphalen, "Microstomia caused by swallowing of caustic soda: report of a case," *The Journal of Contemporary Dental Practice*, vol. 4, no. 4, pp. 91–99, 2003.

[4] C. Seel, H. D. Hager, A. Jauch, G. Tariverdian, and J. Zschocke, "Survival up to age 10 years in a patient with partial duplication 6q: case report and review of the literature," *Clinical Dysmorphology*, vol. 14, no. 1, pp. 51–54, 2005.

[5] M. De Benedittis, M. Petruzzi, G. Favia, and R. Serpico, "Oro-dental manifestations in Hallopeau-Siemens-type recessive dystrophic epidermolysis bullosa," *Clinical and Experimental Dermatology*, vol. 29, no. 2, pp. 128–132, 2004.

[6] G. Aren, Z. Yurdabakan, and I. Özcan, "Freeman-Sheldon syndrome: a case report," *Quintessence International*, vol. 34, no. 4, pp. 307–310, 2003.

[7] A. Mirfazaelian, "Use of orthodontic expansion screw in fabricating section custom trays," *Journal of Prosthetic Dentistry*, vol. 83, no. 3, pp. 474–475, 2000.

[8] C. Cura, H. S. Cotert, and A. User, "Fabrication of a sectional impression tray and sectional complete denture for a patient with microstomia and trismus: a clinical report," *Journal of Prosthetic Dentistry*, vol. 89, no. 6, pp. 540–543, 2003.

[9] R. J. Luebke, "Sectional impression tray for patients with constricted oral opening," *The Journal of Prosthetic Dentistry*, vol. 52, no. 1, pp. 135–137, 1984.

[10] O. C. Chikahiro, O. Chika, T. Hosoi, and K. S. Kurtz, "A sectional stock tray system for making impressions," *Journal of Prosthetic Dentistry*, vol. 90, no. 2, pp. 201–204, 2003.

[11] P. S. Baker, R. L. Brandt, and G. Boyajian, "Impression procedure for patients with severely limited mouth opening," *Journal of Prosthetic Dentistry*, vol. 84, no. 2, pp. 241–244, 2000.

[12] S. Winkler, P. Wongthai, and J. T. Wazney, "An improved split-denture technique," *The Journal of Prosthetic Dentistry*, vol. 51, no. 2, pp. 276–279, 1984.

[13] J. A. Whitsitt and L. W. Battle, "Technique for making flexible impression trays for the microstomic patient," *The Journal of Prosthetic Dentistry*, vol. 52, no. 4, pp. 608–609, 1984.

[14] M. A. Aramany, "Basic principles of obturator design for partially edentulous patients. Part I: classification," *The Journal of Prosthetic Dentistry*, vol. 40, no. 5, pp. 554–557, 1978.

44

Unilateral Maxillary First Molar Extraction in Class II Subdivision: An Unconventional Treatment Alternative

J. W. Booij[1] and Christos Livas[2]

[1]*Private Practice, Schelluinsevliet 5, 4203 NB Gorinchem, Netherlands*
[2]*Department of Orthodontics, University of Groningen, University Medical Center Groningen, Hanzeplein 1,*
 Triadegebouw, Ingang 24, 9700 RB Groningen, Netherlands

Correspondence should be addressed to Christos Livas; c.livas@umcg.nl

Academic Editor: Gilberto Sammartino

The asymmetrical intra-arch relationship in Class II subdivision malocclusion poses challenges in the treatment planning and mechanotherapy of such cases. This case report demonstrates a treatment technique engaging unilateral extraction of a maxillary first molar and Begg fixed appliances. The outcome stability and the enhancing effect on the eruption of the third molar in the extraction segment were confirmed by a 4-year follow-up examination.

1. Introduction

Class II subdivision malocclusion is a dentofacial deformity, estimated to account for up to 50% of Class II malocclusions [1]. It possesses characteristics of both Class I and Class II malocclusion resulting in asymmetry between the right and the left sides of the dentition. Depending on the location of asymmetry, unilateral mechanics is performed to achieve distalization of the mesially positioned maxillary first molar or protraction of the opposing segment. Asymmetrical headgear, coil springs coupled with Class II elastics or TADs [2], fixed functional appliances [3], or asymmetrical premolar extraction patterns [4, 5] are commonly applied in growing patients to correct the Class II occlusion on the affected side.

A less typical treatment strategy combining single extraction of a maxillary first molar and Begg light-wire appliances showed favourable outcomes in terms of occlusion, facial profile, and midline esthetics on average in 2.5 years after appliance removal [6].

This case report describes the orthodontic management of a Class II subdivision patient treated with the abovementioned protocol.

2. Case Report

A 14-year-old female was diagnosed with Class II subdivision malocclusion on the right side and a maxillary-to-facial midline discrepancy of 2 mm (Figures 1 and 2). During the intake, the patient expressed her concerns in complying with extraoral anchorage devices, cumbersome orthodontic accessories, or intermaxillary elastics for a long period. Clinical examination revealed fully erupted maxillary second molars and persistent 55, 74, and 75. With the exception of 48, no tooth agenesis was confirmed by the orthopantomogram (Figure 3). To meet the patient's demands, extraction of the right maxillary first molar was proposed instead.

Before extracting 16 and persistent deciduous molars, bands with 6 mm single 0.022-inch round buccal tubes and palatal sheaths were placed on 17 and 26. After a healing period of 3 weeks, Begg brackets were placed on the anterior maxillary and mandibular teeth. To prevent second molar rotation, a transpalatal arch (TPA) was inserted. Second molar anchorage was reinforced by anchor bends on a customized 0.016-inch premium plus pull-straightened Australian archwire (Wilcock, Whittlesea, Australia) mesial of

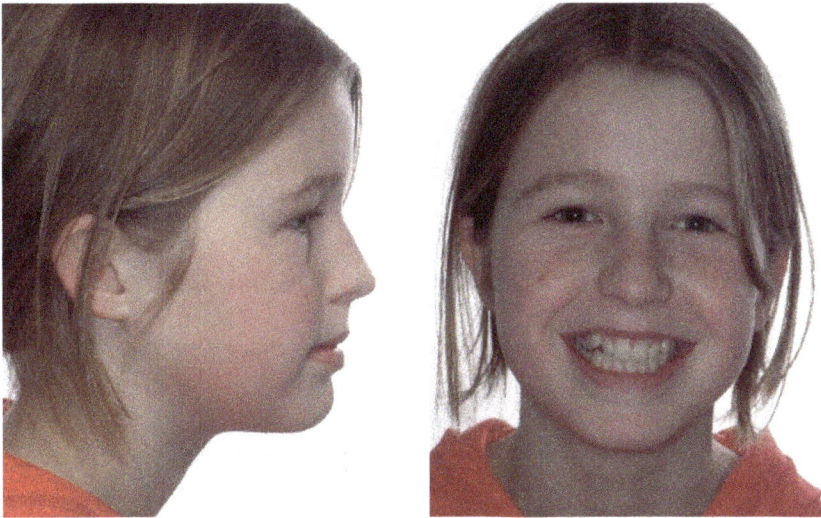

FIGURE 1: Pretreatment extraoral photographs.

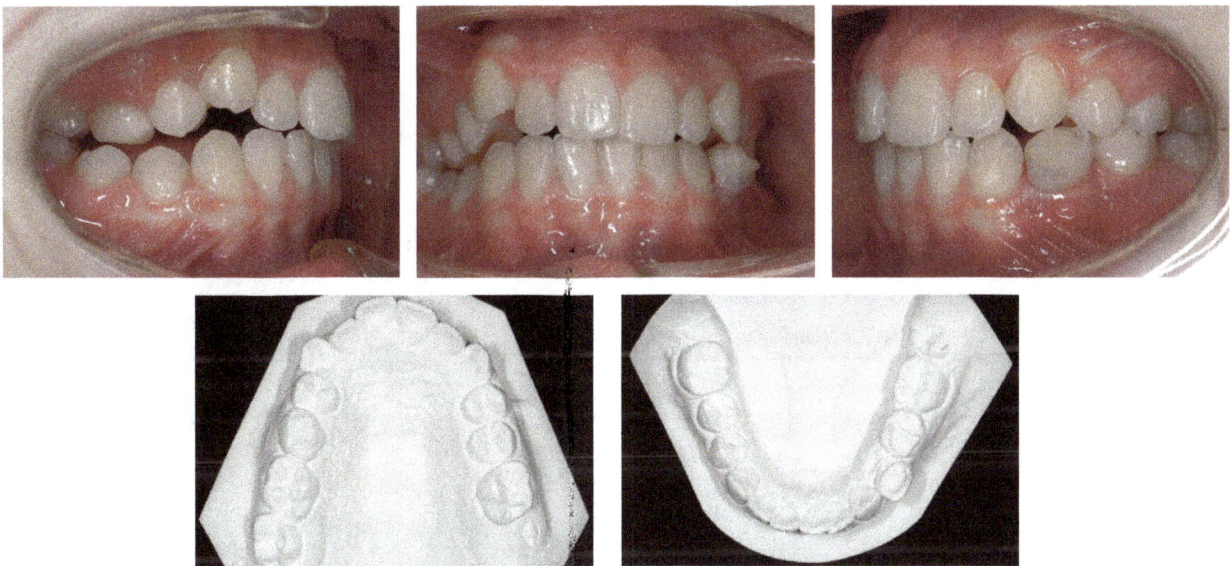

FIGURE 2: Pretreatment intraoral photographs and study casts (occlusal view).

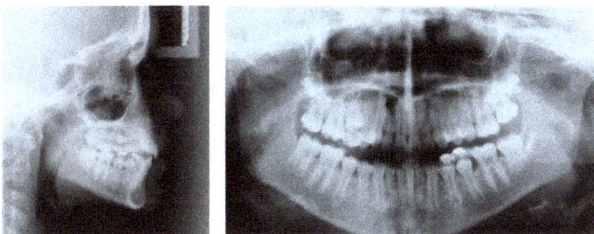

FIGURE 3: Pretreatment radiographs.

the molar tube to counteract unwanted mesial movement of 16 into the extraction space (Figure 4(a)). High hat lock pins (TP Orthodontics, Westville, IN, USA) were placed on maxillary canines and partially bent mesially to receive light 8 mm horizontal elastics (5/16 inches) on the Class II buccal segment extending to the buccal hook on the maxillary second molar band (Figures 4(a)–4(c)). The patient was instructed to replace the Class I elastics on a weekly basis. By bending circle-shaped loops mesial to the canine brackets, controlled retraction of the anterior teeth was achieved. Visits were scheduled 6- to 8-week intervals. The initially malpositioned 12 was engaged to the archwire until adequate space had been created by canine distalization (Figures 4(b) and 4(c)). After 6 months, Class I premolar occlusion was achieved, the premolars were also bonded with light-wire brackets, and Class II elastic wear was instructed for night-time. After alignment of the maxillary premolars, the 0.016-inch starting wire was replaced by a 0.018-inch premium

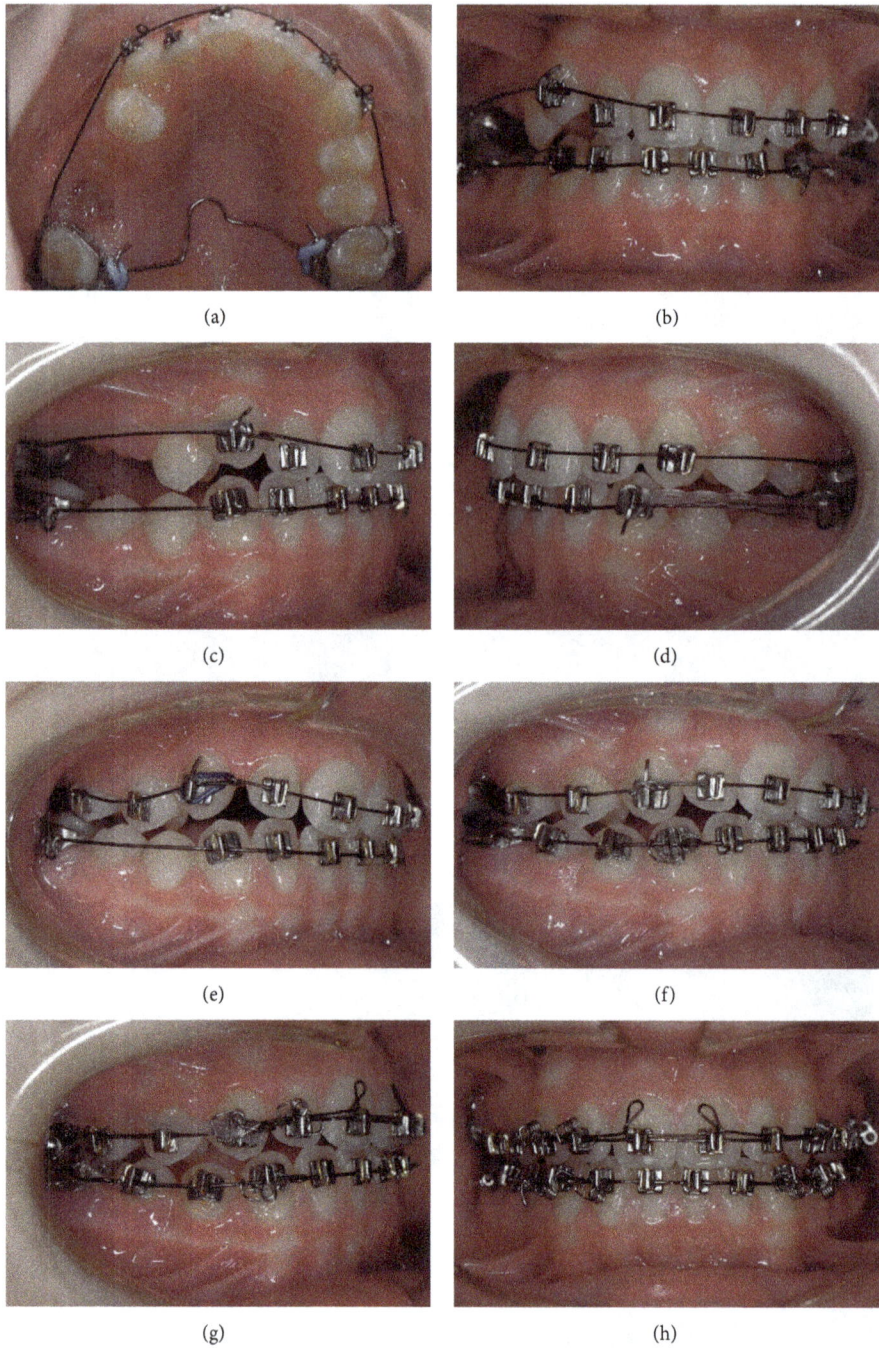

(a)

(b)

(c)

(d)

(e)

(f)

(g)

(h)

FIGURE 4: (a–d) Class II correction on the right side using TPA anchorage and horizontal elastics. In this phase, premolars were not bonded to facilitate sliding mechanics. (e-f) After achieving Class I premolar relationship, the remaining teeth were bonded. (g) Space closure with elastic power chain. (g, h) Torque correction by means of a customized two-spur torque auxiliary of 0.014-inch regular wire and uprighting springs on the maxillary canine brackets.

plus archwire (Wilcock). Additionally, an individual two-spur torque auxiliary of 0.014-inch regular wire (Wilcock) was inserted in the anterior maxillary region to produce proper palatal root torque. For the same reason, uprighting springs (TP, La Porte, Indiana, USA) were fixed in the vertical slots of the canine brackets (Figures 4(g) and 4(h)). Closure of

the residual extraction spaces in the maxillary right buccal segment was carried out with elastic power chains. In the final treatment stage, adjustments were made in the archwires and uprighting springs independently for each tooth for detailed finishing. Completing treatment, canine-to-canine retainers made of multistranded wire were bonded in both arches.

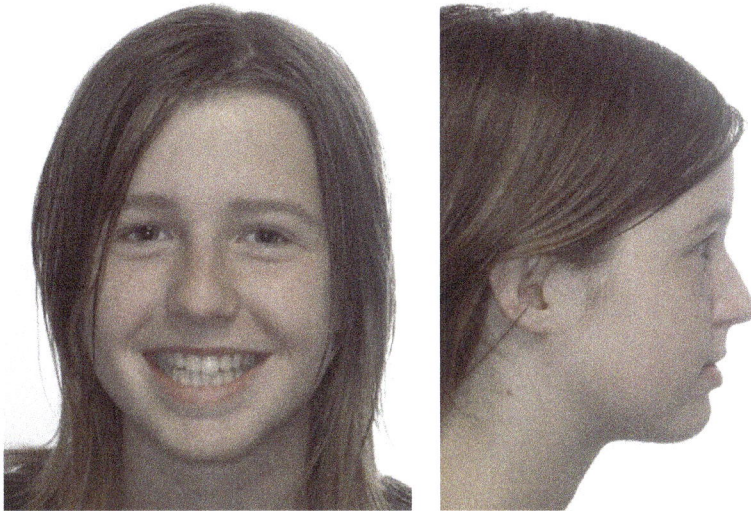

FIGURE 5: Posttreatment extraoral photographs.

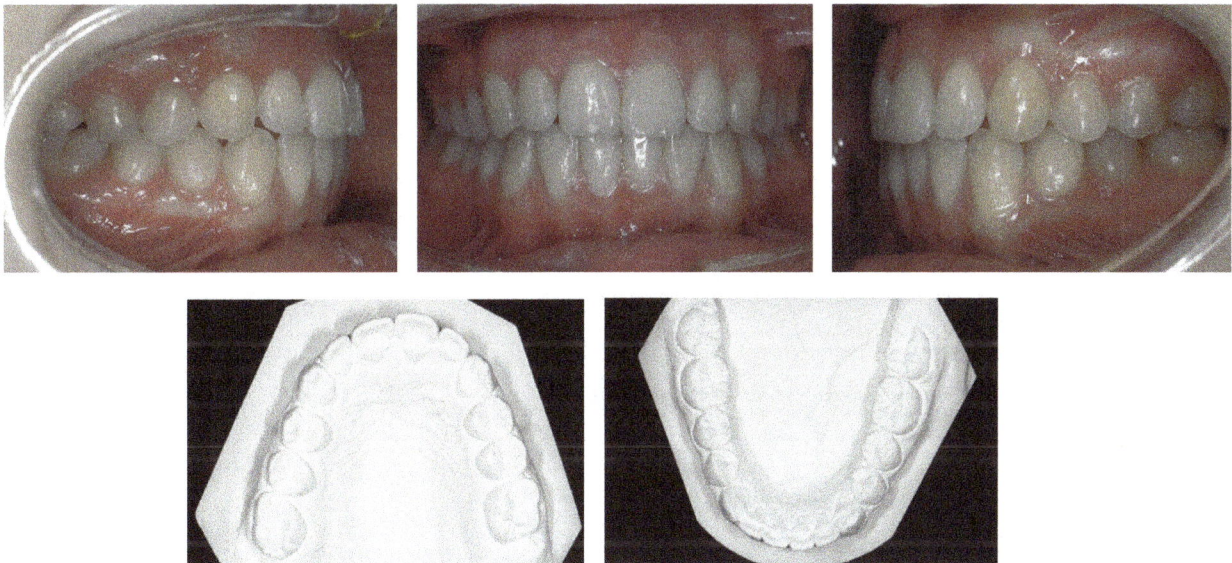

FIGURE 6: Posttreatment intraoral photographs and study casts (occlusal view).

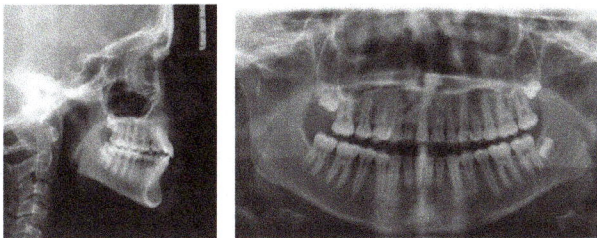

FIGURE 7: Posttreatment radiographs.

The active treatment lasted 26 months. Class I occlusion, tooth alignment, and midline correction were maintained for 4 years after appliance removal (Figures 6 and 9). Anterior

tooth retraction did not compromise the soft tissue profile (Figures 5 and 8). Eruption of 18 was accelerated reaching occlusal contact with the antagonist, while the contralateral molar remained unerupted (Figures 7 and 10).

3. Discussion

Our Class II subdivision technique led to good occlusal and esthetic outcomes, which were preserved for 4 years after active treatment had been completed. Besides stable end results in the long term [6], a positive effect on the axial inclination of maxillary third molars was demonstrated in Class II subdivision cases treated with unilateral maxillary first molar extraction and low friction fixed appliances [7]. Maxillary third molars in the extraction side became 3.1–3.4

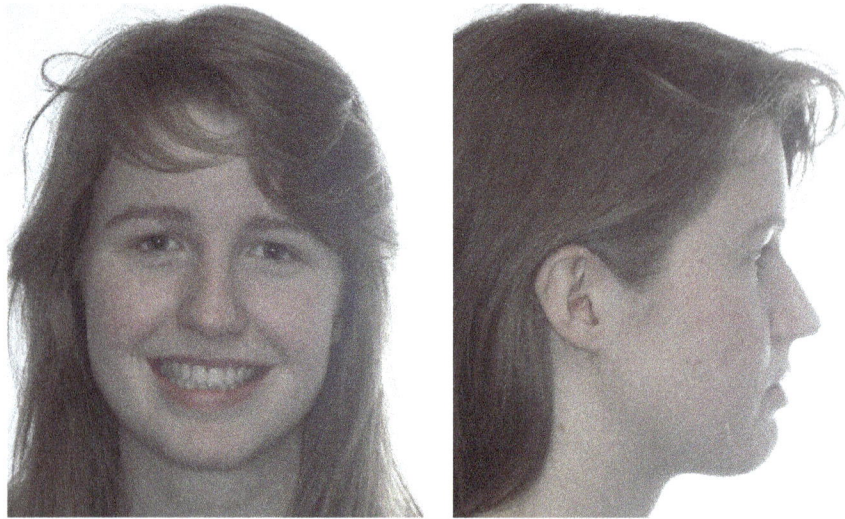

FIGURE 8: Four-year follow-up extraoral photographs.

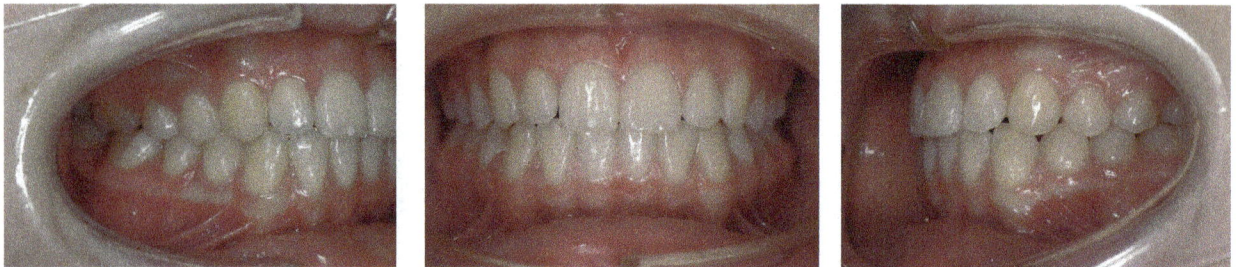

FIGURE 9: Four-year follow-up intraoral photographs.

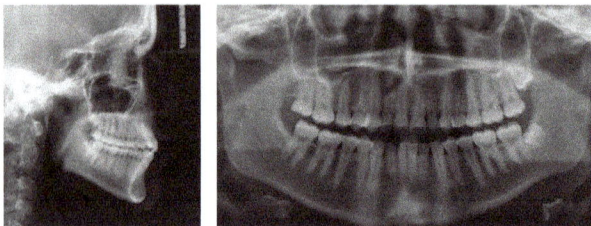

FIGURE 10: Four-year follow-up radiographs.

times more upright than the contralateral teeth [7]. Likewise in this case report, eruption of the maxillary third molar in the extraction segment was strikingly enhanced.

Patient cooperation was restricted to oral hygiene measures and once-per-week replacement of elastics, which may render this method suitable for patients with poor compliance [8]. Modification of this treatment method with bilateral extraction of maxillary first molars has been previously described as "less-compliance therapy" [8].

Longer treatment duration has been observed in asymmetric premolar extraction protocols [4, 5] compared to orthodontic therapy with either unilateral maxillary first molar extraction [6] or Herbst and fixed appliances [3].

Nonetheless, with respect to the end molar occlusion, Class III in the original Class I side may be expected in Class II subdivision patients treated with fixed functional appliances [3].

Without doubt, the popularity of Begg or similar techniques declined dramatically during the last 30 years [9]. However, orthodontic mechanics including application of light elastic forces, anchorage bends, or delayed bonding of premolars during space closure may be integrated in the philosophy of contemporary straight-wire techniques.

Premolar extraction schemes are prescribed by orthodontists in the United States in 85% of extraction cases [9]. From the ethical point of view, a decision to electively extract healthy premolar teeth for orthodontic purposes may not be warranted in cases with compromised first molars. As a general rule, presence of extensive caries lesions, large restorations, endodontic or periodontal problems, or hypoplastic enamel should be taken into account when extraction treatment has been chosen. The first permanent molar has the shortest caries-free survival under the age of 8 years [10]. It also represents the most caries prone tooth in children older than 11 years [11]. In addition to this, first molars can suffer from developmental enamel hypomineralisation of unknown aetiology often affecting permanent incisors. Lately published rates vary between 4.2 and 21.4% depending on the country and examination method [12–14]. Prognosis of endodontics in multirooted teeth may be also questionable. In this context, the first molar has been reported as the most commonly extracted tooth due to endodontic complications [15]. Under such circumstances and in presence of fully erupted maxillary second molars, well-formed third molar at the Class II buccal segment, maxillary dental asymmetry, and fairly aligned mandibular arch, extraction of a maxillary first molar may be a viable option in treating asymmetrical Class II malocclusion cases.

4. Conclusion

This 4-year follow-up case report indicates that unilateral extraction of a maxillary first molar in selected cases might be a rewarding treatment alternative in Class II subdivision subjects and especially in those with compliance issues.

Competing Interests

The authors declare that they have no competing interests.

References

[1] D. A. Sanders, P. H. Rigali, W. P. Neace, F. Uribe, and R. Nanda, "Skeletal and dental asymmetries in Class II subdivision malocclusions using cone-beam computed tomography," *American Journal of Orthodontics and Dentofacial Orthopedics*, vol. 138, no. 5, pp. 542.e1–542.e20, 2010.

[2] C. Livas, "Mini-implant anchorage in a unilateral Class II patient," *Journal of Clinical Orthodontics*, vol. 46, no. 5, pp. 293–298, 2012.

[3] N. C. Bock, B. Reiser, and S. Ruf, "Class II subdivision treatment with the Herbst appliance," *The Angle Orthodontist*, vol. 83, no. 2, pp. 327–333, 2013.

[4] G. Janson, E. A. Dainesi, J. F. C. Henriques, M. R. de Freitas, and K. J. R. S. de Lima, "Class II subdivision treatment success rate with symmetric and asymmetric extraction protocols," *American Journal of Orthodontics and Dentofacial Orthopedics*, vol. 124, no. 3, pp. 257–264, 2003.

[5] G. Janson, N. C. Branco, J. F. Morais, and M. R. Freitas, "Smile attractiveness in patients with Class II division 1 subdivision malocclusions treated with different tooth extraction protocols," *European Journal of Orthodontics*, vol. 36, no. 1, pp. 1–8, 2014.

[6] C. Livas, N. Pandis, J. W. Booij, C. Katsaros, and Y. Ren, "Long-term evaluation of Class II subdivision treatment with unilateral maxillary first molar extraction," *The Angle Orthodontist*, vol. 85, no. 5, pp. 757–763, 2015.

[7] C. Livas, N. Pandis, J. W. Booij, D. J. Halazonetis, C. Katsaros, and Y. Ren, "Influence of unilateral maxillary first molar extraction treatment on second and third molar inclination in Class II subdivision patients," *The Angle Orthodontist*, vol. 86, no. 1, pp. 94–100, 2016.

[8] J. W. Booij, A. M. Kuijpers-Jagtman, and C. Katsaros, "A treatment method for Class II division 1 patients with extraction of permanent maxillary first molars," *World Journal of Orthodontics*, vol. 10, no. 1, pp. 41–48, 2009.

[9] R. G. Keim, E. L. Gottlieb, D. S. Vogels, and P. B. Vogels, "2014 JCO study of orthodontic diagnosis and treatment procedures. Part 1. results and trends," *Journal of Clinical Orthodontics*, vol. 48, no. 10, pp. 607–630, 2014.

[10] J. E. Todd and T. Dodd, "Children's dental health in the United Kingdom 1983: a survey carried out by the social survey division of OPCS, On behalf of the United Kingdom health departments," in *Collaboration with the Dental Schools of the Universities of Birmingham and Newcastle Editions*, Stationery Office, 1st edition, 1985.

[11] J. Suni, H. Vähänikkilä, J. Päkkilä, L. Tjäderhane, and M. Larmas, "Review of 36,537 patient records for tooth health and longevity of dental restorations," *Caries Research*, vol. 47, no. 4, pp. 309–317, 2013.

[12] R. Balmer, J. Toumba, J. Godson, and M. Duggal, "The prevalence of molar incisor hypomineralisation in Northern England and its relationship to socioeconomic status and water fluoridation," *International Journal of Paediatric Dentistry*, vol. 22, no. 4, pp. 250–257, 2012.

[13] T. P. Martínez Gómez, F. Guinot Jimeno, L. J. Bellet Dalmau, and L. Giner Tarrida, "Prevalence of molar-incisor hypomineralisation observed using transillumination in a group of children from Barcelona (Spain)," *International Journal of Paediatric Dentistry*, vol. 22, no. 2, pp. 100–109, 2012.

[14] M. Grošelj and J. Jan, "Molar incisor hypomineralisation and dental caries among children in Slovenia," *European Journal of Paediatric Dentistry*, vol. 14, no. 3, pp. 241–245, 2013.

[15] N. E. Tzimpoulas, M. G. Alisafis, G. N. Tzanetakis, and E. G. Kontakiotis, "A prospective study of the extraction and retention incidence of endodontically treated teeth with uncertain prognosis after endodontic referral," *Journal of Endodontics*, vol. 38, no. 10, pp. 1326–1329, 2012.

45

Cone Beam Computed Tomographic Evaluation and Diagnosis of Mandibular First Molar with 6 Canals

Shiraz Pasha, Bathula Vimala Chaitanya, and Kusum Valli Somisetty

Department of Conservative Dentistry and Endodontics, Sri Rajiv Gandhi College of Dental Sciences, Bangalore 560032, India

Correspondence should be addressed to Bathula Vimala Chaitanya; dr.vimalayashwanth@gmail.com

Academic Editor: Luis M. J. Gutierrez

Root canal treatment of tooth with aberrant root canal morphology is very challenging. So thorough knowledge of both the external and internal anatomy of teeth is an important aspect of root canal treatment. With the advancement in technology it is imperative to use modern diagnostic tools such as magnification devices, CBCT, microscopes, and RVG to confirm the presence of these aberrant configurations. However, in everyday endodontic practice, clinicians have to treat teeth with atypical configurations for root canal treatment to be successful. This case report presents the management of a mandibular first molar with six root canals, four in mesial and two in distal root, and also emphasizes the use and importance of Cone Beam Computed Tomography (CBCT) as a diagnostic tool in endodontics.

1. Introduction

Precise study of the morphology of human teeth is required for the successful treatment with the objective of providing better oral health and restoring stomatognathic functions [1]. The mandibular first molar usually has 2 roots, occasionally 3. Further, there are generally 2 canals in the mesial root and one or 2 in the distal root. Vertucci and Williams [2] were the first persons to report the presence of middle mesial canal in the mandibular 1st molar and since then there were many case reports published showing the presence of mandibular molars with aberrant root canal morphology. In a radiographic study of extracted teeth Goel et al. reported that mandibular first molars had three mesial canals in 13.3% of specimens, four mesial canals in 3.3% specimens, and three distal canals in 1.7% of specimens [3]. It has been postulated that secondary dentin apposition during tooth maturation would form dentinal vertical partitions inside the root canal cavity creating root canals and the third root canal is also created by this process. Such third canals are situated mainly between the two main root canals, the buccal and lingual root canals [4].

This case report presents the management of the 1st mandibular molar with six root canals, four in mesial and two in distal root canal confirmed by CBCT.

2. Case Presentation

A 30-year-old male patient with nonsignificant medical history reported to our department with a chief complaint of pain in right mandibular region. On history taking there were episodes of intermittent pain for the past 15 days. Pain was moderate in nature, nonradiating, aggravates on taking sweets and chewing foods, and relieves on taking medication. On clinical examination a deep carious lesion was seen with respect to 46. Exaggerated response was observed during pulp testing with electric pulp tester and lingering pain was observed with cold pulp test compared to contralateral teeth. IOPAR revealed radiolucency involving enamel, dentin, and pulp with no periapical changes in relation to 46 (Figure 1). It was diagnosed as acute irreversible pulpitis. Root canal treatment was decided and explained to the patient. After securing local anesthesia (2% lignocaine, inferior alveolar

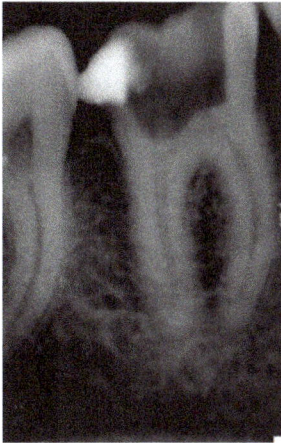

FIGURE 1: Pre-op X-ray.

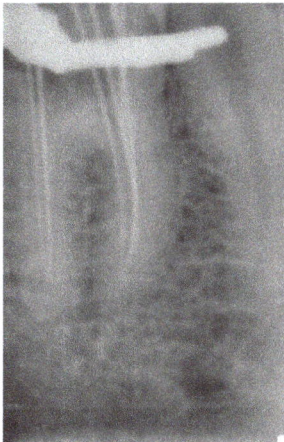

FIGURE 2: IOPA showing 4 mesial canals.

nerve block on the right side) rubber dam was applied and endodontic treatment was initiated. After gaining the proper access four canals were located, two in the mesial and two in the distal. It was evident under magnification that the MB and ML were placed well apart with an isthmus joining two canals. Hence, the possibility of MM canal should be anticipated in the isthmus. On exploration with DG-16 probe, we found 2 additional canals between MB and ML (Figure 5). IOPAR revealed one MM joining the MB canal and another joining the ML canal in the middle third. To confirm this we advised a CBCT of the right mandibular molar. CBCT revealed four canals in the mesial root and two canals in distal root (Figures 3 and 4). Access was refined and orifices were enlarged using orifice openers. The working length was determined with radiographic technique and apex locator (Figure 2). Both the mesial and distal canals were enlarged up to the size of 25/6% taper (M two, VDW) followed by an intracanal medication with calcium hydroxide and chlorhexidine was placed for 1 week. At the 3rd appointment, master cone was selected (Figure 6) and obturation was performed using cold

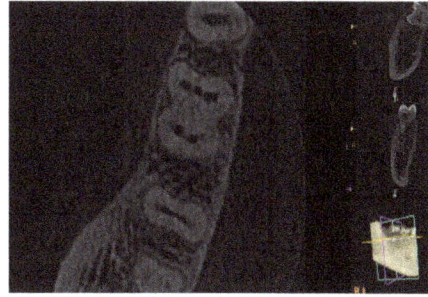

FIGURE 3: CBCT image showing 4 canals in mesial root.

lateral compaction technique and AH-plus root canal sealer. Figure 7 shows the IOPAR immediately after obturation.

3. Discussion

The complicated and diverse root canal system poses a challenge to successful diagnosis and treatment. The incidence rates of MM canal are between 1 and 15% [5]. In most of the cases, middle/extra canals are hidden by a dentinal projection in the mesial and distal aspect of pulp chamber walls, and this dentinal growth is usually located between the two main canals. Pomeranz et al. [6] in their study found that about 12 out of 100 molars had MM canals. They classified them into Fin, confluent and independent. In a similar study done by de Pablo et al. [7] confirms the presence of MM canal in 2.6% mandibular first molars. Gulabivala et al. [8] described a four-canal pattern, but existing as two canals, in Burmese population. Newer diagnostic methods such as computerized tomography (CT) scanning greatly facilitate access to the internal root canal morphology. One of the most important advantages of CBCT is that operator can have a look at slices of tooth of interest [9]. Other diagnostic tools such as multiple preoperative radiographs, use of sharp explorer, ultrasonic tips, staining the chamber floor with 1% methylene blue dye, performing the sodium hypochlorite "champagne bubble test," and visualizing canal bleeding points which are all important aids in locating root canal orifices are used to find out the additional canals present [5]. Also the use of operating microscope has revolutionized the practice of endodontics by allowing the clinicians to visualize the canal more efficiently [10]. Suspicion about a MM canal should always be anticipated when isthmus is clinically evident. The groove between MB and ML is a potential area to be addressed and the access should be modified for effective disinfection of root canal system. The clinicians should always suspect the possibility of additional canals in patients who are 40 years and above. Mandibular first molar with four canals in mesial root has been reported in literature thrice which makes our case report unique and worth mentioning to understand the complexity of root canal system of mandibular first molar.

4. Conclusion

Prognosis of the endodontic treatment on a long term is severely compromised due to the failure to locate and clean

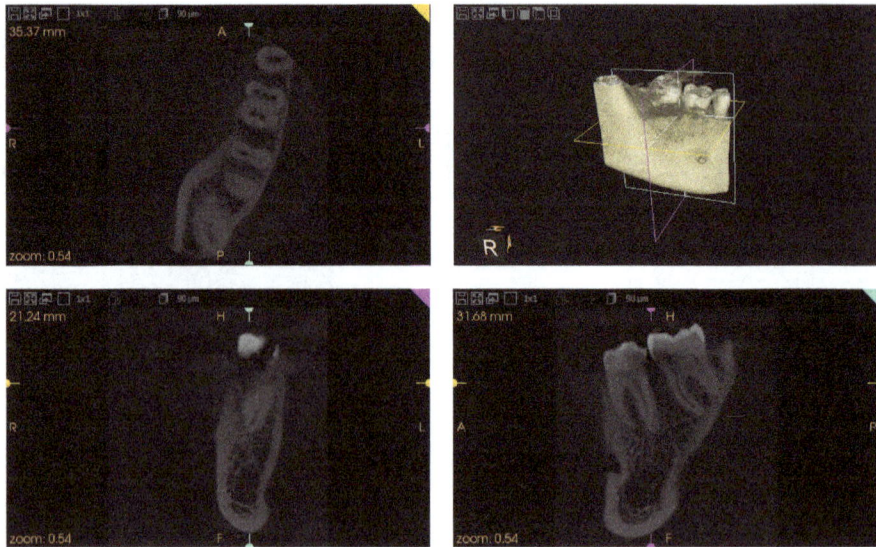

FIGURE 4: CBCT image showing 4 canals in mesial root.

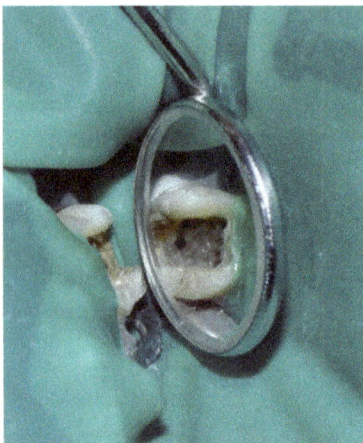

FIGURE 5: Intraoral image showing 6 canals.

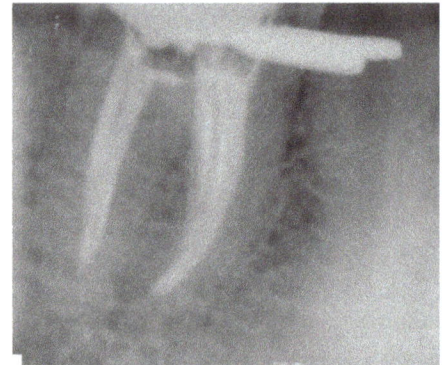

FIGURE 6: Master cone selection.

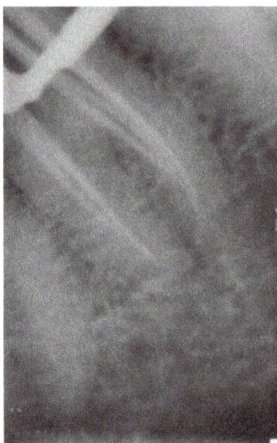

FIGURE 7: IOPAR after obturation.

extra canals. This management is quite challenging. With good knowledge, the will to search, and the magnification and modern imaging techniques, the success rates can be improved. Our case report describes a successful management of a mandibular molar with 6 canals.

Conflict of Interests

The authors declare that there is no conflict of interests regarding the publication of this paper.

References

[1] R. Bains, K. Loomba, A. Chandra, A. Loomba, V. K. Bains, and A. Garg, "The radix entomolaris: a case report," *Endodontic Practice Today*, vol. 3, no. 2, pp. 121–125, 2009.

[2] F. J. Vertucci and R. G. Williams, "Root canal anatomy of the mandibular first molar," *Journal of the New Jersey Dental Association*, vol. 45, no. 3, pp. 27–28, 1974.

[3] N. K. Goel, K. S. Gill, and J. R. Taneja, "Study of root canals configuration in mandibular first permanent molar," *Journal of the Indian Society of Pedodontics and Preventive Dentistry*, vol. 8, no. 1, pp. 12–14, 1991.

[4] A. Martínez-Berná and P. Badanelli, "Mandibular first molars with six root canals," *Journal of Endodontics*, vol. 11, no. 8, pp. 348–352, 1985.

[5] F. J. Vertucci, "Root canal morphology and its relationship to endodontic procedures," *Endodontic Topics*, vol. 10, no. 1, pp. 3–29, 2005.

[6] H. H. Pomeranz, D. L. Eidelman, and M. G. Goldberg, "Treatment considerations of the middle mesial canal of mandibular first and second molars," *Journal of Endodontics*, vol. 7, no. 12, pp. 565–568, 1981.

[7] Ó. V. de Pablo, R. Estevez, M. P. Sánchez, C. Heilborn, and N. Cohenca, "Root anatomy and canal configuration of the permanent mandibular first molar: a systematic review," *Journal of Endodontics*, vol. 36, no. 12, pp. 1919–1931, 2010.

[8] K. Gulabivala, T. H. Aung, A. Alavi, and Y.-L. Ng, "Root and canal morphology of Burmese mandibular molars," *International Endodontic Journal*, vol. 34, no. 5, pp. 359–370, 2001.

[9] F. B. Barletta, S. R. Dotto, M. D. Reis, R. Ferreira, and R. M. Travassos, "Mandibular molar with five root canals," *Australian Endodontic Journal*, vol. 34, no. 3, pp. 129–132, 2008.

[10] W. P. Saunders and E. M. Saunders, "Conventional endodontics and the operating microscope," *Dental Clinics of North America*, vol. 41, no. 3, pp. 415–428, 1997.

46

Reattachment of Coronal Tooth Fragment: Regaining Back to Normal

B. Vishwanath, Umrana Faizudin, M. Jayadev, and Sushma Shravani

Department of Conservative Dentistry & Endodontics, Panineeya Dental College, Hyderabad 60, India

Correspondence should be addressed to M. Jayadev; jayadev311@gmail.com

Academic Editors: I. Anic, Y.-K. Chen, and E. F. Wright

Dental trauma is such a situation wherein the patient is affected both socially and psychologically. During their first dental visit, these patients with trauma are in pain and need emergency treatment. Such patients are quite apprehensive because of impaired functions, esthetics, and phonetics. The prime objective while handling such cases is successful pain management with immediate restoration of function, esthetics, and phonetics. The advances in adhesive dentistry have allowed dentists to use the patient's own fragment to restore the fractured tooth. Reattachment is such an ultraconservative technique which provides safe, fast, and esthetically pleasing results. This paper discusses fragment reattachment technique and presents a clinical case of complicated crown fracture.

1. Introduction

Traumatic tooth fractures are the common reason for seeking dental care. Most dental injuries occur between 2 and 3 years and between 8 and 12 years of age; they are more common in boys than in girls because of their active involvement in extracurricular activities [1–3]. The most frequent causes of trauma are falls; bicycle, motorcycle, and car accidents; sports activities; collision with other people and objects; and domestic violence fights and physical assault [4, 5]. Prevalence of trauma to maxillary incisors accounts for about 37%; this is because of their anterior positioning and protrusion caused by the eruptive pattern [6, 7]. Coronal fracture is the frequent type of dental trauma in the permanent dentition [8, 9]. Eighty percent of traumatized incisors have fracture line proceeding in an oblique direction from labial to lingual aspect [7, 10].

Anterior teeth trauma of a young patient is a tragic experience, which requires immediate attention not only because of damage to dentition but also because of the psychological impact it may have on the patient and parents. Various methods and techniques were employed to restore fractured teeth which include pin retained resin, orthodontic bands, stainless steel crowns, porcelain jacket crowns, and complex ceramic restorations [11, 12]. However all these restorations require significant tooth preparation and were not esthetically adequate; moreover they cannot be used in an emergency esthetic situation [13, 14].

The first case report on reattachment of a fractured incisor fragment was published by Chosack and Eidelman in 1964 in which the complicated tooth fracture was managed by endodontic therapy followed by a cast post and core [15]. The use of acid etch technique for the reattachment of fractured fragment was first reported by Tennery [6]. Similar cases were also reported by Starkey [16] and Simonsen [8]. The success of reattachment depends on certain factors like the site of fracture, size of fractured remnants, periodontal status, pulpal involvement, maturity of the root formation, biological width invasion, occlusion, time material used for reattachment, use of post, and prognosis [17]. Reattachment is a way to restore the natural shape, contour, translucency, surface texture, occlusal alignment, and color of the fragment along with a positive emotional and social response from the patient to the preservation of natural tooth structure, and it is also an economical and a conservative procedure [8, 18–23].

2. Case Report

A 23-year-old male patient reported to the Department of Conservative Dentistry and Endodontics, Panineeya Mahavidyalaya Institute Of Dental Sciences And Research

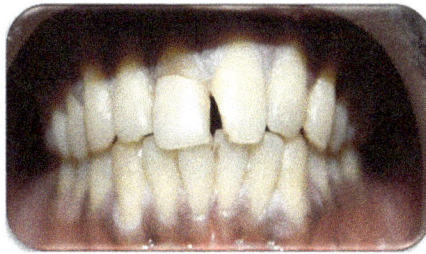

FIGURE 1: Preoperative photograph.

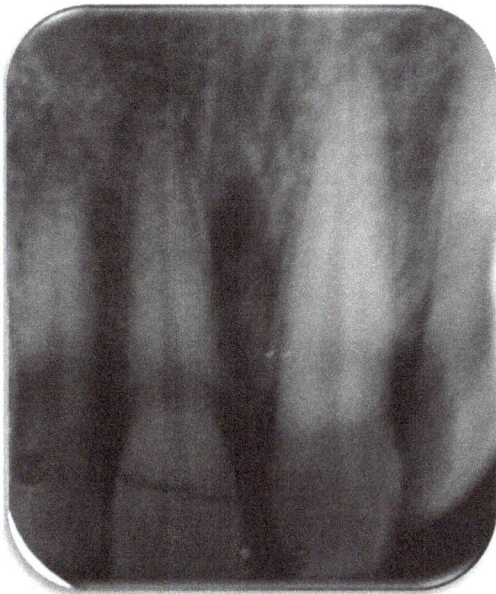

FIGURE 2: Preoperative radiograph.

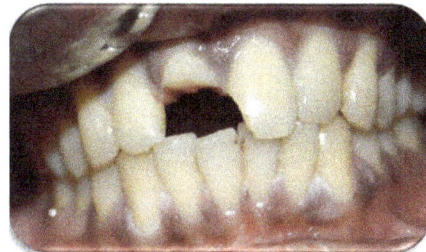

FIGURE 3: After fragment removal.

Centre, Hyderabad, India, with the chief complaint of broken upper front tooth following trauma three days ago which occurred due to a motorcycle accident (Figure 1).

Clinical examination revealed horizontal fracture in the middle third region of the right maxillary incisor involving enamel and dentin with exposure of the pulp and the fractured fragment being loosely attached to the tooth. The fracture was not evident palatally. Left maxillary incisor showed mesioangular incisal chipping. Soft tissue examination showed laceration of the upper lip.

A periapical radiographic examination revealed an oblique fracture labiopalatally; the root formation was complete with no extrusion of the tooth (Figure 2). The patient expressed the desire to maintain the tooth and restore it, as it is economical compared to an indirect restoration. A detailed explanation about the treatment plan was given to the patient, which included endodontic treatment, and then reattachment of the tooth crown using a fiber post and informed consent is taken from the patient.

Local anesthesia was administered followed by the removal of the fractured segment completely and preserved

in physiological saline solution in order to prevent dehydration and discoloration of the tooth fragment (Figures 3 and 4). Following a detailed examination, the fit of the fragment was checked. Working length was established with the help of radiograph followed by the biomechanical preparation by step back technique, with the master file being 45 k-file. Irrigants like 2.5% sodium hypochlorite and saline solution were used during the preparation alternately. The root canal was dried with paper points and obturated using lateral condensation technique with gutta percha (Dentply Maillefer, Ballaigues, Switzerland) and AH plus sealer (Maillefer, Dentply, Konstanz, Germany) (Figure 5). After completion of the endodontic treatment, the root canal was prepared for the post placement by removing the gutta percha from the coronal two-thirds of the canal with peeso reamers (drill size 2) (Figure 6). Bevels are placed on the tooth and the fractured fragment, in order to enhance the retention. The fibre post (Dentply Tulsa, Johnson city, US) was tried in the canal and adjusted to the desired length (Figure 7). Space was also prepared in the pulp chamber of the fractured crown fragments for receiving the coronal portion of the post and also the core. The alignment of the coronal fragment was verified with the post in situ. The root canal was then etched with 37% ortho phosphoric acid, rinsed, and blot-dried with paper points, and bonding agent was applied. The post was then luted in the canal using dual cured resin luting cement (Ivoclar Vivadent). The inner portion of the coronal fragment was similarly etched and bonded to the tooth using flowable composite resin (Ivoclar Vivadent) after proper shade matching. The tooth was polished with polishing disc (Figure 8).

Occlusion was verified and postoperative instructions are given to the patient in order to prevent any loading of the anterior teeth. Clinical and radiographic examinations were

(a)

(b)

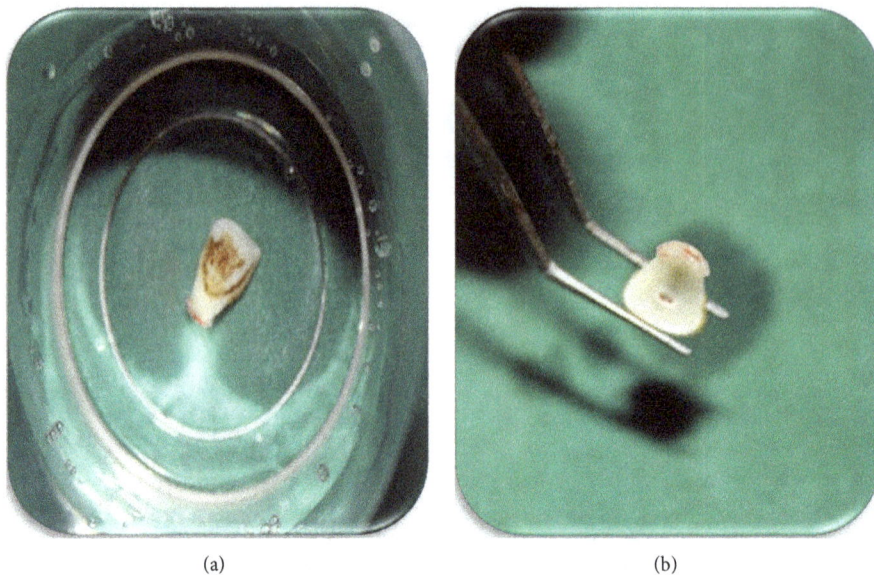

FIGURE 4: Fracture fragment.

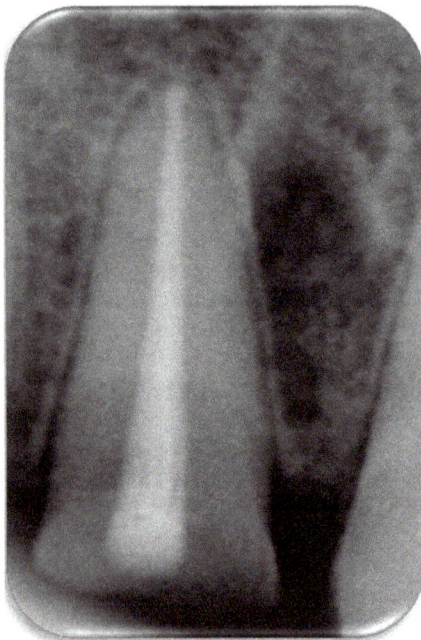

FIGURE 5: Obturation.

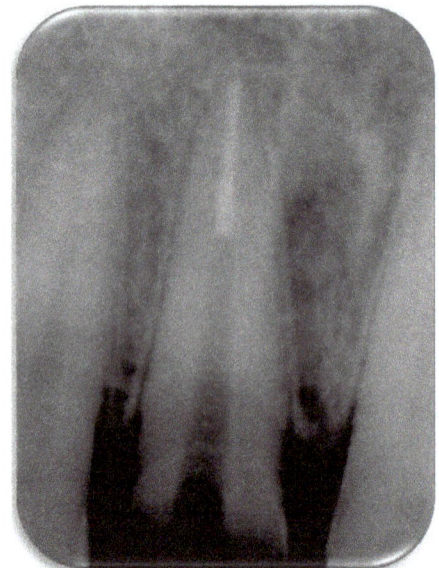

FIGURE 6: Post space preparation.

carried out after 1 month, 3 months, and 6 months and the tooth responded favorably.

3. Discussion

Studies have shown that one out of every four persons under the age of 18 will sustain a traumatic anterior crown fracture [24, 25]. Whenever the fracture fragment is available reattachment should be the first choice of treatment [26, 27]. In recent years due to remarkable advancements of adhesive systems and resin composites, it is now possible to achieve excellent results with reattachment of tooth fragments provided that the biological factors, materials, and techniques are logically assessed and managed [28]. As with the conventional restoration, restorative success depends on proper case selection, strict adherence to sound principles of periodontal and endodontic therapies, and the techniques and materials for modern adhesive dentistry [29–31]

In the present case of complicated crown fracture requiring endodontic therapy, the fractured fragment was available and reattachment of the fragment with fiber post is performed. The use of the natural tooth substance offers

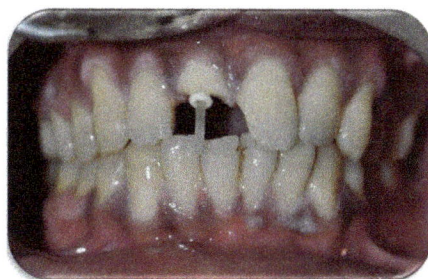

FIGURE 7: Post placement.

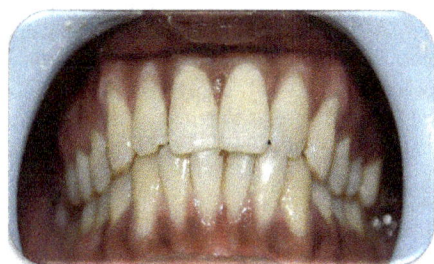

FIGURE 8: Postoperative photograph.

a conservative, esthetic, and economical option that provides good and long lasting esthetics, restores function, results in a positive psychological response, and is certainly a simple procedure. Adhesive post is used as it has the potential for increased retention, is more flexible, and has modulus of elasticity approximately same as dentin, and when bonded with resin cement it distributes forces evenly along the root [32].

The most common complication of post and core system is debonding [33]; another reason for failure is root fracture [34]. Restoration with cast metal posts can cause wedging forces coronally that may result in irreversible failure because of fracture of an already weakened root [35]. Whereas fiber-reinforced composite resin post has demonstrated negligible root fracture. Studies have indicated that dentin-bonded resin post-core restorations provide significantly less resistance to failure than cemented custom cast posts and cores [36, 37]. In addition, the fiber-reinforced posts are used with minimal preparation because it uses the undercuts and surface irregularities to increase the surface area for bonding, thus reducing the possibility of tooth fracture during function or traumatic injury [38].

The clinician must consider that a dry and clean working field and proper use of bonding protocols and bonding materials are the key to achieve success in adhesive dentistry. Reattachment failures occur as a result of new trauma or parafunctional habits, so fabrication of a mouth guard and patient education about treatment limitations enhance clinical success [39].

With all traumatic injuries, followup is of critical importance and the patient should be followed for 3, 6, and 12 months and yearly for 5 years [40]. At these follow-up visits esthetics, tooth mobility, and periodontal status should be confirmed both clinically and radiographically.

4. Conclusion

Because of larger incidence of trauma to dental tissues and their supporting structures, it is important to have proper knowledge of the techniques available and their indications, along with risk benefit ratio. The reattachment of the tooth fragment is possible only when the fragment is available and can be improved with different adhesive techniques and restorative materials. The main concern is to educate the population to preserve the fractured fragment and seek immediate dental care.

References

[1] American Academy of Pediatric Dentistry Council on Clinical Affairs, "Guidelines on management of acute dental trauma," *Pediatric Dentistry*, vol. 30, pp. 175–183, 2008-2009.

[2] P. C. S. Filho, P. S. Quagliatto, P. C. Simamoto Jr., and C. J. Soares, "Dental trauma: restorative procedures using composite resin and mouthguards for prevention," *Journal of Contemporary Dental Practice*, vol. 8, no. 6, pp. 89–95, 2007.

[3] C. M. Forsberg and G. Tedestam, "Etiological and predisposing factors related to traumatic injuries to permanent teeth," *Swedish Dental Journal*, vol. 17, no. 5, pp. 183–190, 1993.

[4] *Textbook and Color Atlas of Traumatic Injuries to the Teeth*, Andreasen J. O., Andreasen F. M., Andersson L., Eds., Blackwell Munksgaard, Copenhagen, Denmark, 4th edition, 2007.

[5] J. C. M. Castro, W. R. Poi, T. M. Manfrin, and L. G. Zina, "Analysis of the crown fractures and crown-root fractures due to dental trauma assisted by the Integrated Clinic from 1992 to 2002," *Dental Traumatology*, vol. 21, no. 3, pp. 121–126, 2005.

[6] T. N. Tennery, "The fractured tooth reunited using the acid-etch bonding technique," *Texas Dental Journal*, vol. 96, no. 8, pp. 16–17, 1988.

[7] A. Reis, A. D. Loguercio, A. Kraul, and E. Matson, "Reattachment of fractured teeth: a review of literature regarding techniques and materials," *Operative Dentistry*, vol. 29, no. 2, pp. 226–233, 2004.

[8] R. J. Simonsen, "Restoration of a fractured central incisor using original tooth fragment," *The Journal of the American Dental Association*, vol. 105, no. 4, pp. 646–648, 1982.

[9] J. O. Andreasen and F. M. Andreasen, *Textbook and Color Atlas of Traumatic Injuries to the Teeth*, pp. 216–256, Mosby Year Book, St. Louis, Mo, USA, 3rd edition, 1994.

[10] N. Joshi, N. Shetty, and M. Kundabala, "Immediate reattachment of fractured tooth segment using dual cure resin," *Kathmandu University Medical Journal*, vol. 6, no. 23, pp. 386–388, 2008.

[11] A. A. Badami, S. M. Dunne, and B. Scheer, "An in vitro investigation into the shear bond strengths of two dentine-bonding agents used in the reattachment of incisal edge fragments," *Endodontics & Dental Traumatology*, vol. 11, no. 3, pp. 129–135, 1995.

[12] M. G. Buonocore and J. Davila, "Restoration of fractured anterior teeth with ultraviolet-light-polymerized bonding materials: a new technique," *The Journal of the American Dental Association*, vol. 86, no. 6, pp. 1349–1354, 1973.

[13] J. O. Andreasen, "Buonocore memorial lecture. Adhesive dentistry applied to the treatment of traumatic dental injuries," *Operative Dentistry*, vol. 26, no. 4, pp. 328–335, 2001.

[14] P. Goenka, S. Dutta, and N. Marwah, "Biological approach for management of anterior tooth trauma: triple case report," *Journal of Indian Society of Pedodontics and Preventive Dentistry*, vol. 29, no. 2, pp. 180–186, 2011.

[15] A. Chosack and E. Eidelman, "Rehabilitation of a fractured incisor using the patient's natural crown. Case report," *Journal of Dentistry for Children*, vol. 31, pp. 19–21, 1964.

[16] P. E. Starkey, "Reattachment of a fractured fragment to a tooth—a case report," *Journal of the Indian Dental Association*, vol. 58, no. 5, pp. 37–38, 1979.

[17] C. P. K. Wadhwani, "A single visit, multidisciplinary approach to the management of traumatic tooth crown fracture," *British Dental Journal*, vol. 188, no. 11, pp. 593–598, 2000.

[18] L. N. Baratieri, S. M. Júnior, A. C. Cardoso, and J. C. D. Filho, "Coronal fracture with invasion of the biologic width: a case report," *Quintessence International*, vol. 24, no. 2, pp. 85–91, 1993.

[19] R. J. Simonsen, "Traumatic fracture restoration: an alternative use of the acid etch technique," *Quintessence International*, vol. 10, no. 2, pp. 15–22, 1979.

[20] J. Santos and J. Bianchi, "Restoration of severely damaged teeth with resin bonding systems: case reports," *Quintessence International*, vol. 22, no. 8, pp. 611–615, 1991.

[21] R. D. Trushkowsky, "Esthetic, biologic, and restorative considerations in coronal segment reattachment for a fractured tooth: a clinical report," *The Journal of Prosthetic Dentistry*, vol. 79, no. 2, pp. 115–119, 1998.

[22] F. C. S. Chu, T. M. Yim, and S. H. Y. Wei, "Clinical considerations for reattachment of tooth fragments," *Quintessence International*, vol. 31, no. 6, pp. 385–391, 2000.

[23] K. Arapostathis, A. Arhakis, and S. Kalfas, "A modified technique on the reattachment of permanent tooth fragments following dental trauma. Case report," *Journal of Clinical Pediatric Dentistry*, vol. 30, no. 1, pp. 29–34, 2005.

[24] J. O. Andreasen and J. J. Ravn, "Epidemiology of traumatic dental injuries to primary and permanent teeth in a Danish population sample," *International Journal of Oral Surgery*, vol. 1, no. 5, pp. 235–239, 1972.

[25] S. Petti and G. Tarsitani, "Traumatic injuries to anterior teeth in Italian schoolchildren: prevalence and risk factors," *Endodontics and Dental Traumatology*, vol. 12, no. 6, pp. 294–297, 1996.

[26] A. Belchema, "Reattachment of fractured permanent incisors in school children (review)," *Journal of IMAB*, vol. 14, no. 2, pp. 96–99, 2008.

[27] Y. Yilmaz, C. Zehir, O. Eyuboglu, and N. Belduz, "Evaluation of success in the reattachment of coronal fractures," *Dental Traumatology*, vol. 24, no. 2, pp. 151–158, 2008.

[28] P. Vashisth, M. Mittal, and A. P. Singh, "Immediate reattachment of fractured tooth segment: a biological approach," *Indian Journal of Dental Research and Review*, pp. 72–74, 2012.

[29] F. M. Andreasen, U. Steinhardt, M. Bille, and E. C. Musksgaard, "Bonding of enamel-dentin crown fragments after crown fracture. An experimental study using bonding agents," *Endodontics & Dental Traumatology*, vol. 9, no. 3, pp. 111–114, 1993.

[30] G. Cavalleri and N. Zerman, "Traumatic crown fractures in permanent incisors with immature roots: a follow-up study," *Endodontics & Dental Traumatology*, vol. 11, no. 6, pp. 294–296, 1995.

[31] M. N. Lowey, "Reattachment of a fractured central incisor tooth fragment," *British Dental Journal*, vol. 170, no. 8, article 285, 1991.

[32] P. Lokesh and M. Kala, "Management of mild-root fracture using MTA and fiber post to reinforce crown—a case report," *Indian Journal of Dental Research and Review*, vol. 3, pp. 32–36, 2008.

[33] A. Torbjörner, S. Karlsson, O. Dr, and P. A. Ödman, "Survival rate and failure characteristics for two post designs," *The Journal of Prosthetic Dentistry*, vol. 73, no. 5, pp. 439–444, 1995.

[34] E. Asmussen, A. Peutzfeldt, and T. Heitmann, "Stiffness, elastic limit, and strength of newer types of endodontic posts," *Journal of Dentistry*, vol. 27, no. 4, pp. 275–278, 1999.

[35] A. S. Deutsch, J. Cavallari, B. L. Musikant, L. Silverstein, J. Lepley, and G. Petroni, "Root fracture and the design of prefabricated posts," *The Journal of Prosthetic Dentistry*, vol. 53, no. 5, pp. 637–640, 1985.

[36] R. T. Beg, M. W. Parker, J. T. Judkins, and G. B. Pelleu, "Effect of dentinal bonded resin post-core preparations on resistance to vertical root fracture," *The Journal of Prosthetic Dentistry*, vol. 67, no. 6, pp. 768–772, 1992.

[37] B. Akkayan and T. Gülmez, "Resistance to fracture of endodontically treated teeth restored with different post systems," *The Journal of Prosthetic Dentistry*, vol. 87, no. 4, pp. 431–437, 2002.

[38] K. C. Trabert, A. A. Caputo, and M. Abou-Rass, "Tooth fracture—a comparison of endodontic and restorative treatments," *Journal of Endodontics*, vol. 4, no. 11, pp. 341–345, 1978.

[39] F. M. Andreasen, J. G. Norén, J. O. Andreasen, S. Engelhardtsen, and U. Lindh-Strömberg, "Long-term survival of fragment bonding in the treatment of fractured crowns: a multicenter clinical study," *Quintessence International*, vol. 26, no. 10, pp. 669–681, 1995.

[40] A. Rajput, I. Ataide, and M. Fernandes, "Uncomplicated crown fracture, complicated crown-root fracture, and horizontal root fracture simultaneously treated in a patient during emergency visit: a case report," *Oral Surgery, Oral Medicine, Oral Pathology, Oral Radiology and Endodontology*, vol. 107, no. 2, pp. e48–e52, 2009.

47

Chairside Fabrication of an All-Ceramic Partial Crown Using a Zirconia-Reinforced Lithium Silicate Ceramic

Sven Rinke,[1,2] **Anne-Kathrin Pabel,**[1] **Matthias Rödiger,**[2] **and Dirk Ziebolz**[3]

[1]*Dental Practice, 63456 Hanau, Germany*
[2]*Department of Prosthetics, University Medical Center Göttingen, 37075 Göttingen, Germany*
[3]*Department of Cariology, Endodontology and Periodontology, University of Leipzig, 04103 Leipzig, Germany*

Correspondence should be addressed to Sven Rinke; rinke@ihr-laecheln.com

Academic Editor: Jamil A. Shibli

The chairside fabrication of a monolithic partial crown using a zirconia-reinforced lithium silicate (ZLS) ceramic is described. The fully digitized model-free workflow in a dental practice is possible due to the use of a powder-free intraoral scanner and the computer-aided design/computer-assisted manufacturing (CAD/CAM) of the restorations. The innovative ZLS material offers a singular combination of fracture strength (>370 Mpa), optimum polishing characteristics, and excellent optical properties. Therefore, this ceramic is an interesting alternative material for monolithic restorations produced in a digital workflow.

1. Introduction

Providing a tooth-colored restoration in only one appointment is the main goal of the chairside concept with computer-aided design/computer-assisted manufacturing (CAD/CAM) technology, which was first realized with the introduction of the CEREC-system [1]. The CEREC-system evolved through a combination of numerous software and hardware upgrades since its launch more than 30 years ago [2]. Meanwhile, the CAD/CAM of dental restorations has become an established fabrication process, especially for all-ceramic solutions [1–4].

Long-term survival rates for CAD/CAM-fabricated inlays and onlays appear to be similar to traditional restorations [5]. The survival possibility of CEREC-generated restorations fabricated from machinable feldspathic porcelain (Vita MK II, Vita Zahnfabrik, Bad Säckingen, Germany) was reported to be approximately 97% for 5 years and 90% for 10 years [5, 6]. For observational periods of up to 17 years, a survival rate of 88.7% was calculated [7]. The most frequent reason for failure was a ceramic fracture (62%) followed by tooth fractures (14%) and caries (19%). To overcome this limitation, new materials with improved fracture strength (e.g., lithium disilicate ceramics (Ls2)) >350 MPa were introduced

for the manufacturing of extended CAD/CAM restorations (partial crowns and full coverage crowns) in the posterior region [8]. Reich and Schierz (2013) assessed the clinical performance of chairside-generated lithium disilicate crowns during an observational period of 4 years [9]. The failure-free rate was 96.3% after 4 years according to Kaplan-Meier analysis. This is comparable with the survival rates reported for posterior metal-ceramic crowns and conventional heat-pressed crowns made from lithium disilicate ceramics [10].

Recent material-related research focuses on the development of CAD/CAM materials offering improved mechanical strength, combined with adequate translucency, and time-saving fabrication [11]. Recently, a new group of machinable ceramics for CAD/CAM techniques has been launched: zirconia-reinforced lithium silicate (ZLS) ceramics (Celtra Duo, Dentsply DeTrey, Konstanz, Germany; Suprinity, Vita Zahnfabrik, Bad Säckingen, Germany). Both materials are supported by CEREC version 4.2 and above. Pursuant to the manufacturers, the mechanical properties of these materials range between 370 and 420 MPa. The addition of 8–10 wt% zirconium oxide leads to an improved strength [12]. After crystallization, the material has a homogeneous texture (mean grit size: approximately 0.5–0.7 μm). The formed crystals are 4 to 8 times smaller than lithium disilicate crystallites. ZLS-ceramics consist of a dual microstructure: the first component is very fine lithium metasilicate with lithium disilicate crystals (average size: 0.5–0.7 μm). This is the main difference from Ls2 ceramics, which only contain lithium disilicate crystals. The second component is the glassy matrix containing 10% zirconium oxide in solution. The result is a very fine microstructure that allows a high flexural strength while at the same time providing a high percentage of glassy matrix, thus leading to good optical, milling, and polishing properties [12].

Currently, the ZLS-ceramics are sold as Suprinity (Vita Zahnfabrik) and Celtra Duo (Dentsply DeTrey) for chairside as well as lab site processing. The zirconia-reinforced silicate ceramic Vita Suprinity is a precrystallized ceramic material. Accordingly, the CAM processing is comparable with lithium disilicate ceramic materials (crystallization firing after milling to achieve the final density). However, the ZLS variation Celtra Duo (Dentsply DeTrey) is a finally crystallized ceramic. This is especially suitable for chairside application, as the final workpiece is available after a milling time of only 10 to 22 minutes. The milled restorations have a flexural strength of 210 MPa. An additional stain and glaze firing will increase the material's flexural strength to 370 MPa [13]. Thus, the final crystallized ZLS variations offer an up-to-date combination of short processing times and high stability. These properties especially allow the chairside fabrication of all-ceramic restorations in the posterior region.

Meanwhile, the mechanical, bonding, and optical properties of these final crystallized ZLS-ceramics (i.e., Celtra Duo) were tested in comparative university-based in vitro studies [13–16]. These tests revealed a fracture strength and a marginal adaptation comparable to the clinically well-proven lithium disilicate (Ls2) glass ceramics [13]. Moreover, under in vitro conditions, the wear and volumetric loss for the glaze-fired ZLS-ceramic Celtra Duo was not significantly different from human enamel [15]. The in vitro evaluation of the bonding properties showed an encouraging bonding performance of the Celtra Duo crowns when pretreated as recommended by the manufacturer (hydrofluoric acid etching), being sufficient to withstand intraoral chewing forces during mastication [16].

This case report describes a treatment with monolithic ceramic restorations which are fabricated from ZLS-ceramics (Celtra Duo Dentsply DeTrey, Konstanz, Germany), in a fully digitized workflow with a powder-free intraoral scanner (CEREC Omnicam, Sirona Bensheim, Germany) and a practice-based milling system (CEREC MCXL, Sirona, Bensheim, Germany).

2. Case Presentation

A 62-year-old man presented with a need for restorative treatment of the lower left second premolar. The existing cast gold inlay showed an insufficient fitting accuracy, and repeated clinical intervention had been necessary due to loss of retention (Figure 1). The tooth was vital; a systematic periodontal treatment led to a stable overall periodontal situation. The patient wanted a replacement of the cast gold

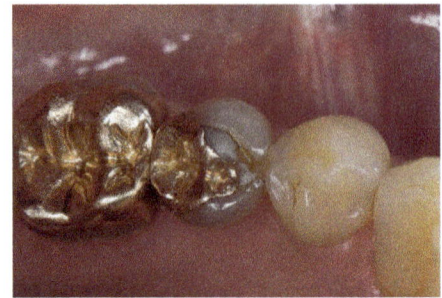

FIGURE 1: Insufficient cast gold inlay on a lower second premolar.

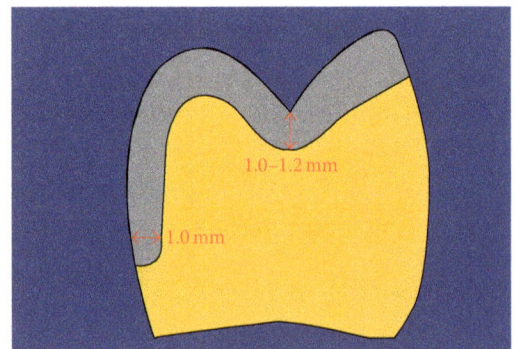

FIGURE 2: Minimum material thickness recommended for all-ceramic partial crowns fabricated from zirconia-reinforced lithium silicate (ZLS) ceramics.

restoration with a chairside fabricated all-ceramic partial crown. For the fabrication process of the monolithic partial crown with the CEREC-system, a fully crystallized ZLS-ceramic (Celtra Duo, Dentsply DeTrey, Konstanz, Germany) was used.

At the beginning of the second clinical appointment, shade selection using a conventional shade guide (Vitapan classic, Vita Zahnfabrik, Bad Säckingen, Germany) was performed. After the application of local anesthetics (Sopira Heraeus Kulzer, Hanau, Germany), the existing inlay restoration was detached, and the caries were removed. A core build-up was placed adhesively (Core-Up OptiMix, Kaniedenta, Herford, Germany). Due to the large defect and the thin remaining buccal wall (thickness < 1.5 mm), the tooth needed a ceramic partial crown. Preparation was performed according to the recommendations of Ahlers et al. (2009) [17], avoiding sharp edges. A minimum material thickness of 1.2 to 1.0 mm in the occlusal area was maintained. The preparation limit was carried out as a shoulder preparation with internal rounded line angle and a cutting depth of 1.0 mm (Figure 2).

Prior to digital impression taking, two layers of non-impregnated retraction cords (sizes 00 and 1) (UltraPak, Ultradent Products, Cologne, Germany) were placed. A V-shaped pack was created by putting a second cord with a larger diameter directly over the first, thus providing a physical lateral displacement of the tissues (Figure 3). The retraction cords were left in the sulcus while the tooth was air-dried. Due to the mainly supragingival preparation, no

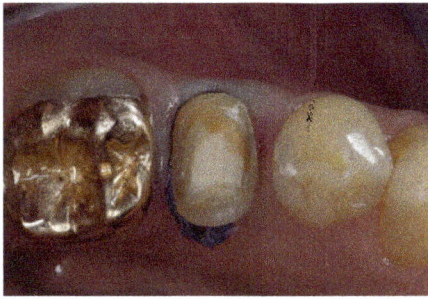

FIGURE 3: Finished preparation with retraction cords placed.

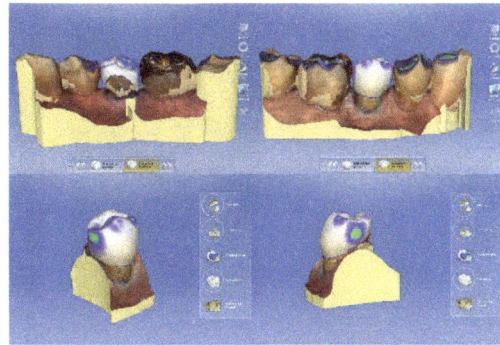

FIGURE 5: Adjustment of the occlusal and proximal contacts.

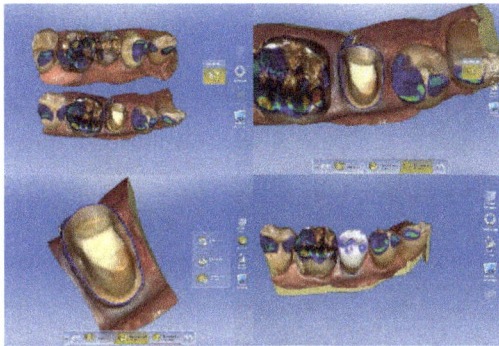

FIGURE 4: Intraoral scans with marked preparation line and design suggestion generated with the CEREC software (version 4.2).

further preparation steps were necessary to take the digital impression. Intraoral scanning was performed with powder-free technology by using a CEREC Omnicam (CEREC Omnicam Sirona Bensheim, Germany). The CEREC Omnicam is a true-color high-resolution 3D intraoral camera using white LEDs as a light source. The 3D calculations were based on triangulation measurement.

First, the lower left quadrant of the mandible was scanned and then data in the upper left quadrant were collected. When the patient closed into an intercuspal position, a buccal scan was taken. The system implemented the digital registration to create a 3D occlusion relation (Figure 4).

In the next step, the virtual models were adjusted, and the preparation limit was marked and edited. After the determination of the insertion path and the model axis, the automated design of the restoration was started (Figure 4). For the design of the partial crowns, the design feature "Biogeneric Individual" was selected. For this design suggestion made by the software, the neighboring teeth are analyzed, and the program extrapolates the naturally created morphology for the design of the restoration. Proximal and occlusal contact strength was set to 25 μm. Spacer thickness was reduced to 50 μm, and the minimum occlusal thickness was adjusted to the material specific value (1000 μm). Finally, the design suggestion was slightly modified regarding position and size with the respective design tool. Furthermore, the proximal contacts were slightly enlarged (Figure 5). Based on the mainly automated design of the biogeneric feature,

the time needed for the design process can be shortened to 5 minutes or less for a single-tooth restoration.

The restoration was then milled as a full-contour monolithic partial crown from a finally crystalized ZLS-ceramic using a practice-based compact milling unit (CEREC MCXL, Sirona, Bensheim, Germany) in a wet grinding process (Figures 6(a) and 6(b)).

The Celtra Duo material type HT (high translucency) in Vita shade A3 was selected to create a pronounced chameleon effect when milling the partial crown. Depending on the size of the restoration, the milling process takes between 10 and 14 minutes.

After machining the restorations, first, the fixation bar of the restoration was removed with water-cooled diamond instruments. Then, the occlusal surfaces were reworked using the same fine-grit size instrument (8390.314.016, Gebr. Brasseler, Lemgo, Germany).

Afterwards, the complete restoration was carefully prepolished with diamond-impregnated polyurethane instruments (94020C.204.040. Gebr. Brasseler, Lemgo, Germany) (Figures 7(a) and 7(b)).

The intraoral try-in of the restoration including internal adjustment and the adjustment of the proximal contacts were the next steps. After the correct fit of the restoration was achieved, the patient was asked to bite down very carefully. Then, the occlusal contacts were marked with articulation paper (Figures 8(a) and 8(b)). Selective adjustment could be performed with water-cooled fine diamond instruments (8390.314.016, Gebr. Brasseler, Lemgo, Germany). When fabricating posterior Celtra Duo crowns and partial crowns, glaze firing is recommended, as this step increases the final stability from 210 to 370 MPa, thus matching the mechanical strength reported for long-term evaluated lithium disilicate ceramics.

The restoration was cleaned by using a steam jet unit and subjected to a first glaze firing process at 820°C (heating rate 55°C/min, hold time 1:30 min) that was combined with an individual staining of the restoration (Celtra Universal Stain & Glaze, Dentsply DeTrey, Konstanz, Germany). It is necessary to coat the entire surface with the glazing material to obtain a uniform glossy finish (Figure 9).

In the present case, an additional glaze firing was performed at 770°C (heating rate 55°C/min, hold time 1:30 min)

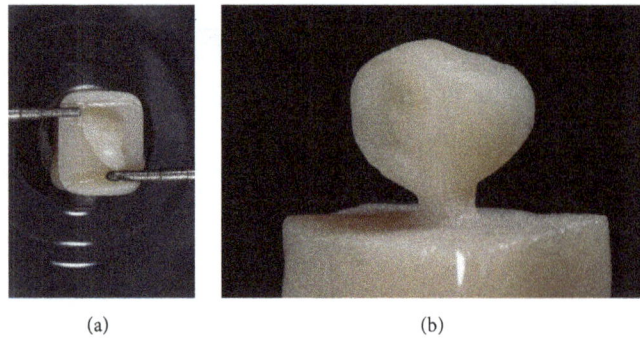

(a)   (b)

FIGURE 6: Wet grinding process of the partial crown using the CEREC MXCL (Sirona Bensheim, Germany) unit.

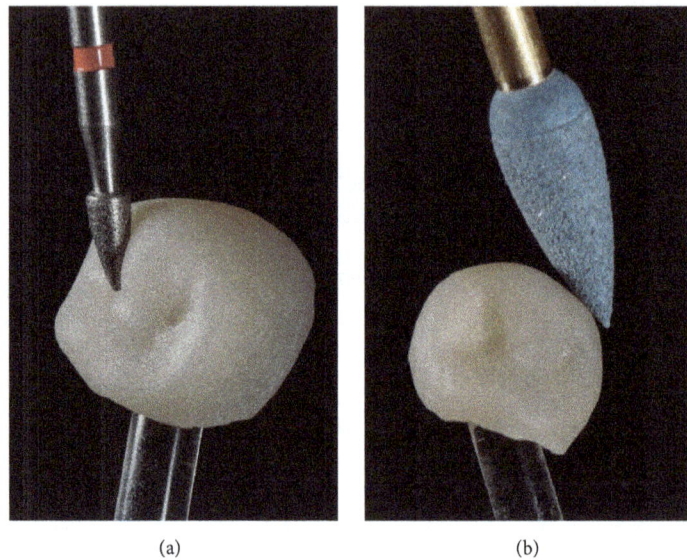

(a)   (b)

FIGURE 7: Postprocessing of the occlusal surface and prepolishing using a diamond-impregnated polyurethane polisher.

to accentuate the shade. The restoration was then mirror-finished with diamond-impregnated polyurethane instruments (94020F.204.040. Gebr. Brasseler, Lemgo, Germany) at moderate speed (not exceeding 8,000 rpm) and using a diamond polishing paste (Direct Dia Paste, Shofu Dental, Ratingen, Germany) (Figure 10).

One hour after impression taking, the restoration was ready for a final esthetic try-in with a try-in gel (Calibra Try-In Paste, Dentsply DeTrey, Konstanz, Germany) to verify the fitting accuracy and the correct match of shade.

Only minor occlusal adjustments of the proximal contacts with diamond-impregnated polyurethane instruments were needed at this stage. The adjusted areas were repolished using a diamond polishing paste (e.g., Direct Dia Paste, Shofu Dental, Ratingen, Germany). The paste is best applied with a nylon brush without water cooling at max. 5,000 rpm.

Before adhesive luting, the surfaces of the restoration that should be bonded were conditioned with 5% hydrofluoric acid (Vita Ceramics Etch, Vita Zahnfabrik, Bad Säckingen, Germany) for 30 seconds (Figure 11(a)).

Then, all acid residues were removed by thoroughly rinsing the restorations with water (a stained etching gel allows a better control of the cleansing). The etched restorations were then dried, and a silane material (Calibra Silane, Dentsply DeTrey, Konstanz, Germany) was applied (residence time: 1 minute) (Figure 11(b)).

After cleaning the tooth with pumice and a chlorhexidine solution, it was isolated with rubber dam. 37% phosphoric acid was applied for 30 seconds to condition the enamel, while the exposed dentine was etched for 15 seconds. However, adjacent teeth should be protected with cellophane matrices before applying the etching gel. In case of unintentional conditioning of the proximal surfaces of adjacent teeth, the cement excess on these surfaces will affect further processing.

A dual-curing one-step adhesive (XP Bond & Self-Curing Activator, Dentsply DeTrey, Konstanz, Germany) was applied on teeth and restoration surfaces and air-thinned. A thin layer of a dual-curing transparent resin cement (Calibra automix transparent, Dentsply DeTrey, Konstanz, Germany) was applied to the preparation immediately; the restoration

(a)

(b)

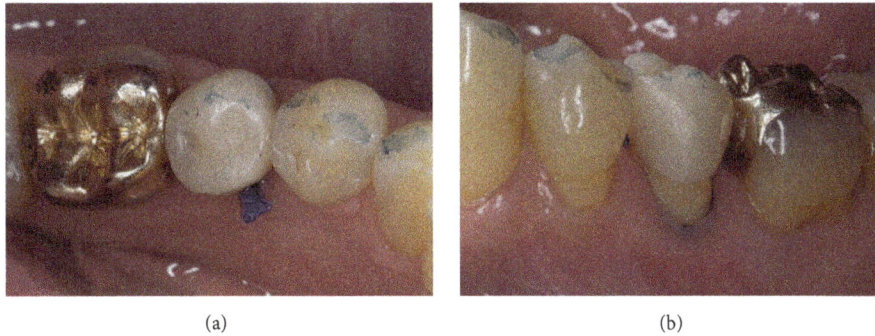

FIGURE 8: Try-in of the prepolished partial crown.

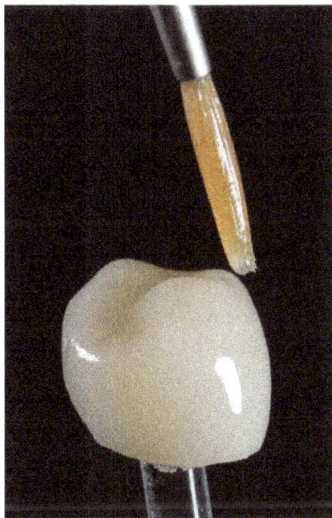

FIGURE 9: Application of the glazing material.

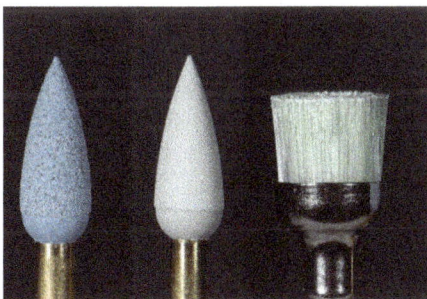

FIGURE 10: Instruments and material for the mirror finish of the restoration.

instruments and the already mentioned 2-stage diamond-impregnated polishers (Figures 13(a) and 13(b)). Two weeks after cementation, the patient was reexamined and reported no postoperative sensitivity. The restorations had a good shade adaptation and postoperative tissues were healthy.

3. Discussion

Since the 1980s, computer-aided design and computer-aided manufacturing (CAD/CAM) have been employed in the chairside fabrication of all-ceramic restorations, especially for inlays and onlays [1, 2].

The launch of new intraoral scanning devices, as well as reliable new high-strength ceramic materials, has likewise been observed by dentists and dental technicians [4, 8, 11]. Several publications have indicated that digital techniques can replace conventional workflows for at least single-tooth restorations and short-span fixed partial dentures (FPDs) [3–7]. As one major advantage of the digital workflow, the time needed for occlusal and internal adjustments is shorter than for restorations fabricated in the conventional workflow [1, 3, 4]. This is supported by the clinical experience documented in the present case report, with only minor adjustments of the proximal and occlusal contacts which took less than 3 minutes.

Four further developments are crucial for the chairside fabrication process, as follows.

3.1. Intraoral Scanner. Earlier scanning systems required the time-consuming application of a scanning powder. With the introduction of powder-free scanning systems like the one applied in the present case report, the scanning process is simplified and shortened [2–4]. This is a very important factor in reducing the total fabrication time in a chairside process [4].

3.2. Automated Design. A high level of accuracy is needed in the design process to exactly reproduce internal as well as occlusal and proximal surfaces to enable a model-free production of an all-ceramic restoration [1, 3]. This is a precondition to avoid time-consuming intraoral adjustments or, in the worst case scenario, a remake of the restoration. With the current version of the CEREC software (4.xx), the design

was then seated. The resin cement was precured for 3–5 seconds on both the lingual and the buccal side. Excess cement in the proximal areas was removed with an explorer and dental floss. The luting agent was now finally light-cured for 40 seconds on each side of the restoration (buccal/occlusal/lingual) (Figure 12). Now, the occlusal contacts were checked and adjusted where necessary. The margins were finished and polished with fine-grit size diamond

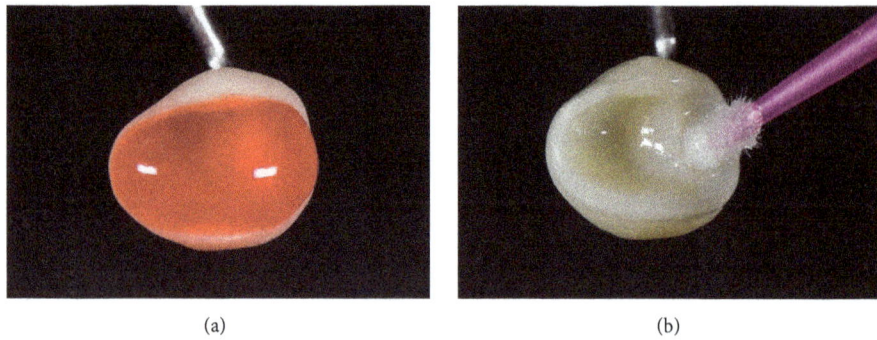

(a)   (b)

FIGURE 11: Conditioning of the ceramic restoration using 5% hydrofluoric (Vita Ceramics Etch, Vita Zahnfabrik, Bad Säckingen, Germany) acid and a silane coupling agent (Calibra Silane, Dentsply DeTrey, Konstanz, Germany).

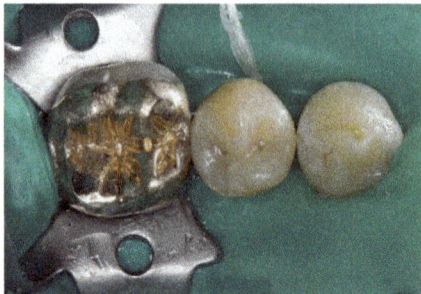

FIGURE 12: Adhesive cementation of the restoration after rubber dam application.

process has become simpler and more intuitive [2–4]. Especially for single-tooth restorations, only minor corrections by the operator are needed to modify the design templates of the software and to reach a design that meets the clinical needs regarding anatomic shape, occlusal contacts, and fitting accuracy [3]. The required time for the design of a single-tooth restoration is less than 5 minutes in the majority of cases.

3.3. Reduced Fabrication Time. An essential requirement for the successful integration of chairside procedures is to shorten the fabrication time as much as possible [1, 3]. Apart from a simple intraoral scanning procedure and an automated design, this is provided by the time-effective milling of the ceramic material [11]. With the material used in the present case report, a partial crown is milled within 12–14 minutes using the CEREC MXCL milling unit. Compared to other materials offering a comparable fracture strength, no crystallization firing is needed, as the final strength can be achieved with a glaze firing [11, 12]. This reduces the fabrication time to approximately 30–40 minutes [9, 11].

3.4. Innovative Materials. Due to their combination of strength and translucency, ZLS-ceramics offer ideal preconditions for the fabrication of monolithic restorations that are only characterized by staining [8, 11]. First in vitro studies comparing the translucency of various ceramic materials revealed a higher translucency of the ZLS-ceramic Celtra Duo

compared to IPS e.max CAD in the polished state (38% versus 34%) [14]. The pronounced translucency of the material increases the so-called chameleon effect and improves the shade adaption. This effect is supported by the findings of the present clinical case report. The omission of ceramic veneering eliminates the risk of veneering ceramic fractures [2, 12]. Due to its special microstructure, this material group is easy to polish [11, 12]. All these material properties are of clinical benefit for chairside restorations. Nevertheless, at this time the material is available only in monochromatic CAD/CAM blocks, covering in parts the Vitapan classical shade range (A1–A3.5 and B2). For crowns and partial crowns, the generation of a tooth-like gradient in the shades from the cervical to the incisal area requires the use of stains in an additional firing cycle. Apart from enlarging the range of monochromatic blocks, covering the complete Vitapan shades (A–D), the fabrication of polychromatic CAD/CAM blocks with an opaque core surrounded by a translucent layer could be a meaningful innovation. This could reduce the necessity of a separate staining procedure as well as the fabrication time.

In the present study, the ZLS-ceramic was conditioned by an etching process with 5% hydrofluoric acid for 30 seconds. Based on the findings of an in vitro investigation, this pretreatment ensures a bonding strength comparable to the well-known lithium disilicate ceramics in combination with dual-curing composite cements and self-adhesive cements [16]. An alternative pretreatment by air-abrasion with 50 μm aluminous oxide cannot be recommended, as this procedure only leads to 50% of the bonding strength determined for a pretreatment with hydrofluoric acid and silane application [16].

Nevertheless, it is a limitation of these new materials that data from clinical studies are missing. Moreover, financial investments for intraoral scanners, CAD software, and the milling unit are high in comparison with conventional workflows, despite considerable progress in the further development of digital workflows [3].

4. Conclusions

ZLS-ceramics offer a good combination of high strength and outstanding optical properties. As the materials can be milled in their finally crystallized state, they are interesting for

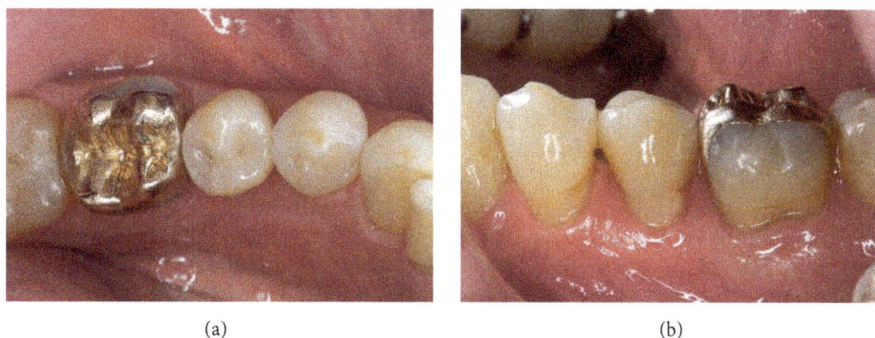

(a)   (b)

FIGURE 13: Clinical situation two days after adhesive cementation.

the time-saving chairside fabrication of monolithic restorations in load-bearing areas that require a fracture strength of >350 MPa (partial crowns and full crowns). However when using ZLS-ceramics, the material specific processing instructions should be strictly observed, even though ZLS-ceramics show a positive combination of properties that were confirmed in several laboratory studies. This is especially important regarding the necessary minimum wall thickness and required adhesive luting. Results from additional clinical studies are required to validate the positive results from these initial clinical experiences.

Conflict of Interests

Sven Rinke has received lecture fees from Dentsply DeTrey, Konstanz, Germany. The other authors declare that there is no conflict of interests regarding the publication of this paper.

References

[1] D. Fasbinder, "Using digital technology to enhance restorative dentistry," *Compendium of Continuing Education in Dentistry*, vol. 33, no. 9, pp. 666–672, 2012.

[2] D. J. Poticny and J. Klim, "CAD/CAM in-office technology: innovations after 25 years for predictable, esthetic outcomes," *Journal of the American Dental Association*, vol. 141, supplement 2, pp. 5S–9S, 2010.

[3] K. Baroudi and S. N. Ibraheem, "Assessment of chair-side computer-aided design and computer-aided manufacturing restorations: a review of the literature," *Journal of International Oral Health*, vol. 7, no. 4, pp. 96–104, 2015.

[4] S. Ting-shu and S. Jian, "Intraoral digital impression technique: a review," *Journal of Prosthodontics*, vol. 24, no. 4, pp. 313–321, 2015.

[5] J.-G. Wittneben, R. F. Wright, H.-P. Weber, and G. O. Gallucci, "A systematic review of the clinical performance of CAD/CAM single-tooth restorations," *International Journal of Prosthodontics*, vol. 22, no. 5, pp. 466–471, 2009.

[6] D. J. Fasbinder, "Clinical performance of chairside CAD/CAM restorations," *Journal of the American Dental Association*, vol. 137, pp. 22S–31S, 2006.

[7] T. Otto and D. Schneider, "Long-term clinical results of chairside Cerec CAD/CAM inlays and onlays: a case series,"

International Journal of Prosthodontics, vol. 21, no. 1, pp. 53–59, 2008.

[8] R. W. K. Li, T. W. Chow, and J. P. Matinlinna, "Ceramic dental biomaterials and CAD/CAM technology: state of the art," *Journal of Prosthodontic Research*, vol. 58, no. 4, pp. 208–216, 2014.

[9] S. Reich and O. Schierz, "Chair-side generated posterior lithium disilicate crowns after 4 years," *Clinical Oral Investigations*, vol. 17, no. 7, pp. 1765–1772, 2013.

[10] S. Pieger, A. Salman, and A. S. Bidra, "Clinical outcomes of lithium disilicate single crowns and partial fixed dental prostheses: a systematic review," *Journal of Prosthetic Dentistry*, vol. 112, no. 1, pp. 22–30, 2014.

[11] I. Denry and J. R. Kelly, "Emerging ceramic-based materials for dentistry," *Journal of Dental Research*, vol. 93, no. 12, pp. 1235–1242, 2014.

[12] S. Krüger, J. Deubener, C. Ritzberger, and W. Höland, "Nucleation kinetics of lithium metasilicate in ZrO_2-bearing lithium disilicate glasses for dental application," *International Journal of Applied Glass Science*, vol. 4, no. 1, pp. 9–19, 2013.

[13] V. Preis, M. Behr, S. Hahnel, and M. Rosentritt, "Influence of cementation on in vitro performance, marginal adaptation and fracture resistance of CAD/CAM-fabricated ZLS molar crowns," *Dental Materials*, vol. 31, no. 11, pp. 1363–1369, 2015.

[14] D. Awad, B. Stawarczyk, A. Liebermann, and N. Ilie, "Translucency of esthetic dental restorative CAD/CAM materials and composite resins with respect to thickness and surface roughness," *The Journal of Prosthetic Dentistry*, vol. 113, no. 6, pp. 534–540, 2015.

[15] C. D'Arcangelo, L. Vanini, G. D. Rondoni, and F. De Angelis, "Wear properties of dental ceramics and porcelains compared with human enamel," *The Journal of Prosthetic Dentistry*, vol. 115, no. 3, pp. 350–355, 2016.

[16] R. Frankenberger, V. E. Hartmann, M. Krech et al., "Adhesive luting of new CAD/CAM materials," *International Journal of Computerized Dentistry*, vol. 18, no. 1, pp. 9–20, 2015 (German).

[17] M. O. Ahlers, G. Mörig, U. Blunck, J. Hajtó, L. Pröbster, and R. Frankenberger, "Guidelines for the preparation of CAD/CAM ceramic inlays and partial crowns," *International Journal of Computerized Dentistry*, vol. 12, no. 4, pp. 309–325, 2009.

Permissions

List of Contributors

Dawasaz Ali Azhar
Department of Oral Medicine and Radiology, College of Dentistry, King Khalid University, Abha, Saudi Arabia

Mohammad Zahir Kota
Department of Oral Surgery, College of Dentistry, King Khalid University, Abha, Saudi Arabia

Sherif El-Nagdy
Department of Oral Pathology, Faculty of Dentistry, Mansoura University, Dakahliya, Egypt

Hisham Y. El Batawi
Pediatric Dentistry, SharjahUniversity City, P.O. Box 27272, Sharjah,UAE
Correspondence should be addressed to Hisham Y. El Batawi

Kokoro Nagata, Kasumi Shimizu, Chu Sato, HiroshiMorita, YoshihiroWatanabe and Toshiro Tagawa
Departments of Oral andMaxillofacial Surgery, andClinicalSciences, Medical Life Science Mie UniversityGraduate School of Medicine, 2-174 Edobashi, Tsu, Mie 514-8507, Japan

Dilek Helvacioglu-Yigit and Seda Aydemir
Department of Endodontics, Faculty of Dentistry, University of Kocaeli, 41190 Kocaeli, Turkey

Sujatha Govindrajan, J. Muruganandhan,1 Shaik Shamsudeen and Nalin Kumar
Department of Oral and Maxillofacial Pathology, Sri Venkateswara Dental College and Hospital,Thalambur, Chennai 603103, India

M. Ramasamy
Department of Orthodontics, Sri Venkateswara Dental College and Hospital,Thalambur, Chennai 603103, India

and Srinivasa Prasad
Department of Oral and Maxillofacial Surgery, Sri Venkateswara Dental College and Hospital,Thalambur, Chennai 603103, India

Sanjeev Joshi
Department of Prosthodontics Including Crown and Bridge & Implantology, Himachal Institute of Dental Sciences, Paonta Sahib, Himachal Pradesh 173025, India

Sucheta Bansal
Department of Oral and Maxillofacial Pathology, Himachal Institute of Dental Sciences, Paonta Sahib, Himachal Pradesh 173025, India

Mayur S. Bhattad, M. S. Baliga and Ritika Kriplani
Department of Pedodontics and Preventive Dentistry, Sharad Pawar Dental College and Hospital, Sawangi 442001, Wardha, Maharashtra, India

Andrea Enrico Borgonovo, Andrea Marchetti, Virna Vavassori and Dino Re
Istituto Stomatologico Italiano, Department of Oral Rehabilitation, School of Oral Surgery, University of Milan, via Pace, 21, 20122Milan, Italy

Rachele Censi
Department of Implantology and Periodontology III, Istituto Stomatologico Italiano, Milan, Italy

Ramon Boninsegna
Department of Clinical and Experimental Sciences, University of Brescia, Italy

Prathima Sreenivasan
Department of Oral Medicine and Radiology, Kannur Dental College, Anjarakkandy, Kannur, Kerala 670612, India

Faizal C. Peedikayil
Department of Pedodontics, Kannur Dental College, Anjarakkandy, Kannur, Kerala 670612, India

Sumal V. Raj
Department of Oral Medicine and Diagnostic Radiology, Sri Sankara Dental College, Akathumuri, Varkala, Kerala 695318, India

Manasa Anand Meundi
Department of Oral Medicine and Radiology, Dayananda Sagar College of Dental Sciences, Shavige Malleshwara Hills, Kumaraswamy Layout, Bangalore 560078, India

R. Ebru Tirali and S. Burcak Cehreli
Department of Pediatric Dentistry, Faculty of Dentistry, Baskent University, 11. Sokak No. 26, Bahcelievler, 06490 Ankara, Turkey

Cagla Sar
Department of Orthodontics, Faculty of Dentistry, Baskent University, Ankara, Turkey

Ufuk Ates
Department of Oral and Maxillofacial Surgery, Faculty of Dentistry, Baskent University, Ankara, Turkey

Metin Kizilkaya
Private Practice, 34100 Istanbul, Turkey

Neslihan FJmGek, Ali KeleG and Elçin TekJn Bulut
Department of Endodontics, Faculty of Dentistry, InonuUniversity, 44280 Malatya, Turkey

Hemant Shakya, Vikram Khare, EnaMathur andMansi Chouhan
Department of Oral Medicine and Radiology, Mahatma Gandhi Dental College & Hospital, Jaipur 302022, Rajasthan, India

Nilesh Pardhe
Department of Oral & Maxillofacial Pathology, Mahatma Gandhi Dental College & Hospital, Jaipur 302022, Rajasthan, India

Bansari A. Bhuta, Archana Yadav, Rajiv S. Desai and Shivani P. Bansal
Department of Oral Pathology, Nair Hospital Dental College, Dr. A. L. Nair Road, Mumbai, Maharashtra 400 008, India

Vipul V. Chemburkar and Prashant V. Dev
Department of Radiology, Topiwala National Medical College & B. Y. L. Nair Hospital, Mumbai 400008, India

K. Radhakrishnan Nair, Anoop N. Das and Manoj C. Kuriakose
Department of Conservative Dentistry and Endodontics, Azeezia College of Dental Sciences and Research, Kollam 691537, India

Nandakumar Krishnankutty
Department of Periodontics, Azeezia College of Dental Sciences and Research, Kollam 691537, India

Leandro Berni Osório
Stomatology Department, Pediatric Dentistry, School of Dentistry, Federal University of Santa Maria, 97015-370 Santa Maria, RS, Brazil
Department of Orthodontics, Pontificia Universidade Cat´olica do Rio Grande do Sul, 90619-900 Porto Alegre, RS, Brazil

Vilmar Antonio Ferrazzo
Stomatology Department, Orthodontics, School of Dentistry, Federal University of Santa Maria, 97015-370 Santa Maria, RS, Brazil

Geraldo Serpa
Stomatology Department, Radiology, School of Dentistry, Federal University of Santa Maria, 97015-370 Santa Maria, RS, Brazil

and Kívia Linhares Ferrazzo
OralMedicine and Oral Pathology, School of Dentistry, Franciscan University Center, 97015-370 SantaMaria, RS, Brazil

Mansoor Shariff and Mohammed M. Al-Moaleem
Prosthodontic Department, College of Dentistry, King Khalid University, P.O. Box 3263, Abha 61471, Saudi Arabia

NasserM. Al-Ahmari
College of Dentistry, King Khalid University, P.O. Box 3263, Abha 61471, Saudi Arabia

Jafar Abdulla Mohamed Usman
Subsitutive Dental Sciences, College of Dentistry, King Khaled University, P.O. Box 3263, Abha 61471, Saudi Arabia

Anuroopa Ayappan
Department of Prosthodontics, Sree Mookambika Institute of Dental Sciences, Kulashekaram, India

Dhanraj Ganapathy
Derartment of Prosthodontics, Saveetha Dental College, Chennai, India

Nilofer Nisha Nasir
Department of Conservative Dentistry and Endodontics, Rajah Mutthiah Dental College, Annamalai University, Chidambaram, Tamilnadu, India

Radhika Chopra, MohitaMarwaha, Payal Chaudhuri and Kalpana Bansal
Department of Pedodontics and Preventive Dentistry, SGT Dental College & Research Institute, Budhera 123505, Gurgaon, Haryana, India

and Saurabh Chopra
Department of Pediatrics, Subharti Medical College, Meerut 250005, India

Shruti Tandon, Abdul Ahad, Arundeep Kaur and Farrukh Faraz
Department of Periodontics and Oral Implantology, Maulana Azad Institute of Dental Sciences, Bahadur Shah Zafar Marg, New Delhi 110002, India

Zainab Chaudhary
Department of Oral and Maxillofacial Surgery, Maulana Azad Institute of Dental Sciences, Bahadur Shah Zafar Marg, New Delhi 110002, India

Padma Pandeshwar
Sri Venkateshwara Dental College and Hospital, Kariyappanahalli, Anekal Road, Bannerughatta, Bangalore 560083, India

Jayanthi
Oral Medicine, Diagnosis and Radiology, Bangalore Institute of Dental Sciences, Lakkasandra, Wilson Garden, Bangalore, India

K. and D.Mahesh
Dayananda Sagar College of Dental Sciences, Shivage Malleshwara Hills, Kumarswamy Layout, Bangalore, India

Neeta Bagul, G. S. Mamatha and Aditi Mahalle
Department of Oral Pathology and Microbiology, Dr. D. Y. Patil Dental College and Hospital, Pimpri, Pune 411018, India

Mohammed Nadershah
1Department of Oral and Maxillofacial Surgery, Boston Medical Center, Boston University, 850 Harrison Avenue, Boston, MA 02118, USA

Ahmad Alshadwi
Oral and Maxillofacial Surgery Department, Boston Medical Center, Boston University, 100 East Newton street, Boston, MA 02118, USA

Andrew Salama
Boston Medical Center, Boston University, 850 Harrison Avenue, Boston, MA 02118, USA

Maximilian Krüger and Maximilian Moergel
Department of Oral and Maxillofacial Surgery-Plastic Surgery, Johannes Gutenberg University of Mainz, Medical Center, Augustusplatz 2, 55131 Mainz, Germany

Torsten Hansen
Institute of Pathology, University of Mainz, Medical Surgery, Langenbeckstraße 1, 55131 Mainz, Germany

Adrian Kasaj
Department of Operative Dentistry and Periodontology, Johannes Gutenberg-University, Augustusplatz 2, 55131 Mainz, Germany

Yukiko Kusuyama, Shino Okada, KenWakabayashi and Noritami Takeuchi
Department of Dentistry and Oral Surgery, Matsubara Tokushukai Hospital, 7-13-26 Amamihigashi, Matsubara-shi, Osaka 580-0032, Japan

Yoshiaki Yura and KenMatsumoto
Department of Oral and Maxillofacial Surgery II, OsakaUniversity, Graduate School of Dentistry, Osaka 565-0871, Japan

S. Gokkulakrishnan and Satish Kumaran
1Department of OMFS, Institute of Dental Science Bareilly, Bareilly 243006, India

Ashish Sharma
Department of OMFS, Kothiwal Dental College & Research Centre, Moradabad, India

P. L. Vasundhar
Department of OMFS, Sri Sai College of Dental Surgery, Srikakulam, India

Basavaraj T. Bhagawati, Manish Gupta and Gaurav Narang
Department of Oral Medicine and Radiology, Shree Bankey Bihari Dental College, Masuri, Ghaziabad, Utta Pradesh-201302, India

Sharanamma Bhagawati
Department of Periodontology, Shree Bankey Bihari Dental College, NH-24, Masuri, Ghaziabad, Utta Pradesh-201302, India

Carla Vecchione Gurgel, Ana Lídia Soares Cota, Tatiana Yuriko Kobayashi, Salete Moura Bonifácio Silva, Maria Aparecida AndradeMoreira Machado and Daniela Rios
Department of Pediatric Dentistry, Orthodontics and Public Health, Bauru School of Dentistry, University of São Paulo, São Paulo, Brazil

Daniela Gamba Garib and Thais Marchini Oliveira
Department of Pediatric Dentistry, Orthodontics and Public Health, Bauru School of Dentistry, University of São Paulo, São Paulo, Brazil
Hospital for the Rehabilitation of Craniofacial Anomalies, University of São Paulo, São Paulo, Brazil

Rizwan Ali Shivji, Vaibhav D. Kamble and Mohd. Atif Khan
Department of Prosthodontics, VSPM Dental College and Research Centre, Nagpur, India

K. L. Ferrazzo
School of Dentistry, Franciscan University Center, Andradas Street, 1614, 97010-032 Santa Maria, RS, Brazil

L. B. Osório and V. A. Ferrazzo
Department of Stomatology, School of Dentistry, Federal University of Santa Maria, Floriano Peixoto Street, 1184, 97015-372 Santa Maria, RS, Brazil

A. N. Sulabha
Department of Oral Medicine and Radiology, Al-Ameen Dental College and Hospital, Athani Road, Karnataka, Bijapur 586108, India

C. Sameer
Department of Oral and Maxillofacial Surgery, Al-Ameen Dental College and Hospital, Karnataka, Bijapur 586108, India

Pietro Fusari,Matteo Doto and Matteo Chiapasco
Unit of Oral Surgery, Department of Health Sciences, San Paolo Hospital, University of Milan, Via Beldiletto 1/3, 20142 Milan, Italy

Roopak Bose Carlos, Mohan Thomas Nainan, Shamina Pradhan, Roshni Sharma and Shiny Benjamin
Department of Conservative Dentistry and Endodontics, Vydehi Institute of Dental Sciences and Research Centre, No. 82, EPIP Area, Whitefield, Bangalore 560066, India Rajani Rose
Dental Solutions, 157, 4th Main, BEML layout, Off ITPL Road,Thubarahalli, Bangalore 560066, India

Archana Singh, Ankita Singh, Rajul Vivek, T. P. Chaturvedi, Pankaj Chauhan and Shruti Gupta
Department of Prosthodontics, Faculty of Dental Sciences, Institute of Medical Sciences, Banaras Hindu University, Varanasi 221005, India

José Alcides Arruda, Pâmella Álvares, Luciano Silva, Antônio Caubi, Marcia Silveira and Ana Paula Sobral
Faculdade de Odontologia de Pernambuco, Universidade de Pernambuco, Avenida General Newton Cavalcante, 1650 Aldeia dos Camar´as, 54753-020 Camaragibe, PE, Brazil

Eugênia Figueiredo
Hospital da Restauração, Avenida Governador Agamenon Magalhães, S/N, Derby, 52010-040 Recife, PE, Brazil

Leorik Silva
Universidade Federal do Rio Grande do Norte, Campus Universitário Lagoa Nova, P.O. Box 1524, 59078-970 Natal, RN, Brazil

Farhin Katge, SajjadMithiborwala and Thejokrishna Pammi
Department of Pedodontics & Preventive Dentistry, Terna Dental College, Sector 22, Plot No. 12, Nerul (W), Navi Mumbai 400706, Maharashtra, India

Nabil Khzam,1 David Bailey
DB Dental, Corner Tydeman & Pensioner Guard Roads, Perth,WA 6159, Australia

Helen S. Yie
Irwin Dental Centre, Irwin Barracks, Perth,WA 6010, Australia

Mahmoud M. Bakr
General Dental Practice, School of Dentistry and Oral Health, Griffith University, Gold Coast, QLD 4222, Australia

Giorgio Lombardo, Jacopo Pighi, Giovanni Corrocher, Anna Mascellaro and Pier Francesco Nocini
Clinic of Dentistry and Maxillofacial Surgery, University of Verona, Piazzale Ludovico Antonio Scuro 10, 37100 Verona, Italy

effrey Lehrberg
Department of Biomaterials, Implant Dentistry Centre, 501 Arborway, Jamaica Plain, Boston, MA 02130, USA

JMauroMarincola
Universidad de Cartagena, Avenida del Consulado, Calle No. 30, No. 48-152, Cartagena, Bol'ıvar, Colombia

Vamsi Krishna CH, K.Mahendranadh Reddy, Nidhi Gupta, Y.Mahadev Shastry', N. Chandra Sekhar, Venkat Aditya and G. V. K. Mohan Reddy
Department of Prosthodontics, Sri Sai College of Dental Surgery, Kothrepally, Vikarabad 501101, India

FareediMukram Ali
Department of Oral and Maxillofacial Surgery, SMBT Dental College and Hospital, Sangamner, Maharashtra 422608, India

Kishor Patil
Department of Oral Pathology and Microbiology, SMBT Dental College and Hospital, Sangamner, Maharashtra 422608, India

Sanjay Kar
Department of Oral and Maxillofacial Surgery, Mansarovar Dental College, Hospital & Research Centre, Bhopal, Madhya Pradesh 462001, India

Atulkumar A. Patil
Department of Dentistry, Dr. Vaishampayan Memorial Government Medical College, Solapur, Maharashtra, India

Shabeer Ahamed
Department of Periodontics, Malabar Dental College, Edapal, Kerala 679578, India

Kapoor Sonali, Agrawal Vineet Suresh, Patel Abhishek and Patel Jenish
Department of Conservative and Endodontics, M. P. Dental College and Hospital, Vadodara 390011, India

Murat Ulu, EFatih Gunhan and Huseyin Akcay
Department of Oral and Maxillofacial Surgery, Faculty of Dentistry, Izmir Katip Celebi University, 35640 Izmir, Turkey

lif Tarim Ertas and Meral Yircali Atici
Department of Oral and Maxillofacial Radiology, Faculty of Dentistry, Izmir Katip Celebi University, 35640 Izmir, Turkey

Christos Livas
Department of Orthodontics, University of Groningen, University Medical Center Groningen, Hanzeplein 1. Postbus 30.001, 9700 RB Groningen,The Netherlands

Suryakant C. Deogade
Department of Prosthodontics, Hitkarini Dental College & Hospital, Jabalpur, Madhya Pradesh 482005, India

J. W. Booij
Private Practice, Schelluinsevliet 5, 4203 NB Gorinchem, Netherlands

Christos Livas
Department of Orthodontics, University of Groningen, University Medical Center Groningen, Hanzeplein 1, Triadegebouw, Ingang 24, 9700 RB Groningen, Netherlands

Shiraz Pasha, Bathula Vimala Chaitanya and Kusum Valli Somisetty
Department of Conservative Dentistry and Endodontics, Sri Rajiv Gandhi College of Dental Sciences, Bangalore 560032, India

B. Vishwanath, Umrana Faizudin, M. Jayadev and Sushma Shravani
Department of Conservative Dentistry & Endodontics, Panineeya Dental College, Hyderabad 60, India

Anne-Kathrin Pabel
Dental Practice, 63456 Hanau, Germany

Sven Rinke
Dental Practice, 63456 Hanau, Germany
Department of Prosthetics, University Medical Center Göttingen, 37075 Göttingen, Germany

Matthias Rödiger
Department of Prosthetics, University Medical Center Göttingen, 37075 Göttingen, Germany

Dirk Ziebolz
Department of Cariology, Endodontology and Periodontology, University of Leipzig, 04103 Leipzig, Germany

Index

www.ingramcontent.com/pod-product-compliance
Lightning Source LLC
Chambersburg PA
CBHW061248190326
41458CB00011B/3615